Surgically Shaping Children

Recent and Related Titles in Bioethics

Joseph S. Alper, Catherine Ard, Adrienne Asch, Jon Beckwith, Peter Conrad, and Lisa N. Geller, eds. *The Double-Edged Helix: Social Implications of Genetics in a Diverse Society*

Nancy Berlinger. *After Harm: Medical Error and the Ethics of Forgiveness*

Audrey R. Chapman and Mark S. Frankel, eds. *Designing Our Descendants: The Promises and Perils of Genetic Modifications*

Grant R. Gillett. *Bioethics in the Clinic: Hippocratic Reflections*

John D. Lantos. *The Lazarus Case: Life-and-Death Issues in Neonatal Intensive Care*

Carol Levine and Thomas H. Murray, eds. *The Cultures of Caregiving: Conflict and Common Ground among Families, Health Professionals, and Policy Makers*

Erik Parens, Audrey R. Chapman, and Nancy Press, eds. *Wrestling with Behavioral Genetics: Science, Ethics, and Public Conversation*

Mark A. Rothstein, Thomas H. Murray, Gregory E. Kaebnick, and Mary Anderlik Majumder, eds. *Genetic Ties and the Family: The Impact of Paternity Testing on Parents and Children*

Thomas H. Murray, consulting editor in bioethics

Surgically Shaping Children

Technology, Ethics, and the Pursuit of Normality

Edited by

ERIK PARENS

Senior Research Scholar
The Hastings Center
Garrison, New York

The Johns Hopkins University Press
Baltimore

The Johns Hopkins University Press
2715 North Charles Street
Baltimore, Maryland 21218-4363
www.press.jhu.edu

Library of Congress Cataloging-in-Publication Data
Surgically shaping children : technology, ethics, and the pursuit
of normality / edited by Erik Parens.
p. ; cm.
Includes bibliographical references and index.
ISBN 0-8018-8305-9 (hardcover : alk. paper)
1. Children—Surgery—Moral and ethical aspects. 2. Abnormalities,
Human—Moral and ethical aspects. 3. Surgery, Plastic—Moral
and ethical aspects. 4. Children—Surgery—Decision making.
5. Decision making in children.
[DNLM: 1. Reconstructive Surgical Procedures—ethics—Child.
2. Achondroplasia—surgery—Child. 3. Biomedical Technology—ethics.
4. Cleft Palate—surgery—Child. 5. Genitalia—abnormalities—Child.
6. Social Perception—Child. wo 600 s961 2006] I. Parens, Erik, 1957–
RD137.S846 2006
617.9′8—dc22   2005027618

A catalog record for this book is available from the British Library.

To my parents,
Rachel and Henri Parens,
who balanced shaping and letting be
as well as any child could wish

CONTENTS

List of Contributors   *ix*

Acknowledgments   *xi*

Introduction: *Thinking about Surgically Shaping Children*   *xiii*
ERIK PARENS

PART I   PERSONAL NARRATIVES ABOUT APPEARANCE-
NORMALIZING SURGERY

1 Twisted Lies: *My Journey in an Imperfect Body*   3
SHERRI G. MORRIS

2 Do I Make You Uncomfortable? *Reflections on Using Surgery
to Reduce the Distress of Others*   13
CASSANDRA ASPINALL

3 My Shoe Size Stayed the Same: *Maintaining a Positive Sense of Identity
with Achondroplasia and Limb-Lengthening Surgeries*   29
EMILY SULLIVAN SANFORD

4 The Seduction of the Surgical Fix   43
LISA ABELOW HEDLEY

PART II   TECHNOLOGY AND THE PURSUIT OF NORMALITY

5 Concepts of Technology and Their Role in Moral Reflection   51
JAMES C. EDWARDS

6 Emily's Scars: *Surgical Shapings, Technoluxe, and Bioethics*   68
ARTHUR W. FRANK

7 Thoughts on the Desire for Normality   90
EVA FEDER KITTAY

PART III   THE SURGICAL CONTEXT

8 To Cut or Not to Cut? *A Surgeon's Perspective
on Surgically Shaping Children*   113
JEFFREY L. MARSH

9 What's Special about the Surgical Context?   125
WENDY E. MOURADIAN

10 Are We Helping Children? *Outcome Assessments
in Craniofacial Care*   141
WENDY E. MOURADIAN, TODD C. EDWARDS, TARI D. TOPOLSKI,
NICHOLA RUMSEY, AND DONALD L. PATRICK

PART IV   CHILDREN AND PARENTS DECIDING ABOUT
APPEARANCE-NORMALIZING SURGERY

11 Who Should Decide and How?   157
PRISCILLA ALDERSON

12 The Power of Parents and the Agency of Children   176
HILDE LINDEMANN

13 "In Their Best Interests": *Parents' Experience
of Atypical Genitalia*   189
ELLEN K. FEDER

14 Toward Truly Informed Decisions
about Appearance-Normalizing Surgeries   211
PAUL STEVEN MILLER

15 Appearance-Altering Surgery, Children's Sense of Self,
and Parental Love   227
ADRIENNE ASCH

16 What to Expect when You Have the Child You Weren't Expecting   253
ALICE DOMURAT DREGER

Index   267

PRISCILLA ALDERSON, Ph.D., Professor of Childhood Studies, Social Science Research Unit, Institute of Education, University of London, London, England

ADRIENNE ASCH, Ph.D., Edward and Robin Milstein Professor of Bioethics, Yeshiva University—Wurzweiler School of Social Work, New York, New York

CASSANDRA ASPINALL, M.S.W., L.I.C.S.W., Social Worker, Craniofacial Center, Children's Hospital and Regional Medical Center, Seattle, Washington

ALICE DOMURAT DREGER, Ph.D., Visiting Associate Professor of Medical Humanities and Bioethics, Feinberg School of Medicine, Northwestern University; Director of Medical Education, Intersex Society of North America, Chicago, Illinois

JAMES C. EDWARDS, Ph.D., Professor of Philosophy, Department of Philosophy, Furman University, Greenville, South Carolina

TODD C. EDWARDS, Ph.D., Research Scientist and Affiliate Assistant Professor, Department of Health Services, University of Washington, Seattle, Washington

ELLEN K. FEDER, Ph.D., Assistant Professor, Department of Philosophy and Religion, American University, Washington, DC

ARTHUR W. FRANK, Ph.D., Professor, Department of Sociology, University of Calgary, Calgary, Alberta, Canada

LISA ABELOW HEDLEY, J.D., Children of Difference Foundation, New York, New York

EVA FEDER KITTAY, Ph.D., Professor, Department of Philosophy, State University of New York, Stony Brook, New York

HILDE LINDEMANN, Ph.D., Associate Professor, Department of Philosophy, Michigan State University, East Lansing, Michigan

JEFFREY L. MARSH, M.D., Clinical Professor or Surgery, Plastic & Reconstructive, University School of Medicine, Saint Louis, Missouri; Director, Pediatric Plastic Surgery, St. John's Mercy Medical Center, Saint Louis, Missouri; Medical Director, Cleft Lip/Palate and Craniofacial Deformities Center, St. John's Mercy Medical Center, Saint Louis, Missouri

PAUL STEVEN MILLER, LL.B., Professor, University of Washington School of Law, Seattle, Washington

SHERRI G. MORRIS, J.D., lawyer, San Diego, California

WENDY E. MOURADIAN, M.D., M.S., Associate Clinical Professor of Pediatrics, Pediatric Dentistry and Health Services, University of Washington, Seattle, Washington

DONALD L. PATRICK, Ph.D., M.S.P.H., Professor and Director, Social and Behavioral Sciences Program, Department of Health Services, School of Public Health and Community Medicine, Seattle, Washington

NICHOLA RUMSEY, M.S.C., Ph.D., Professor of Appearance and Health Psychology, Centre for Appearance Research, University of the West of England, Bristol, United Kingdom

EMILY SULLIVAN SANFORD, B.A., English teacher, Oskar Lernt Englisch, Inc., Berlin, Germany

TARI D. TOPOLSKI, Ph.D., Research Scientist and Affiliate Assistant Professor, University of Washington, Seattle, Washington

This book is the product of a project undertaken by The Hastings Center and funded by the National Endowment for the Humanities (RZ-20715). We live in a time where there is precious little support for projects that bring people together to think about complex ethical and social questions. For the opportunity to think together about the meaning of using one new means to pursue the ancient end of shaping children, I and the Surgically Shaping Children working group are deeply grateful to the National Endowment for the Humanities.

In addition to the contributors to this volume, five others generously gave their time and insights to the ongoing working-group process: Jeffrey Blustein (Albert Einstein College of Medicine), Dena S. Davis (Cleveland-Marshall College of Law), Joel Frader (Northwestern University Medical School), Gregory Kaebnick (The Hastings Center), and Thomas H. Murray (The Hastings Center).

When we did not have the expertise we needed within the working group, we sought and received the help of a distinguished roster of consultants, including Ian A. Aaronson (Medical University of South Carolina), Cheryl Chase (Intersex Society of North America), Philip Gruppuso (Brown University), Nathan Ionascu (New York Medical College), Eric Juengst (Case Western Reserve University), William G. Reiner (University of Oklahoma Health Sciences Center), David L. Rimoin (UCLA School of Medicine), and Ronald P. Strauss (University of North Carolina School of Dentistry).

Running such a project requires the efforts of many people. Thanks first to The Hastings Center's librarian, Chris McKee, who tirelessly and insightfully facilitates our research. Thanks also to Michael Khair, Samantha Stokes, Alissa Lyon, and Stacy Sanders, for their research assistance. Without the technical support of Ylber Ibrahimi, neither this project nor much else would happen here at the Center. Thanks also to Vicki Peyton, whose administrative assistance was indispensable in getting this book to the Johns Hopkins University Press.

An anonymous reader for the Johns Hopkins University Press made insightful observations, which I hope she or he will think strengthened this volume. Finally, thanks so much to Wendy Harris at the Johns Hopkins University Press, who, from the very beginning of our research project, supported our effort to create this book. Without Wendy's care and patience, this volume would not now be in your hands.

Thinking about Surgically Shaping Children

ERIK PARENS

This volume explores the ethical questions that arise when surgery is used to make children look more normal. It grows out of The Hastings Center's Surgically Shaping Children project, which is, as it were, the child of two other Hastings Center projects I have had the privilege to direct.

The first of those projects, on prenatal testing and disability rights, took up the ethical questions that emerge when we selectively abort fetuses shown by prenatal genetic tests to carry disabling traits (Parens and Asch 2000). More specifically, that project (funded by the Ethical, Legal, and Social Implications of the Human Genome Project [ELSI] program at the National Institutes of Health) investigated the disability community's critique of such testing. While the project gave me a deep appreciation of that critique, it also gave me an appreciation of just how heterogeneous are the disabling conditions we can test for (from Tay Sachs to extra fingers)—and of just how difficult it can be to make useful generalizations about "disabling conditions." In addition to making me want to continue to engage the disability community's arguments, that project made me think it would help to narrow the focus and begin to investigate particular cases.

Thus, our Surgically Shaping Children project (funded by the National Endowment for the Humanities) took up three cases, which are themselves heterogeneous. The first case involves surgeries to make children's ambiguous or atypical genitalia look more normal; many adults with such atypical anatomies refer to themselves as intersexed. The second involves surgeries to lengthen the legs of children who have achondroplasia; adults with achondroplasia refer to themselves as dwarfs or Little People. Originally, I thought that our third case would consider surgeries to make the features of children with Down syndrome look more normal. Because it turns out that fewer and fewer of those surgeries are being done, however, we decided to concentrate on another set of craniofacial surgeries: those done on cleft lips and palates. Though I didn't know it at the time, as I explain below, going from a controversial to a non-controversial class of surgeries would turn out to complicate—and thereby deepen—our reflections. For that change in course, I am deeply indebted to Dr. Wendy Mouradian, a member of our project's working group.

The other "parent" of the Surgically Shaping Children project was our Enhancing Human Traits project (also funded by the National Endowment for the Humanities), which explored the ethical debates that surround efforts to use medical technologies to improve human traits and capacities (Parens 1998). Surgical breast enlargement was one of the classic examples circulating in the background of the project. Another was the use of Prozac to improve normal moods—or, in Peter Kramer's famous phrase, to make some people feel "better than well" (Kramer 1993). Indeed, we often spoke in that project as if the central question was, What are the ethical costs of various efforts to make us *better than normal?* But that formulation of the project's central question, with images of shallow and greedy social climbers in the background, failed to identify what I now see as that project's primary concern.

That concern was not about persons pursuing frivolous ends or unfair social advantages, as real and important as those concerns may be. It was about pressures on persons to transform the bodies—and thereby the selves—they were thrown into the world with. From that angle, giving tall girls hormones to slow their growth was and is every bit as worrisome as giving short boys hormones to enhance theirs. In one formulation, the worry was about individuals becoming different from who they really were—or, as some would put it, "inauthentic."[1] As Carl Elliott saw before I did (Elliott 2003), my fundamental concern was about how we are using these technologies to transform human identities.

The Surgically Shaping Children project brings that concern about using technology to transform identities front and center. We weren't talking about advantage-seeking social climbers. Instead, we were talking about parents and children, who hoped that more normal appearance would improve psychosocial functioning. They hoped that transforming children's bodies could transform how those children are experienced by, and thus experience, others and the world.

Moreover, insofar as this project was about children, it forced me and the working group to face one of the deep tensions at the root of many if not all of the debates regarding what we might call "self-shaping technologies." Parents have two fundamental obligations. One is to let their children be, to let them unfold according to their own desires and capacities. The other parental obligation is to shape children, to promote their flourishing or psychosocial functioning.

Whereas during our Enhancement project I could forget or ignore the obligation to transform ourselves in some circumstances to achieve some ends, I could no longer forget or ignore it in our Surgically Shaping Children project. No matter how firmly we believe in the obligation to allow our children to unfold in their own way, we cannot ignore our obligation also to shape them.

This book explores that tension between the obligations to let children be and to shape them. Given the depth of that tension, and given the heterogeneity of the facts of the different cases, at the end of the day, our Surgically Shaping Children working group could agree on only one unsurprising but nonetheless important conclusion: based on respect for persons, individuals (whether children alone, parents alone, or children and parents together) must be helped to make truly and fully informed decisions. But at the beginning of the day, all those involved in making such decisions, especially parents, need to be helped to reflect on what life with atypical anatomies is—and is not—like. And they need to be helped to explore that fundamental tension between their obligation to shape their children and their obligation to let their children unfold in their own way. This book aims to promote such "beginning-of-the-day" reflection. The ideal of truly informed decision making is as easy to invoke as it is difficult to achieve.

The Structure of the Volume

Our project pursued three intertwined strands of inquiry, each of which can be glimpsed in the phrase *surgically shaping children.* Most generally, we were interested in the large conceptual, ethical, and social issues that arise when we use technology to *shape* ourselves, to make ourselves look more normal. To help us from straying too far from the world of flesh-and-blood persons making life-altering decisions, we limited our conversation to one mode of technological shaping: *surgery* (as opposed to, say, pharmacology or genetics). In another effort to keep us from straying too far, we limited ourselves to talking about surgeries that arise when the potential patient is a child. Thus our attention to the surgical shaping of *children.*

All three of those strands are visible in each of the four major parts of the book. Part I offers narratives from people whose views about appearance-normalizing surgery grow out of their experience as a person with (or parent of a person with) an atypical anatomy. Going from the particular to the general, Part II offers broader theoretical reflections on the meaning of using technology to fulfill our desire to look more normal. Part III provides reflections about the surgical context from medical professionals involved in the delivery and improvement of surgical care. The final part offers reflections and ultimately practical advice about how parents, children, and medical professionals can improve decision making about appearance-normalizing surgeries.

In the spirit of affirming a wide variety of ways of being, this volume includes essays in a variety of formats: from personal narratives and scholarly essays to those about the need for new data and about how to promote truly informed decisions. The contributions are not only written by people with a variety of lay and academic backgrounds, but by people with different perspectives: from those who are highly skeptical about the value of appearance-normalizing surgeries to those whose livelihoods depend on delivering such surgeries. For all of their differences, all of the authors are ultimately grappling with the same basic question regarding the ethical and social implications of surgically shaping children.

Part I. Personal Narratives about Appearance-Normalizing Surgery

When we began our project, I asked surgeons who try to normalize the appearance of children with atypical genitalia to put me in touch with persons who were glad to have had the surgeries. I was told that such people had moved on with their lives and had no desire to draw attention to an anatomical difference that no longer existed. Although that account is surely plausible, surgeons themselves are increasingly aware of the need to collect data to support it (Sytsma 2004).

As Alice Dreger, Cheryl Chase, and the Intersex Society of North America have amply and painfully shown, however, myriad children born with atypical genitalia who have had such surgeries are outraged and do want to talk. Many of these now-grown children have already written eloquently not only about how those appearance-normalizing surgeries deprived them of sexual sensation, but about the agonizing psychological pain caused by the secrecy and shame that have attended their surgeries (Dreger 1999).

Indeed, children with intersex conditions can suffer the excruciating consequences of secrecy and shame even when they are not subjected to surgeries aimed at making their genitalia look more normal. Sherri G. Morris, author of the first essay in this collection, was born with an intersex condition called androgen insensitivity syndrome. She was raised and always experienced herself as a woman, but didn't find out until she was in law school that she had been born with a male karyotype (XY) and male gonads (testes). Even though Morris was not subjected to the sorts of appearance-normalizing surgery that have deprived many intersexed people of sexual sensation, she did have surgery as an infant to remove her testes. When she entered puberty, she was told that surgeons had removed her "twisted ovaries." As Morris observes, it was not the physiological effects of androgen insensitivity syndrome that caused her suffering. Rather, it was "the realization that I had been told lies by those from whom I had a right to expect the truth—my parents." Secrecy, silence, lies, and shame produced suffering so great that she considered suicide.

To her great good fortune and the reader's, Morris found out the truth about her condition and, as we're often told it can, it set her free. Her message resonates throughout this volume: if children with atypical bodies are assured of their caretakers' unconditional love, if those children are helped to understand the facts about their bodies, and if, whenever possible, they are included in decisions about the treatment of their own bodies, they will be fine.

Unfortunately, even when families intend to express unconditional love, they don't always succeed. In her essay, Cassandra Aspinall writes as a person affected with cleft lip and palate, as the parent of an affected child, and as a social worker who helps families manage the care of children with craniofacial differences. Aspinall describes what it was like to learn from her own grandmother that she was "different"—and that that wasn't okay. When she was four, Aspinall sat on her grandmother's lap and tried to interpret her palpable sadness:

> [My grandmother] wanted to tell me it was okay that I was different. She traced her finger over the upper line of my lip and began to talk about the fact that my lip was not like most people's, but that that was okay. She told me that because my upper lip already had what was called a Cupid's Bow, I would not have to "paint on" that sort of look the way she did with lipstick. I remember I had trouble understanding what she was talking about. She seemed upset, but I didn't know why. I wanted to make her feel better, but I didn't share her sadness about my face or myself.

In hindsight, Aspinall sees that her grandmother was sad at the thought of her granddaughter being rejected *by others*. Perhaps her grandmother worried about her prospects for finding love. Though her grandmother was worried about the harmful and wrongful reactions of others, Aspinall got the impression that something was wrong with *her*. As she writes, "It is strange that [my grandmother's] desire to protect me from harm had the unintentional consequence of making me feel bad, of actually causing me harm."

Thus Aspinall approaches one of the project's core questions: What are the costs to the child when the surgery's primary purpose is not to make the child feel better, but to make others feel better about the child? Should an affected person who feels fine about her body change her body to make others feel better? To her credit, Aspinall does not ignore the respect in which how others feel about us affects how we ultimately feel about ourselves. But she makes vivid the respect in which the surgeries we were talking about were done more for others than for the children whose bodies were being altered. She never shies away from the complexity of these questions. She does not argue against parents deciding for their children in all cases. Indeed, she says explicitly that she has never regretted that she received primary cleft lip surgery, even though that surgery was *not* about repairing physiological function, but was about improving her appearance (and thereby her psychosocial functioning). *And* she wants to invite us to think about whether anatomically typical persons should change their views rather than requiring anatomically atypical persons to change their bodies.

If there is increasing agreement that parents should *not* decide for children about surgeries to normalize atypical genitalia and widespread agreement that in our imperfect world parents *should* decide for children about primary surgeries to repair cleft lips and palates, the nature of the agreement about surgeries to normalize short limbs falls somewhere in between. In most cases, there are medical reasons to wait until the child is almost in her teens before doing these surgeries. Even if there were not, however, given the trade-offs, reasonable parents would wait for their child to be old enough to share in the conversation about the surgery.

Or so Emily Sullivan Sanford suggests in her essay. When she wrote the story of her life before, during, and after surgeries to lengthen her short arms and legs, Sanford was still a college student. With honesty and insight, she gives an account of how, in spite of the pain and long-term undesirable side effects associated with the surgeries, she is glad to have endured them.

As Sanford's essay makes clear, she comes from a family who loved her deeply and sought to support her in whatever decisions she made. As the essay also makes eminently clear, a huge part of why she can look back and be glad about the surgery she underwent is that she was allowed to decide for herself. That is, she decided for herself to the extent that any of us ever does. She does not imagine that we make decisions alone, and is perfectly frank about the fact that her parents invited her to consider the surgeries. But she draws a stark contrast between her own situation and that of children whose parents presume to choose *for* their children. She writes:

> During one clinical check-up, I felt chills down my back and anger in my cheeks as I heard a mother confer with the surgeon about limb-lengthening for her 7-year-old daughter. "Children can't make the decision of course," she smiled, "they're too young." I pitied her daughter immediately because, although I was sitting in a wheelchair similar to the one to which she would also soon be confined, I had brought myself there.

Again, to her great credit, Sanford does not ignore any of the inconvenience, pain, or long-term physiological costs that attended her decision to have the surgeries. Nor does she seem to have any need or desire to deny that she was born with achondroplasia. As the title to her essay emphasizes, the surgeries did not change her shoe size.

From a young woman who decided with her parents for limb-lengthening surgeries, we turn in the next essay to a parent who, with her husband, has struggled with decisions about possible surgeries for their daughter. With marvelous frankness and clarity, lawyer and documentary filmmaker Lisa Abelow Hedley writes about the depth of her desire that her daughter LilyClaire, who is a dwarf, appear more normal—and about the depth of her commitment to protect her daughter against "those marauding, seductive, and unattainable notions of normalcy."

When LilyClaire is 7 years old, surgeons face Hedley and her husband with a difficult choice. Because they believe that LilyClaire is not old enough to decide for herself, Hedley and her husband engage in a sometimes excruciating process of deciding what is in her best interests. Specifically, they have to decide whether, in addition to subjecting LilyClaire to a surgery that will straighten the bowing in her legs (and thereby prevent cartilage degeneration), they will also subject her to an additional six months of treatment to lengthen her legs by 2 to 4 inches.

The goal of preventing cartilage degeneration is straightforwardly medical; it aims to promote what we might call normal *physiological* functioning. The goal of adding height, on the other hand, is primarily *psychosocial*. Of course, for anyone who rejects dualist conceptions of the relationship between the physical and the psychical (the body and the mind), the distinction between physiological and psychosocial aims is fuzzy. Improved physiological functioning usually has positive psychosocial effects, and improved psychosocial functioning can have positive physiological effects. It's a continuous loop.

But in practice, in thinking about and choosing among interventions, parents and children make distinctions. Using fuzzy and unstable distinctions seems to beat the alternative of abandoning the effort to think critically about the options. In the end, Hedley and her husband decide *for their daughter* the question about the intervention to achieve the physiological aim. And they decide to let their daughter decide *for herself* the question about the intervention to achieve the psychosocial goal. As powerful as is "the seduction of the surgical fix," she and her husband elect to wait to let Lily-Claire decide for herself about the extra 2 to 4 inches.

Part II. Technology and the Pursuit of Normality

Philosopher James C. Edwards invites us in his essay to step far back and to reflect on the meaning of using technology to shape ourselves and our children. On one well-known view, technology is a morally neutral tool that we can put to whatever ends we desire. On the alternative, Heideggerian view that Edwards explicates, however, technology is anything but neutral. It is "a particular way of revealing things." It "lets things be seen—in a particular way; it reveals them as having a particular character, a particular Being." According to Heidegger, what is characteristic of the technological way of revealing things is that things are "set upon" and "challenged forth." The result is that "everywhere everything is ordered to stand by, to be immediately on hand, indeed to stand there just so that it may be on call for a further ordering." Such ordering aims at making things useful for whomever needs them, whenever she might need them. Thus the aim is to erase the particularity of such things, to make them as "anonymous and interchangeable" as possible, so that they will be available for our further ordering. As Edwards puts it, "The characteristic kind of thing brought to light by the practices of technology is *Bestand*, 'standing reserve,' 'stock.'"

Heidegger's deepest worry is not that this way of revealing turns coffee mugs or toothbrushes into "anonymous and interchangeable markers in a great game of economic ordering." Rather, his worry is that "*we ourselves* sooner or later come to see ourselves as *Bestand*." Which brings us to how Heidegger's thinking bears on our project's inquiry. About our efforts to shape children's bodies with surgery, Edwards asks: "Are we (with the best of intentions, of course) treating that child's body (and life) as *Bestand*, as raw material to be shaped so as to fit our (and presumably her) sense of what is 'natural,' 'normal,' and 'orderly'? And if we are, is anything wrong with that?" Edwards's answer is that we should not attempt to offer a general answer to those questions. He suggests that, instead, we should help those facing decisions about surgically shaping children to engage those questions. He urges us to try to remember that what seems like "common sense"—Of course good parents seek to make their children's bodies look more normal!—is in fact a particular view that depends on a particular way of being in the world. He does not argue against surgery, but for thinking.

The next essay, "Emily's Scars,"[2] by sociologist Arthur W. Frank, helps the reader to step back in a slightly different direction and to consider the different approaches of those who consider bioethical questions in general—and questions about surgical shapings in particular. Frank calls the first approach or framework consumer-protection bioethics. This sort of approach accepts the presuppositions of consumerism. According to Frank, those who adopt it aim to help people "to know exactly what is being delivered at what cost and with what risk." The ethical standards of protectionist bioethics require medical professionals "to be responsible salespeople [who then leave] the choice to patient-consumers."

The approach that Frank calls Socratic, however, assumes that we can and should talk about more than cost and safety. It assumes the importance of the sorts of "beginning-of-the-day" reflections I mentioned above. As Frank puts it, Socratic bioethics calls attention to connections: "connections between practices, so that people recognize how one practice reinforces another, and also connections between people, breaking down the idea that any decision can be strictly *individual*, insofar as that word suggests that one person's decision does not affect how another person chooses."

Consumer-protection bioethics does not in principle preclude Socratic bioethics;

indeed, this volume offers essays engaged in both bioethical modes. But Frank worries that in North American culture today, consumer-protection bioethics increasingly dominates, and we forget some of the questions posed by Socratic bioethics: questions about, for example, how one individual's "particular trouble relates to others' troubles, and how their proposed solutions might cause others more trouble."

Like the other members of the working group, Frank does not hope that we can draw lines between surgeries that deserve some bioethical seal of approval and ones that do not. Indeed, in his chapter, he emphasizes how Emily Sullivan Sanford (whose narrative appears in Part I) both chose surgery to lengthen her legs to look more normal *and* refused surgery to remove the scars caused by the limb-lengthening surgeries she underwent. Instead of drawing lines, Frank is calling for the sort of dialogue that would allow families to engage in real reflection about the meaning of their actions for themselves and others.

Perhaps one of the most Socratic of questions regards the desire for normality itself: Why do parents and/or children so badly want normal appearance that they are willing to subject their own or their children's healthy bodies to surgery? That question might seem slightly mad. Again, if common sense tells us anything, it is that normal appearance is fervently to be desired. Yet that is the question that Eva Feder Kittay generously agreed to explore in her chapter.

Drawing on her experience as a child with an abnormal past and as the mother of a now-grown child with an abnormal body, Kittay's analysis begins from a careful consideration of the elusive meanings of *normal*. She shows that the concept of normality is integrally tied to the notion of desirability. What is desirable and thought normal "is intrinsically a social concept, in much the same way that language is, and like language, norms cannot be private." On the one hand, insofar as those concepts regarding who is normal (and thus desirable) and who is abnormal (and undesirable) are social, they are powerful and hard to displace. On the other, as she writes: "It is possible to establish new norms, to alter existing norms, just as language itself can break into dialects, or can alter by the addition of new terms and new concepts." Kittay argues that insofar as the desire for normality is the desire for recognition, community, and self-respect—and most deeply is the desire to be loved—it is our responsibility to speak in new dialects, to establish new norms, which make such recognition, community, self-respect, and love possible for all of us.

Like Edwards and Frank, Kittay does not argue for or against appearance-normalizing surgery. She does, however, argue for understanding what motivates us when we consider such surgeries. In the end, she invites us to believe that we can learn to see children with atypical anatomies as normal every bit as much as we can learn a new language dialect.

Part III. The Surgical Context

My colleagues and I are exceedingly lucky to have persuaded Jeffrey L. Marsh to write up his reflections, which were based on his experience in our working group and as a surgeon who performs craniofacial surgeries like the ones that Cassandra Aspinall describes in her contribution to this volume. Marsh not only performs these surgeries in this country, but also travels around the globe to perform them at no cost to children whose families cannot afford them.

In his chapter, Marsh stands by the principle he has worked by for the past twenty-five years, that "the goal of treatment is to minimize the stigmata of the deformity so that the individual can enter adult life as if the deformity had not happened." *And* he also engages in critical reflections on his own practice and on that of his colleagues, who treat children with conditions that do not involve the face. He explores, for example, why he thinks that using surgery to correct cleft lip and palate is similar to, and importantly different from, surgery to lengthen the legs of children with achondroplasia and surgery to make ambiguous genitalia look more normal. In addition to offering insights regarding the psychology of surgeons and families and regarding naïve conceptions of the difference between the psychosocial and physical aims of surgery, he also acknowledges the dearth of data to justify appearance-normalizing surgeries that purport to improve psychosocial functioning.

In the end, Marsh makes a statement that may surprise some observers of the normalization debates. He writes that, before his presentation to our working group, "I had not appreciated the tension between the goal of making a child look more normal and the goal of affirming a wide variety of human appearance." Some of us humanists could say something that would no doubt sound equally surprising to some of Dr. Marsh's colleagues: "Until Dr. Marsh's presentations, many of us had not fully appreciated the relief that can come to a child and family when the appearance of a child with a cleft lip and palate is 'normalized.'" Perspective, perspective, as James Edwards reminds us in his essay; all seeing is perspectival.

"What's Special about the Surgical Context?" was written by craniofacial specialist and pediatrician Wendy E. Mouradian and explores some of the challenges that are especially acute for children and parents facing decisions about appearance-normalizing surgeries. According to Mouradian, among the salient features of the context are the uncertain and subjective nature of the quality-of-life outcomes these surgeries aim to achieve; the fact that the patients are children; and the vulnerability of patients and families in their relationship with surgeons.

To the question regarding the vulnerability of families in the surgical context,

Mouradian brings the sort of insight that perhaps only can grow out of personal experience. To help the reader consider the nature of vulnerability in general—and the correspondingly great need to place trust in the surgeon—Mouradian tells stories of her own experience. One is about her own still fairly recent experience of being a patient who needed and received a new liver, and about the relationship of trust she developed with her surgeon.

In "Are We Helping Children?" Mouradian and her colleagues from the world of craniofacial care, Todd C. Edwards, Tari D. Topolski, Nichola Rumsey, and Donald L. Patrick, give a detailed account of a concern expressed by Jeffrey Marsh and others; namely, that patient and care provider decision making is constrained by a lack of strong outcomes data to support the conclusion that appearance-normalizing surgeries improve psychosocial functioning. In keeping with what Adrienne Asch says in her essay in this volume, Mouradian and her colleagues observe that "there is no simple correlation between craniofacial appearance and psychosocial outcomes"—and argue that doing surgeries without good evidence of benefit can do harm.

Mouradian and her co-authors do not oppose appearance-normalizing surgeries. Indeed, they are all part of teams that offer such interventions. But, again, they believe that doing surgeries without good evidence of benefit can do harm. They do not for a moment underestimate how difficult it will be to collect such evidence. They do, however, report on already-available evidence and make recommendations about what needs to be done to collect better evidence.

In the meantime, while we wait for such research to be done, Mouradian and colleagues urge that it is critical to provide families with information about *non*surgical means of promoting psychosocial adjustment. Our systems of care, they suggest, need "an ethos that strengthens the psychosocial component of care and focuses more on patient- and family-centered outcome assessments." It would be ironic indeed if, in our efforts to improve psychosocial functioning, we were to forget that nonsurgical, psychosocial tools can at least in some circumstances be effective at improving well-being.

Part IV. Children and Parents Deciding about Appearance-Normalizing Surgery

In 1995 the American Academy of Pediatrics (AAP) issued its influential policy statement, "Informed Consent, Parental Permission, and Assent in Pediatric Practice" (American Academy of Pediatrics 1995). The AAP states that "patients should participate in decision-making commensurate with their development; they should provide assent to care whenever reasonable." Even if children are not capable of giving fully informed *consent,* they should be involved in any decision where their parents give *permission;* that is, if the child is not old enough to give consent but is old enough to participate in the conversation, parents and medical professionals must seek her *assent.*

The authors of the AAP statement were too wise to offer hard-and-fast rules about the ages at which children are old enough to offer informed assent and when they are then old enough to give fully informed consent. They do, however, suggest that "older school-age children" (that is, ages 9 through 12) have the capacity to give assent and that many adolescents "age 14 and older" may have developed the decisional skills necessary to decide for themselves.

Reasonable people will disagree about when children are capable of assent and, later, informed consent. Indeed, reasonable people in our working group disagreed. Sociologist Priscilla Alderson, who has for many years studied children making decisions about surgical treatments, argues in her chapter that parents and medical professionals significantly underestimate the ability of children to decide for themselves. Reviewing evidence that reveals problems in the dominant child development theory, Alderson writes:

> Child development theory has trained us all to think in quite rigid age-stage stereotypes, to tend to hear what we expect the age group to say and be deaf to the children who do not match these prejudices. If we were to truly hear children's voices, we would have to suspend the age-stage theories we rely on for rapid, efficient interactions, and instead enter a "non-ageist" arena . . . [This would involve] the risk of listening to the child instead of the ascribed age level, hearing some children speak in "adult" voices, and exploring with them how far they can and wish to share in making decisions about surgery.

Whereas Alderson emphasizes the underappreciated capacities of children to decide wisely for themselves, philosopher Hilde Lindemann emphasizes the responsibilities of parents to choose wisely for their children. Lindemann describes what she takes to be the "necessarily asymmetrical" power relationship between children, who are physically, emotionally, and socially vulnerable, and parents, who are responsible to keep such children safe, to nurture them, and to "teach them how to live within their society." Lindemann argues that "parents are morally remiss if they do not use the power they have over their children." The bulk of her essay, however, explores some of "the moral dangers that beset parents who contemplate wielding that power by authorizing body-shaping surgery for children with physical anomalies." To get at those dangers, she appeals to the notion of *master narratives:* stories that express ideas that pervade our consciousness so thoroughly that we usually don't recognize that they are products of a particular time and place.

One of her four master narratives is what she calls the narrative of the Scientific Fix: the idea that we can fix anything and everything that we deem broken. Her concern about that narrative is that it sometimes moves parents to forget to teach their children "how to respond to circumstances that are *beyond* their control." As she puts it, "Grace is the virtue of living with what cannot be fixed, resisting fantasies of repair or restitution and accepting the limits of one's own effectiveness. Parents of children with serious physical abnormalities would do well, when considering the power they have over their children, to reflect on the power these narratives have over them."

Like Lindemann, philosopher Ellen K. Feder reflects on the cultural forces that shape parental decisions. Based on her interviews with families, Feder explores the decisions about surgeries to make children with atypical genitalia look more normal. She begins from the simple question, Why would loving parents subject their children to appearance-normalizing surgery, if that surgery puts those children at significant risk for losing sexual sensation—and puts the entire family at risk of suffering from the anxiety and guilt that attend efforts to conceal the child's unusual anatomical difference and history?

To answer that question, Feder turns to Pierre Bourdieu's concept of *habitus*. Akin to Heidegger's concept of the frame (or *Gestell*), which James C. Edwards explores in his essay, and also akin to the concept of the master narrative, which Lindemann explores in hers, Bourdieu's concept of *habitus* is the name for the unseen set of rules we live by, the grid we move in, the structuring structure that orders our lives without our conscious awareness. *Habitus* is the realm of common sense, or "what goes without saying." It is the realm in which we know things like, to paraphrase an ugly saying I heard as a child, "boys have penises, girls have vaginas, and freaks are in the circus."

Feder argues that if we grew more aware that what goes without saying is too often what goes without justification, we might learn to accept genital variation—instead of squandering so many resources on, and causing so much harm in the process of, trying to erase it. At a minimum, she argues, decisions about surgeries to correct the appearance of abnormal-looking genitalia should be made by those whose bodies will be operated on.

While the first two case narratives that Feder reports on are almost exclusively about the physical and psychological trauma that afflict families in which intersex surgeries have been done, the third case she describes offers great hope. It is not that the third family eschews all surgery. It agrees to some. The hope is in one mother coming to believe that "she doesn't have to take on the world to care for her child . . . to make him feel safe and to feel 'normal.'" Instead of focusing her energies on concealing her son's difference, this mother tries to, as Eva Feder Kittay might put it, speak in a new dialect, establish a new norm. This mother decides to create an environment where her child's differences can be seen and accepted—including running around in sprinklers and taking baths with kids whose genitalia look different from his. In the end, this mother exhibits one of the virtues that Hilde Lindemann describes and that Lisa Abelow Hedley exhibited: the wisdom to know when to decide for one's child and when to let her decide for herself, to know when to shape one's child and when to let her be.

The next essay, "Toward Truly Informed Decisions about Appearance-Normalizing Surgeries," was written by legal scholar Paul Steven Miller, who for the duration of our project was a commissioner on the Equal Employment Opportunity Commission. A large part of his chapter is devoted to a succinct discussion of several cases, which required courts to adjudicate among the interests of a child, her parents, and the state, when a surgery aimed at psychosocial (as opposed to physiological) function. That is, these are instances where one party believes that appearance-normalizing surgery is in the child's best interest and another party does not. In the last of those cases, Miller approvingly describes a Colombian court's ruling that the consent of parents for appearance-normalizing surgeries for their intersexed children was invalid. The court determined that the parents were motivated more by "intolerance of their own children's sexual difference" than by a considered view of their children's best interests.

Miller, who is a dwarf, is not unfamiliar with the stigmatization, discrimination, and inconvenience that can go with physical differences. And he is profoundly aware of the extent to which the pain associated with looking different originates in disordered social practices rather than in the disordered bodies of people who look different. He is not arguing against these surgeries tout court. He is, however, arguing for truly informed decisions about appearance-normalizing surgeries. Like the Colombian court, Miller believes that no matter how much parents love their child, they are at risk of harboring "fears, myths, and stereotypes about their child with a disability." Thus, he argues that parents need to "seek out the perspectives of those who live with the trait that the surgery seeks to change." Only if parents learn about the "life experiences, perspectives, and independent judgment of the community of affected adult individuals" will such decisions be truly informed.

From Paul Steven Miller's focus on the law and on promoting fully informed decision making, we turn to Adrienne Asch's essay, which concentrates on the psychological experience of children and invites the reader to consider how appearance-altering surgeries might make children feel about themselves. Asch, who is a bioethicist, trained psychoanalyst, and disability rights theorist, and who lives with blindness, begins her essay, however, by helping the reader to appreciate the power of the argument *for* appearance normalization. She acknowledges that we want our bodies to be attractive to ourselves and to others, and that "we surely do not want our physical selves to prevent other people from knowing the rest of us." Moreover, she acknowledges the full force of the argument that early surgery to make a child look more like what the parent envisioned might help some parents to bond with the child. She understands the argument that appearance-altering surgery could facilitate the sort of parental love that she herself says is essential for the child's sense of well-being.

But Asch is also keen to help the reader to remember that well-being has many determinants—and to help the reader try to put herself in the place of the child. Asch marshals data, for example, which suggest that there is a stronger correlation between how people feel about themselves and their sense of well-being than between how objectively attractive they are and their sense of well-being. While Asch grants the logical possibility that the child might interpret the offer of surgery (or, when older, interpret the fact that his parents submitted him to surgery) to be a sign of parental love, she warns parents and professionals that the child could as easily interpret it as a sign of rejection. Asch offers the words of disability scholar Harilyn Rousso, who, like Paul Steven Miller in his essay, articulates the key role that a disabling trait can have in one's core conception of oneself: "My disability, with my different walk and talk and my involuntary movements, having been with me all of my life, was part of me, part of my identity. With these disability features, I felt complete and whole. My mother's attempt to change my walk, strange as it may seem, felt like an assault on myself, an incomplete acceptance of all of me, an attempt to make me over." Rousso experiences her mother's attempt to alter her behavior as a rejection of her "authentic" self. Asch exhorts us: Try to imagine what it feels like to be a child and to have your parents reject what you take to be a core part of yourself!

Asch grants that if parents decide *with* children to get appearance-altering surgery, that decision "can be an instance of the love that promotes the child's well-being." But, taking her argument to its logical conclusion (which I flesh out below), she argues that parents should not decide *for* children; they should not, on her view, undertake appearance-normalizing surgery before the child is old enough to experience the sense of well-being that goes with being loved in a surgically unaltered state.

Historian of science Alice Domurat Dreger contributes the final essay, "What to Expect when You Have the Child You Weren't Expecting." Dreger is an internationally recognized expert on the history of the treatment of people who are intersexed (as well as on the history of conjoined twins). Proceeding from that expertise, Dreger offers advice to parents who get a child that is different from the "standard-issue kid" they were expecting. Like several of the other authors in this volume, one of her basic messages is, as pediatrician and bioethicist Joel Frader once put it at a project meeting: cool your jets.

In her essay, Dreger fills out that recommendation concerning how parents should approach decisions regarding the offer of appearance-normalizing surgeries: "Wait until the initial shock of all this has worn off, until you can get to know this child—and yourself, as a parent—a little better. Wait until you are well enough to digest the flood of information coming your way. Wait until you get over any sensation of drowning, until you feel steady on your feet, steady enough to ask to talk to more people, including especially parents who have had this kind of experience (even if their child had a different anomaly), and adults who were born with this kind of body." Like Paul Steven Miller in his essay, Dreger suggests that while parents are cooling their jets, they should seek out people who have firsthand knowledge of what life is like with the trait in question.

One of the core beliefs that motivates Dreger's essay (and much of her work, including her latest wonderful book, *One of Us: Conjoined Twins and the Future of Normal*) is that the problems that plague people with atypical anatomies do not begin with those people's bodies, but with the attitudes of those others who treat them badly. From that belief, it follows that we ought to consider changing the minds of those who hold hurtful and mistaken ideas about atypical bodies before we change the bodies of persons with atypical bodies. Such a view has been articulated from many corners over the last couple of decades (Davis 1997), though perhaps nowhere more powerfully than by Dreger.

As someone who has only the greatest regard for that view and the greatest admiration for Dreger, I think it is important to remember an important feature of the intersex case. Far too often, intersex surgeries do *not* achieve the end of more normal appearance and they may rob the patient of sexual sensation (Frader et al. 2004). That is, too often intersex surgeries *fail* to achieve their stated aim. That those surgeries sometimes egregiously fail to achieve normalized appearance and fail to maintain normal sexual function is *not*, however, an argument against surgeries that *succeed* at appearance normalization. If we want to argue against surgeries that would succeed at making a child look more normal, then we have to wage different arguments, for example, along one or more of the lines developed by Adrienne Asch and others: that the surgeries are complicit with suspect or hurtful norms, or that improving appearance does not *really* improve psychosocial functioning, or that these surgeries send to the child the hurtful message that they are not loved just as they are (Asch 1989).

I fear that I and Dreger and many like-minded others sometimes conflate concerns about the surgeries that fail and concerns about the surgeries that succeed. As gratifying as it can feel, it is not fair to let our moral outrage at surgeries that do *not* achieve their stated purpose to stand in for an argument against surgeries that *do* achieve their stated purpose. To our credit, however, our project not only considered a class of surgeries that often fails to achieve its stated aim (that is, intersex surgery), but also considered at length a class of surgeries that usually succeeds at normalizing appearance (that is, cleft lip and palate surgery). (Limb-lengthening surgeries don't have as long or as bad a record as intersex surgeries and don't have as long or as good a record as cleft lip and palate surgeries.)

Our working group unanimously supported waiting for children to be old enough to participate in decisions about risky and painful surgeries that might fail to reliably retain function and produce more normal appearance (for example, surgery for intersex and achondroplasia). With one exception, however, our group did *not* argue that parents should wait to involve children in decisions about primary cleft lip surgery, which carries relatively small risks and achieves its stated purpose. The exception was Adrienne Asch, who, after much struggle and soul searching, concluded that she could not endorse any decision about a purely elective surgery—such as primary cleft lip surgery—that was made by parents alone. The others in the group, however, no matter how great our commitment to letting bodies be, no matter how great our commitment to changing minds instead of bodies, could not get to Asch's conclusion. Perhaps in a world much better than ours, cleft lips would be viewed as one more form of human variation. In this world, however, most of us could not imagine that the dangers Asch fears should outweigh the dangers that can attend having a face with such significantly atypical characteristics. Nonetheless, I and the other members of the working group are grateful to Asch for making her argument and following it to its logical conclusion. Common sense is easy to come by; genuinely different ways of looking at the world are not.

The group's nearly unanimous acceptance of primary cleft lip surgery (surgery that often does not have a physiological aim and succeeds at normalizing appearance) does not in any way detract from the fundamental point made by so many of the contributors to this book: we need to learn new dialects, to be better at letting atypical bodies be. We do need to beware of thinking of our bodies as mere stuff, which we can put to whatever purposes we see fit. We do need to get better at affirming human variation. *And* we must never sacrifice the well-being of real children on the altar of those noble aspirations.

When to say yes or no to appearance-normalizing surgeries should rest with families. Sometimes good parents will decide for children, sometimes they will decide with children, and sometimes they will let their children decide for themselves. Given the particulars of individual cases, ethical logarithms will not be forthcoming. While we can't expect logarithms, we can and should expect better conversations and deeper understanding among all who participate in these decisions. We hope that this book will facilitate those conversations and that understanding.

NOTES

1. I have more recently attempted (Parens 2005) to sympathetically explore how people from different ethical frameworks will view the same enhancement technology as either compromising or promoting authenticity.

2. This is the only essay in the volume that has already been published (*The Hastings Center Report* 34, no. 2 [200]):18–29).

REFERENCES

American Academy of Pediatrics. 1995. Informed consent, parental permission, and assent in pediatric practice. *Pediatrics* 95 (2):314–17.

Asch, A. 1989. Reproductive technology and disability. In *Reproductive Laws for the 1990s,* edited by S. Cohen and N. Taub, 69–124. Clifton, NJ: Humana.

Davis, L. J., ed. 1997. *The Disability Studies Reader.* New York: Routledge.

Dreger, A. D. 1999. *Intersex in the Age of Ethics.* Hagerstown, MD: University Publishing Group.

———. 2004. *One of Us: Conjoined Twins and the Future of Normal.* Cambridge, MA: Harvard University Press.

Elliott, C. 2003. *Better than Well: American Medicine Meets the American Dream.* New York: W. W. Norton.

Frader, J., et al. 2004. Health care professionals and intersex conditions. *Archives of Pediatric and Adolescent Medicine* 158:426–28.

Kramer, P. D. 1993. *Listening to Prozac.* New York: Viking.

Parens, E., ed. 1998. *Enhancing Human Traits: Ethical and Social Implications.* Washington, DC: Georgetown University Press.

———. 2005. Authenticity and ambivalence: Toward understanding the enhancement debate. *The Hastings Center Report* 35 (3):34–41.

Parens, E., and A. Asch, eds. 2000. *Prenatal Testing and Disability Rights.* Washington, DC: Georgetown University Press.

Sytsma, S. 2004. Ethical dilemmas in retrospective studies on genital surgery in the treatment of intersex infants. *Cambridge Quarterly of Healthcare Ethics* 13 (4):394–403.

PART I

PERSONAL NARRATIVES ABOUT APPEARANCE-NORMALIZING SURGERY

CHAPTER ONE

Twisted Lies

My Journey in an Imperfect Body

Sherri G. Morris, J.D.

We are the new couple on the block, our living room skirted by dozens of unpacked cartons. Our neighbors take pity on us, bringing over tuna noodle casserole, cleaning supplies, and paper towels. We have a marriage certificate, a mortgage, one too many small appliances, and a stack of unmailed thank-you notes. I am Sherri, he is Richard. In short, we are typical newlyweds. Typical, that is, except for one tiny detail: in our marriage, there are two Y chromosomes.

Other couples with two Y chromosomes generally started out life as Richard and Richard, not Richard and Sherri. But in my case, I have been Sherri since birth. Indeed, my birth in 1958 was undistinguished, as I appeared to be an ordinary, healthy baby girl.

Approximately two weeks after I was born, however, my pediatrician noticed that my groin area was oddly distended after routine feedings. My medical records from that period show that he concluded that I had some type of hernia, for which he referred my parents to an appropriate surgeon to have it repaired.

When the surgeon began to operate, he discovered what appeared to be two suspicious-looking gonads in my inguinal area. He biopsied one of them, suspecting that they were not ovaries. Lab tests confirmed his suspicion: my gonads were, in fact, testes. My records state that the surgeon then did a buccal smear to check for Barr bodies (which appear only in the cells of genetic females). The test was negative, revealing that I had a Y chromosome.

Even in 1958 my treating physicians understood that this meant that I had been born with a rare genetic disorder, known at the time as testicular feminization syndrome and now known as androgen insensitivity syndrome (AIS). Because of an X-linked androgen receptor defect, my body does not respond to testosterone (in my case, the resistance to androgens is complete), the consequence of which is that during gestation I did not virilize. At the same time, by virtue of having a Y chromosome, I developed testes, which produced anti-Mullerian hormone, dissolving my rudimentary Mullerian ducts. This means that I lack a uterus, fallopian tubes, or a cervix, the normal complement of internal female organs.

At the time I was born (and, disturbingly, even in many places today), it was the common practice to remove the testes at birth, the putative concern being that they have a risk of becoming cancerous. In truth, this risk is virtually nonexistent until well after puberty, but I believe that removing my testes satisfied an equaling compelling psychological need to render my body congruent, particularly given that it must have been profoundly worrisome to my parents to have a female-looking child with male gonads.

Sadly, my parents were not offered any type of emotional counseling to help them parse the distressing fact of having a child labeled, as my medical records show I was, a *pseudo-hermaphrodite.* Instead, my diagnosis was considered a tragic mistake of nature by both my physicians and my parents. Given that I looked normal, however, my parents undoubtedly took solace in that they did not ever have to reveal the truth about my body to friends or relatives, and could keep it a secret even from immediate family members.

Having not had an opportunity to work through their own shame and guilt at having a child born with an intersex condition, my parents were even less able to develop any kind of game plan to disclose the details about such a fact to me. Instead, they were advised by my pediatric endocrinologist to tell me I had a simple hernia when, as a young child, I discovered the abdominal scar just above my pubic region. They were then to say nothing again until the eve of puberty, at which time they should tell me that I had "twisted ovaries," which had been removed at birth to prevent them from becoming cancerous. I'm not convinced that even at that point in my life they would have otherwise said anything, but at puberty I had to start taking hormone replacement therapy (Premarin) and so it became necessary to offer some explanation about why I suddenly needed to visit an endocrinologist and take a daily pill.

I recall the day my mother told me the "twisted ovaries" lie. I remember it not only because I quickly surmised that this meant that I would never be able to have biological children, a devastating blow, but also because the word *cancer* almost eclipsed the rest of the limited information I received. I was worried that my "ovaries" were not removed as a prophylactic measure to prevent cancer, but that I instead actually had cancer and that my parents just weren't telling me the truth.

There are two other significant things about that fateful day when I was 11. It was the only time for the next twenty-five years that there was any mention at all about my medical condition, other than my mother periodically reminding me to fill the prescription for Premarin or telling me that she'd scheduled another appointment with the endocrinologist. For twenty-five years the entire matter was swept under the rug, without any expectation that I would need outside support to help me cope with the fact that I did not have a normal puberty, would never have biological children, and had an abnormally short vagina, a detail conveniently omitted on that day but which I discovered myself at age 14 when out of curiosity I tried to insert a tampon into my vagina.

The other remarkable thing about the "twisted ovaries removed to prevent them from becoming cancerous" lie was that years later, after I met many other women with AIS from many other countries, I learned that this same thing had been told to them. I call it "the lie heard round the world." It is hard to imagine that endocrinologists of every stripe were instructed during their medical education that this lie would yield a better psychological outcome than the truth.

Perhaps it seems strange, but during early adolescence it was not infertility that troubled me the most. Instead, I was crushed not to get my period, as I looked forward to this threshold event since seeing a film in fifth grade describing the wonderful changes that supposedly soon would be happening to my body. Menstruation is a coming-of-age rite for adolescent females, and my friends would inevitably discuss the subject in intimate conversation. "Did you get yours?" became the question-du-jour in seventh grade, and I had to lie, feeling inadequate and ashamed the whole time.

Shortly after starting college, in the pre-AIDS and pre-herpes 1970s, the question shifted to whether I had had sex, a significant topic of conversation for early-stage freshmen of my generation. I started college shortly before my seventeenth birthday, and it was overwhelming to learn that all of my friends were sexually active, while I could not see how I would ever have sex given my anatomical limitations and attendant feelings of being undesirable and unacceptable.

Also during college the plot thickened as I discovered that there was something more going on than just not having ovaries. I was unable to get home to see my endocrinologist one semester, and went to the college infirmary to try to get a prescription for Premarin. I knew this was risky business because questions would be asked before handing me a prescription, but my mother insisted I have a prescription filled and I knew she would make me show her the bottle at my next visit home. I was not prepared, however, for the very first question the college doctor asked me. She inquired whether I had a uterus, perhaps because—as I only understood years later—she wanted to know whether I'd had a hysterectomy and needed just estrogen or also required progesterone.

I had to reveal that I didn't know whether I had a uterus, whereupon she took me into an examining room. I cannot imagine, and do not recall, how she was able to do any kind of examination, because only a child-sized speculum would have fit inside me at the time. Nonetheless, the examination concluded, and she handed me a prescription without telling me anything about my uterus. I was shaking as I steeled myself to inquire about whether I indeed did have one, and she said "no" without further explanation. I left the infirmary with my head spinning, tears streaming down my face as I headed back to my dorm room. It was the last time I ever went to any doctor for any reason other than the flu for the next eighteen years.

Shortly after arriving at law school I found myself studying in the all-night medical school library after the law library closed. It didn't take long for curiosity to get the better of me, and I started rooting around in the stacks of medical texts in search of information about my "twisted ovaries." I suspected that I had not been told the truth—or at least the whole truth—and needed to unearth the particulars about why I had no pubic or underarm or leg hair, why there was a scar running laterally across my bikini line, and why my "ovaries" would have become twisted in the first place.

I began by researching the causes of primary amenorrhea and hit pay dirt fairly quickly, stumbling upon a list of clinical features for a condition then known as testicular feminization syndrome. Any lingering doubts about whether I had reached a correct diagnosis were erased when I saw the accompanying pictures of young female patients (their eyes notably blacked out but their genitals in sharp focus) who had the condition. The stark absence of pubic hair made me confident that I too had this syndrome.

The information I read was both shocking and oddly satisfying. To that point I had always considered myself unequivocally female, even though my inability to menstruate or have children made me feel like "damaged goods." It was a stunning blow to discover that I had XY chromosomes and testes. To my mind at the time, it meant that I wasn't truly female at all, and that in some sense my whole life was a charade.

Yet even in the midst of such angst there was an element of relief. When I was 11 and was told that my "ovaries" had been removed because they were twisted and could have become cancerous, I was left with a lingering fear that I was secretly dying of cancer and that no one was telling me the truth about it. When I realized that my testes had likely been surgically removed in infancy, and this explained the scar above my genitals, it at least quelled such concern about my having cancer.

This newfound information also pieced together the cryptic puzzle of my life into a more understandable whole. Rather than seeing myself as a one-off freak, I felt reassured that this was a known quantity—a condition that had a name and of which I was not the only sufferer.

At the same time, the newly unearthed dark truths about my chromosomes and gonads were too much for me to handle alone. Yet it was impossible for me even to contemplate sharing this information with another living soul. I did what any rational first-year law student would do when confronted with any overwhelming personal obstacle: I tucked the information away into the deep recesses of my mind, put my nose to the grindstone, and made law review instead.

Throughout my 20s and most of my 30s I continued this pattern of overachievement at work and suppression of my terrible personal secret, even to myself. The best way to describe it is to say that I felt painted into a corner from which I could see no way out. Although gregarious by nature, I knew that I could never share the truth about myself with any friend, much less a romantic partner. For that reason I began, and then quickly aborted, relationships with men as I firmly believed that if they saw my absence of pubic hair they would not only recoil in horror, but also ask questions I was unequipped to answer.

There was, to a somewhat lesser extent, a similar isolation from even my female friends. I was afraid that they would discover my nonexistent knowledge about periods, and both marriage and children, topics that inevitably would come up in conversation, seemed completely beyond my reach. I never allowed myself to change in a locker room or anywhere else where someone might catch a glimpse of my juvenile-looking nipples and anomalous genitals. Always, I was left with the overarching sense that if people knew the real truth about me, they wouldn't like me at all. The toll on my self-image was profound.

Ultimately, however, it was neither the discovery of my genetics nor the particulars of the syndrome itself that caused me sustained psychological difficulty. Instead, the realization that I had been told lies by those from whom I had a right to expect the truth—my parents—left me sad and angry in equal measure. This breach of trust communicated to me that there was something shameful and unacceptable about my body even to those from whom I expected unconditional acceptance. Sadly, my parents were acting on the recommendation of my pediatric endocrinologist, who, at best, likely took no more than one or two courses in psychology during his training.

During this same protracted period I found myself rehashing incidents related to the medical management of my case. It was clear that my endocrinologist was uncomfortable with my visits to his office, no doubt because he was an active participant in keeping the truth from me and therefore not only needed to be careful about what he said, but also needed to have fabricated answers at the ready should I ask questions. Rather than fostering a healthy doctor-patient relationship, his communications were stilted and opaque. This meant that even as a later adolescent, I was unable to become an informed and active participant in my care.

But by far the most disturbing of my recollections was of being on an examining table while interns and residents "inspected" me, all the while discussing the particulars of my anatomy in medical jargon I could not understand. Adolescence is an awkward body image time under the best of circumstances, and for those born with any physical anomaly, this awkwardness is undoubtedly compounded. But rather than mitigating my body image challenges, being put on display in this manner made me feel ashamed, freakish, and certainly "unfit for human consumption" in any sexual sense. The loss of control in having others comment and touch my body, while I was expected to lie still and silent, felt to me like rape. This was not done in furtherance of my "treatment," but rather in furtherance of an intern's medical education. Physician training is important, but can such examinations be justified if they leave the patient feeling violated?

Low self-esteem, shame, and isolation are inevitable byproducts of a medical paradigm founded on lying to the patient about her condition, creating an environment in which the patient is discouraged from gaining an understanding of her body, allowing others to inspect and comment on her body, not offering counseling and support to work through the feelings of grief and anger, and keeping the patient isolated from other individuals with whom she shares a common experience. I believe that to provide expert diagnoses and treatment without placing the patient at the center of the protocol is more than just insensitive—it is bad medicine, particularly when patient compliance is necessary. I routinely flushed the pills I had been prescribed (in my case, Premarin) down the toilet, asserting the only control I had over the helplessness I felt. Having received no clear explanation of why I needed this prescription, I wasn't onboard and informed about the consequences of not taking it.

But the incremental harm I was doing to my body by not taking the pills would certainly have been outstripped by the more immediate harm I contemplated doing to myself. The persistent helplessness and hopelessness I felt, compounded by tremendous shame and coupled with the detachment of not having anyone with whom I could share this onerous secret, caused me to give serious consideration to ending my life.

In the back of my mind, however, was a profound and almost desperate wish to meet someone else like myself before I died. Whenever I would hear about someone who couldn't have children, I wondered if she too had "twisted ovaries." Much like an adopted child in search of a biological parent, I would walk down the street and look into people's eyes, wondering if we shared a common genetic link (in this case, the X-linked recessive trait for AIS).

This primordial need to connect with someone who understood what it was like to walk in my shoes might have gone unmet had I not heeded what can only be described as a small voice inside me prompting me to go a medical school library on the morning of December 26, 1994. In the past I had periodically gone to the library in search of information about AIS (as I had come to understand my condition was called), though often left frustrated having found only articles highlighting new research into the androgen receptor gene without any discussion of the psychological challenges faced by patients who lived with this disorder. But on that date my world changed when I stumbled across a letter published in the *British Medical Journal* by another woman with AIS.

The anonymous letter not only recounted a life experience that was hauntingly similar to my own, but also held out the possibility that someday I would meet someone who was like me. That possibility became even more of a reality when, in a later issue of the same journal (which I discovered later that same day), I saw a response to the first letter. This second letter provided information about a newly formed support group, based in the United Kingdom, for women with AIS.

Holding in my hands the telephone number and other contact information for the support group, I had to retire to a nearby study carrel, where I began crying with an intensity I had never before experienced. The best way I can describe it is to say that I had been shipwrecked on an uninhabited island for thirty-five years and in that moment discovered that there was another person on the island and that she had a lifeboat.

The journey from that afternoon in 1994 until the present has been extraordinary. In early 1995 I traveled to the United Kingdom to attend the first organized meeting of the support group. A member of the group graciously offered to meet my plane at Heathrow airport, and there for the first time I stood side by side with someone who knew—knew what it was like to have a body that looked and felt like mine, and knew the same secrecy and silence and lies and shame that had been the hallmarks of my existence. My life in earnest had begun.

Following that initial meeting, I attended several more meetings of the U.K. group, whereupon I established a similar support group in the United States. Having found help for myself, I felt it important to ensure that other women with AIS have access to the same kind of information and support. But there was a second, and perhaps even more important, motivation for forming the group: to ensure that other adolescents not spend years feeling alone and afraid, burdened by a secret and unable to form healthy friendships and romantic attachments.

It was amazing to discover that my life experience, which had felt so abnormal for so many years, was actually quite normal for those who, like me, were born with an intersex condition. To hear other women articulate the same fears and concerns I had was both liberating and reassuring. Ultimately, however, the most important "take-home" message I derived from participating in the group was that I saw the other members as both worthwhile and likeable, and that in turn allowed me to see how someone else might know the truth about my life and not recoil in horror or reject me out of hand.

In time I was able to leverage the strength I derived from participating in the group, sharing for the first time the truth about my having been born intersexed with some close friends. For so many years I had lived in fear that someone would discover that I had AIS; it was almost unimaginable that I would disclose this information about myself voluntarily. Yet there I was telling my friends and seeing that they did not reject me but instead were supportive and encouraging.

An even greater hurdle was the road to a romantic alliance. I had been terrified of allowing anyone to see me naked from the waist down, certain that my absence of pubic hair (this, of course in the days before such a look became fashionable) would itself earmark me as freakish and undesirable. The problem of vaginal hypoplasia weighed heavy on my mind, as I had not pursued any treatment to ameliorate this shortcoming (pun intended).

Armed with both information and a new vigor to deal with the situation, I resumed medical care after having not been to a doctor in more than fifteen years. In the process, I began to take estrogen, and started to use dilators to address my vaginal length problem. Walking into a doctor's office for the first time since I was 17 was, however, no small matter. I literally found myself shaking in the waiting room. For almost the whole of my life since adolescence, I dreaded going to the doctor. I didn't much trust doctors, given that they never told me the truth about having AIS and having been put on "display" for interns and residents.

While I cannot say that my more recent interactions with endocrinologists have always been pleasant, it is a fundamentally different experience to be a patient who knows the truth and is able to be an informed participant in making decisions about her care, something denied me by those doctors who perpetuated the lie about my having "twisted ovaries" and who seemed to have a palpable discomfort in treating me.

After having started to address my medical concerns, and in conjunction with ongoing therapy to sort out my feelings, I was finally able to consider in earnest for the first time embarking on an intimate, sexual relationship.

A few years ago I met my husband, Richard, through a local chapter of Mensa. We initially made contact through a listserv for this local group. Upon joining, I mentioned an enjoyment of classical music and opera. This sparked Richard's interest, and we had a brief on-line exchange following which he ran a Google search on my name, something he was in the habit of doing when he met new friends. Richard got more than he bargained for, as the search yielded a variety of articles about my being intersexed, my involvement with the support group, and my efforts to change how the medical community responds to intersex infants and adults. As it turned out, however, this was not off putting for him, but was a catalyst for us developing a natural openness and intimacy in our relationship.

To find myself married to someone I love, to have a life that is filled with the richness of close friendships, was unimaginable to me just a few short years ago. Those who lied to me about having AIS rationalized to themselves that they were protecting me, yet their actions fostered an atmosphere of shame and secrecy, which in turn communicated to me that the truth about me was unacceptable. The need to be loved and accepted for who we are is fundamental, yet this is denied to someone who is told lies and who receives the message that she is unacceptable through both actions and words.

If my experience speaks to anything, it is the need for the medical community no longer to see being intersexed as a horrible mistake of nature to be corrected, to the maximum extent possible, through surgical and medical intervention. Instead, my experience informs me that a better outcome is possible only if parents of a newborn with AIS or other intersex condition are referred for appropriate counseling so that they can work through any guilt or shame they feel about having an intersexed child. Only in conjunction with such counseling can they make informed choices about their child's care based on what is in the long-term interest of the child rather than making impulsive decisions designed to erase, often through surgical means but equally through lies, such shame and guilt.

At the same time, it is critical that parents be placed in touch with an appropriate support group, not only so that they can listen to the experiences of other adults living with a condition similar to their child's, but also so that they can gather support from other parents who are faced with the same challenges. In this way, their experience can be normalized, and they, in turn, can go on to become a valuable resource for their children, fostering an open and honest dialogue in the process.

Medicine, particularly Western medicine, does an outstanding job of curing illness but still has much to learn about healing. Those who are drawn to medicine as a career are committed to helping their patients and want what is in their patients' long-term best interests. The challenge is that physicians are sometimes overly impressed with new technologies and surgical techniques, losing sight of the fact that there is meaning and purpose to being born "different," and that surgery and secrecy have the potential to invalidate the patient's experience.

If I had a choice, I would not elect to be born without AIS. The challenges I have faced have contributed to who I am. Having AIS is not for me the tragedy my parents and doctors thought it would be. Secrecy and silence have left far deeper scars than my transitory struggle to come to terms with having been born with testes and XY chromosomes. Having met hundreds of other women with AIS, I can say that this has been true for them as well. While these experiences are sometimes dismissed as "anecdotal," I think that the experience of hundreds of individuals, particularly in a relatively small population, should be viewed as instructive if not conclusive.

It is encouraging to see the shift in thinking by physicians who are treating the intersexed children born today. There is a better world ahead for these children, not only as society grows more tolerant, but also because they will have access to important support resources that were not available when I was born. Medicine can play a key role in achieving a better outcome for these individuals—not with a scalpel but with information, options, and a deeper appreciation of their needs.

Do I Make You Uncomfortable?

Reflections on Using Surgery to Reduce the Distress of Others

Cassandra Aspinall, M.S.W.

The music was loud and people were everywhere. I had been to many parties like this before. A guy walked up to me and asked me to dance. After a few dances, we went somewhere quiet to talk. Things were proceeding in the way they typically did for most young adults at any party. But then it happened again. The twist that presents itself when least expected. "I want to kiss you," he said moving his face closer to mine. "Why do you want to kiss me?" I asked, feeling it was an obvious but coy and witty remark. "I want to find out if the inside of your mouth is as different as the outside of your mouth."

I am different, but I often don't remember that I am. I have a bilateral, or two-sided, cleft of my lip and upper gum-line. The cleft extends into my upper gum-line but not into the roof of my mouth (also known as the palate). I was born this way. I am not different to myself, but I am in the eyes of others.

In addition to my life experience as a person with a cleft, I am also a social worker with a master's degree on a team at a tertiary-level hospital that treats children with craniofacial conditions. I work with parents and children throughout the lifespan. I began this job fifteen years ago, before having children. I now have three children and my youngest son was born with a unilateral, or one-sided, cleft of the lip and palate. It is as an affected person, as the parent of an affected child, and as a professional that I will reflect on what it means to be experienced and labeled as different by others, and what it means to use surgery to try to erase or modify such a difference.

Why Parents Want Normalizing Surgeries for Their Children

One of my earliest memories of being perceived as different involves one of my grandmothers. I remember her holding me on her lap when I was about 4 years old.

She wanted to tell me that it was okay that I was different. She traced her finger over the upper line of my lip and began to talk about the fact that my lip was not like most people's, but that that was okay. She told me that because my upper lip already had what was called a Cupid's Bow, I would not have to "paint on" that sort of look the way she did with lipstick. I remember I had trouble understanding what she was talking about. She seemed upset, but I didn't know why. Did my grandmother feel sorry for me? Did she want me to look better so that I would feel better? Or if I looked better would she feel better? I wanted to make her feel better, but I didn't share her sadness about my face or myself.

At such a young age I didn't understand what her or my feelings were about and why they seemed different. But now I have some thoughts on this disconnect between what I think about myself and how others sometimes react to me.

When some people meet me for the first time they may notice the scars on my face and sometimes assume that something bad has happened to me or that something is wrong with me. Over time, these first impressions are moderated by what people learn about who I am beyond what I look like. For the most part people adjust to how I appear and their initial confusion or concern goes away.

While this process may be a natural part of what others often go through when they meet me, I have never had to do it for myself. I have always been who I am. As far as I am concerned, I started out like everyone else and just needed to work on growing up and developing into what I could be. But at a very young age my appearance became an unexpectedly important factor in that process. I believe that appearance concerns become an issue for those of us who are anatomically different much earlier than they do for others. For example, when my grandmother looked at me she imagined what should have been: the smooth lip and the straight nose. She attempted to console me, even though it seemed that it was she, not I, who needed consolation. At the time, I wasn't thinking about who I could have been, but she was.

Later, though, I did begin to think about that. I began to realize that my difference was not like other people's. I couldn't find someone like myself. My sisters could look around and see others like themselves and identify the things about themselves that set them apart. Things like whether they had blonde or brown hair. But hair color did not seem to be a critical part of who they thought they were in the way that my cleft lip had become a central part of who I thought I was. While I intellectually understand why some differences are less defining than others, in my heart I imagine that someday severity of difference will not need to become (even temporarily) a central and therefore potentially defining attribute.

Over the years I have been confused by how and when it is decided that a person's physical difference needs to be changed. Why are some differences tolerated while the decision to change others is almost expected? When a difference is deemed "severe," the question isn't usually "Should something be fixed?" but "When should it be fixed?" But should we always try to make uncommon differences look more normal? If you have an uncommon difference, can you appreciate that as a good thing? Can others ever appreciate it as a good thing?

It often seems to me that people almost fear having a discussion about the motivations behind "normalizing" surgeries. But families deserve to have that discussion. I am often concerned that without an openness to such a conversation, we will miss an important opportunity to understand and affirm human variation. We spend far too much time and energy being suspicious and afraid of what is considered "nonstandard" and assuming that our only job is to figure out how to eliminate "it."

Given that context, maybe it's not so hard to understand that because I look different meeting new people can sometimes make me feel bad or uncomfortable. But the question remains: How could I feel bad with my own grandmother?

Today I can surmise that my grandmother was sad and worried about the prospect of me being rejected *by others*. She was worried about the wrong and hurtful ways others might treat me, even if at the time I thought she was concerned about something that was wrong with me. Her fear that she couldn't protect me made her sad.

It is strange that her desire to protect me from harm had the unintentional consequence of making me feel bad, of actually causing me harm. My grandmother and others like her were putting themselves in my shoes. When they imagined how they would react under the same circumstances, they could only imagine the possibility of rejection. The immediate reaction then was to figure out how to make sure that they could help me to avoid the experience of rejection as much as possible. They could only imagine doing that by eliminating the difference that they felt would lead to someone's difficulty in connecting with me. But eliminating differences associated with cleft lip and palate usually involves having surgery.

This is where time needs to be spent carefully considering the motivations behind surgical change. The relationship between external change and an internal state of mind is very important to assess. Shame is an important part of that relationship. I would never describe myself as someone who is ashamed of who I am. But there have been times in my life when I have been ashamed of how I look. Who we think we are and how we think we look are of course not easy to disentangle. But it is important to give children and their families a chance to try. They deserve a chance to try to distinguish between operations that satisfy the child's desire to bring her appearance more in line with how she sees herself and operations that bring her appearance more in line with how others think she ought to see herself. To start trying to get clear about that distinction, it's important to start asking some simple questions like, What is the problem that is being treated? Whose problem is it? and, Who will benefit?

Parental Efforts to Protect Children Can Backfire

I grew up in a large family. I have two older sisters and two younger brothers. I don't remember my brothers, sisters, or parents reacting in any particular way to how I looked. I developed interests and decided what I liked and did not like to do. I was quiet and smart and kept to myself when I was young.

Outside of my home, I do remember problems with teasing. I remember people calling me big nose, and snot face, and flat face. But despite this I was able to make friends and join groups that shared my interests. The fact that I was teased challenged me but did not define me. I had evidence from my family that I was okay and I believed that there was more to me than my appearance. I remember feeling resentful about how I was treated by the popular kids. But lots of kids were excluded from the popular group.

One thing that truly did set me apart from my siblings and friends was the amount of experience I had with doctors, surgery, and hospitals. My parents had good access to health care and I was able to get surgical, medical, dental, and orthodontic treatment when I needed it. I found this to be both an advantage and a burden. I received attention that other kids didn't. But I also experienced more pain and life disruption. I worried that my treatment affected what our family could do, because of the time and money my parents spent on the treatment of my cleft.

In fact, I remember one day when my mom stopped me from taking a bus downtown. Bankbook in hand, I was ready to empty my account and give the money to my parents to pay for my orthodontic treatment. As guilty as I felt about the cost of my care, I can't recall ever hearing one of my siblings complain about either the time or money it required.

Throughout my childhood my father repeatedly told me that I could do whatever I wanted as long as I worked hard at it. I never got the sense that my appearance would get in the way of anything I might want to achieve. I was aware that I looked different and it might have kept me from some activities for limited amounts of time. But overall I felt safe and cared for. This was not just because I had help and support but also because I was allowed to be who I thought I was becoming.

We moved into a new neighborhood when I was 9 and I had to change schools. This was very hard, as I had to meet new people. But with the support of my family, my disposition, and my varied interests, I think the trauma was reduced. When I was a teen and wanted to look into ways to use makeup to cover up my scars, my mother took me to a salon to find out more about it. She never pressed me on it, nor was she upset when I lost interest in actually doing it.

As a social worker in the clinic, I can say that not all children are as lucky as I was. In some situations, parents are panicked about the appearance of their children and the possibility of them being seen as different. Although all parents can experience this sort of distress at one time or another, some experience it much more than others. When parents have consistent anxiety about their child's appearance, more and more energy gets spent on efforts to decrease difference and avoid social situations that might lead to difficult interactions. Unfortunately, panicked parents can, in their efforts to protect their children, end up creating exactly what they so desperately want to avoid: fear, anxiety, and depression.

Adolescence with a Norm-Challenging Anatomical Difference

All of these issues about appearance only get more complicated with the normal changes that go along with adolescence. Everything is on fire, everything is moving, and no day is the same. Much of this process is spent on trying to prove that you are both like everyone else and not like anyone else. This is a difficult challenge under the best of circumstances, especially in these days of media homogenization and hype. For those of us with norm-challenging anatomies, it is another thing altogether.

In middle school (when I was ages 12 to 14) I attended a large city school. I remember my acute sense of isolation. At that age I was certain that no boy would ever want to date me, not just because of what I looked like but because of my sense that having a "birth defect" marked me as doomed to produce deformed children. I had braces and just had my bone graft (a surgery to implant bone from the body into the upper gum-line to stabilize the gap created by the cleft). From my perspective, neither of these interventions seemed to really help me since they did not fix my appearance. I knew they had to get done but they didn't help me with what I thought were my biggest deficits: my nose and my lip. I was very concerned that they were crooked and scarred.

Every time someone told me "you have beautiful eyes" I was convinced that they told me that because they were afraid that they would let slip out how ugly they really thought I was. Any compliment I got was suspect. I was angry and felt betrayed that I had always been told that I was beautiful no matter what anyone said. All of the folk stories about the importance of what's on the inside made me furious. In the hormonal cauldron of adolescence I remember thinking that those stories were nothing but lies to make children like me feel better. I realized that people found my appearance to be a problem and a barrier to seeing who I really was. How could people in my family have pretended for so long and so effectively about what now seemed to be so blatantly obvious?

My mother attempted to help me. But I didn't make it easy for her. I accused her of lying to me about what I really looked like. I blamed both my parents for "causing" my problem because it was congenital. I would often spend enormous amounts of time attempting to improve my appearance. After I had applied and reapplied makeup, I remember feeling torn between wanting people to notice what I had done and being upset when they did. Being noticed as looking better meant that I looked bad to begin with.

I know I wasn't the only one who struggled in my adolescence, but I felt that my struggles were especially hard because of the nature of my difference, which seemed like such a key element in understanding how others related to me. When I came in contact with others, they seemed to struggle to figure out what they thought of me. As they struggled they seemed to make false assumptions about what I was like. For example, when I was a teenager, I was often asked if the scars on my face were from some sort of accident. This is because when people saw me, they would search for meaning and come up with something that connected with their reality. They often believed that I was like them and then "something happened" and I became different. I admit there were times when I let people believe this. I allowed them to create an identity for me that made sense to them.

The lack of a shared starting place is what seems to complicate someone's ability to develop a good understanding of who I am. If when you look at me you do not recognize part of yourself, then your discomfort may stop you from wanting to connect with me. If this happens with enough frequency and results in enough discomfort, I may seek to change this interaction. I may decide that I want to decrease your sense of being confused about my appearance by making myself appear more like you. I may decide to have surgery to try to relieve your discomfort. Since my adolescence, I have always asked myself: Should I go through surgery to help improve *your impression* of me, when my sense of self-acceptance is not the issue, but your treatment of me is?

Improving your impression of me or your treatment of me might seem like a normal enough reason for me to get surgery. But I am not so sure that this is the only way we should look at improving this type of interaction. Because difference evokes discomfort, should we always jump to looking only at how to eliminate or reduce difference? In my experience, too little time and energy is spent trying to focus on the ways we could increase the understanding and acceptance of difference.

The funny thing is that we all know people who actually experiment with increasing differences in their appearance. Again, traditionally, the most popular time for this sort of experimentation is adolescence. Even if sometimes viewed as risky, activities like body piercing and tattooing are widely seen as acceptable. I often wonder if the rule is that for a difference to be acceptable, it has to be chosen or reversible or hideable.

Having some time ago emerged from adolescence, I now think that having a cleft is an important part of who I am. I did not grow up in spite of my cleft, or separate from my cleft, or only in the context of my cleft. I grew up with it, and it is part of me. I currently have no interest in treating my scars with surgery or cosmetics. At the same time, I don't have a problem with others who choose to change their appearance. I know I am different and that some people feel that I could be "improved." My choice is not a rebellion or an abdication, although people around me may sometimes interpret how I live my life in those ways. I have always found it very difficult to explain how having a cleft contributes to but does not overwhelm my sense of self.

My Life beyond Adolescence and Surgery

I have seen photos of myself before my initial surgery to fix my cleft lip. And I have never regretted that my parents chose those initial surgeries for me. I also have never felt that surgeries done to revise that first surgery should not have been done. But how I look at surgery has changed since I had my last operation, at around the age of 17. At some point, I decided I didn't need to improve my appearance. I also didn't need to look more like someone else who didn't have a cleft. It seemed to me that the benefits of further surgeries no longer outweighed the burdens.

As a young adult, I was almost rigidly against paying any attention to my appearance. Partly that attitude reflected my desire to express and stay true to my unique identity, partly it reflected my growing commitment to feminism. I felt deeply that any move toward appearance improvement would be an admission that my appearance mattered too much. And this admission would somehow lend credence to those who had teased me because I was different. I applied pressure on myself to reject any appearance-enhancing techniques. Rejecting those techniques not only helped to reinforce my view of who I was, but it allowed me to reject those who viewed me differently.

I believe that part of what was going on here was that I was working on sorting out the difference between who I thought I was and who others thought I should be. As time went on I think I became increasingly less worried about what other people saw. But that's not to say that my level of concern about the opinions of others has disappeared. Even today I find myself seesawing between thinking that invasive treatments like surgery wouldn't be too hard to get through and then feeling appalled that I would even consider going "under the knife" just to avoid being noticed as different. The deliberation is neither clean nor easy. How much weight do I really give to what other people think? I find that some people do not understand that despite my abnormality I am not interested in "being improved." When I am feeling my strongest I feel well equipped to deal with these conflicts and come to the conclusion that, if someone cannot overcome their prejudices about my appearance, then it is she, not I, who needs to change. At the same time, is it really weak or vain to think that looking better will improve my life experience? If this seems confusing it's because it is: welcome to my world.

I also believe that others, who may have what are considered to be more significant differences than my own, may weigh the benefits and burdens differently. In those cases, the prejudiced impressions of others typically are not brief, easily changed, or infrequent. It is in these encounters that patients may decide to accept the risk of changing their bodies in order to decrease the psychological pain that their difference as interpreted imposes on them. The key here is that, whenever possible, the affected person has to work through this equation and decide on her own path.

I wish that we lived in a perfect world and it was reasonable to wait for children to decide for themselves about primary cleft surgeries (which aim largely at improving psychosocial—not physiological—functioning). But we don't live in a perfect world, and I am resigned to the fact that loving parents will not question the importance of the initial surgeries that close the primary clefts. But this does not mean that their decision will be easy. Parents wrestle with the physical risks associated with surgery, even if in the end they accept them to achieve "benefits" about which they are ambivalent. I put *benefits* in scare quotes because parents love their children as they are and in an important sense don't see the altered appearance as a benefit. They wish that the unconditional love they have for their child would be shared by the world. But it is not. Without that initial surgery, the child's difference would be greater and so would her distance from others. Is this right or just? No. Is this realistic? Yes. I firmly believe that you can be resigned to the reasonableness of parents giving permission for surgeons to do primary cleft surgeries on their babies—while simultaneously being committed to involving children whenever possible in decisions about appearance-normalizing surgeries. All things considered, the benefits of primary cleft surgery seem to me clear enough to warrant settling for parental permission (as opposed to waiting until later for the child to share in making that decision). But in that respect primary cleft surgeries are different from many secondary cleft surgeries as well as from the other surgeries that are discussed in this volume.

Once we acknowledge that reasonable people will make different decisions about many appearance-normalizing surgeries and that children can and should be involved in many of those decisions, then we are better situated to offer truly helpful clinical insights. Engaging in shared decision making about appearance-normalizing surgeries should ultimately be to the benefit of children, parents, and practitioners alike.

Surgical Decision Making Involving Children

This process of figuring out what I really wanted and helping others do the same has always been challenging. We all exist in a social environment. How I feel about myself will always be influenced by what others think of me. It's not bad to want to improve your appearance. Obviously, making your way through this for yourself is very complex. But the issues become even more difficult when children are involved.

The question at hand is, How do we help families to make these determinations with children? In considering the balancing of benefits and burdens of treating children, the viewpoints of both the child and her parents need to be considered. I appreciate that this process can be time consuming and complex. But I believe that all patients—including children—deserve to consider the actual outcomes that may affect them in both the short and long runs.

As a clinical social worker in a busy surgically oriented clinic, I am charged with helping kids and families work through decisions about surgery. As I help them to make these decisions I see them struggle with the same issues I struggled with. I work with them as I did with myself to figure out what they are truly comfortable with. This involves going through a process of realizing that it is okay to want to improve your appearance because you want to look less different and hope to experience less teasing. It is also okay to admit that you could feel better about yourself if you improve the way you look. What is not okay is to create a situation where you end up making an external change that *only* satisfies *someone else's* view of how you should appear.

These determinations are obviously very complicated to make when you are trying to sort out the issues for yourself. As an adolescent, I experienced them as bewildering and exhausting. And I must also admit that I have never felt confident that any decision I have made is my "final answer." But once a surgery is done, I learn to live with both the benefits and burdens. I can face this reality as an adult, but how do I help to facilitate such decisions for my son?

My Child Is Different Like Me

As I mentioned earlier, my youngest son has a one-sided cleft of his lip and alveolar ridge (upper gum-line) and a submucous cleft of his palate. His cleft was discov-

ered on prenatal ultrasound at around 24 weeks' gestation. This meant that our identification of him as someone with a visible difference started before he was even born.
I got complex ultrasound evaluations during all my pregnancies because of my own
cleft. The discovery that my third child had a cleft of the lip was initially hard for both
me and my husband to adjust to. Given my personal and professional experiences, I
hadn't expected to have a difficult reaction. I had so much information about what to
expect. How could I be upset that I would have a child who would be like me?

What I remember is that all of my negative experiences began to flood back to me.
All of the complications I had seen at the hospital were at the forefront of my mind.
At that time we also found out that my third baby would be another boy. Like many
parents, we had envisioned having a girl to add to our family. My husband said that,
given the circumstances, I should be glad that our third child would be a boy. His
point was that it would be much easier for a boy to be born with a facial difference
than a girl. Having once been a girl with a cleft myself, I was initially devastated by
his comment. But realistically speaking, the appearance of women in American society seems to matter more than the appearance of men. Sad as it is, that fact feels almost primal.

Regardless of the gender issues, parents must be helped to understand that, even
if their child is not born with a life-threatening illness (an isolated cleft is not a life-
threatening diagnosis under most circumstances), bearing a child with an anatomical difference will precipitate what feels like a crisis to the parents. It is impossible to
tell prior to a child's birth how big that crisis will be for these particular parents or
how long it will last. But even in my situation there were adjustments to make and issues to deal with. It is critical to address the parents' shock so that they can be helped
to deal with issues of shame and anxiety.

As I moved through my pregnancy, I acclimated to the reality that my child would
look different. Since I had seen many children with clefts prior to the initial surgery,
I didn't feel the need for any special preparation. However, my husband requested to
see pictures of children with clefts before the initial surgical repair. I understood from
my clinical experience that even with full prenatal preparation there would be some
initial shock when we saw our son for the first time. I had learned not to underestimate the impact of that first face-to-face meeting and not to overestimate the control
I could exert by providing educational information ahead of time.

The only pictures I had of myself prior to my first lip surgery were from the hospital medical records department. My mother didn't have any. Was this because she
was ashamed of me? Was this because she was a busy parent with two older children
to care for? I wasn't really sure. In meeting hundreds of parents who have children
with clefts you rarely meet anyone who does not take pictures of their newborn ba-

bies. But women in my mother's generation did not want before-surgery pictures. They thought such pictures would be too scary to share with their children as they got older or with relatives who did not see the child before the lip surgery. Today parents seem to understand the importance of helping their children to understand where they started. These parents, who are not hobbled by shame, are working to help their children accept themselves.

This prenatal preparation transformed our experience as expectant parents. I was trying to deal with my worry about how my baby would look, but of course not only about that. We were worried that my son might also have other undiscovered problems. But we dealt with what we knew was wrong to get over it and get back to our previous state of happy excitement and anticipation.

The reality is that such preparation can only go so far toward reducing anxiety. Like all parents, I met my son alongside my husband and we loved him. Our love transcended what our eyes saw and our brains registered as different. This is a critical point. Our brains registered him as different and there was a shock. This shock is something we each had and we each had to deal with. It did not last long. But it was as intense a reaction as any you will ever have. No matter how brief it was we carry it with us always. At the time we worried about what others would think when they saw him for the first time. When others saw him, is that how they would feel? Would they look at him and try to make sense of why he looked that way? Would they feel uncomfortable about how he looked? And because they did not deeply love him the way we did, would they abandon him, mistreat him, or mislabel him?

We cried briefly. We thanked God that he was otherwise healthy and covered him with hugs and kisses. After all, he wasn't really different if "different" meant somehow "bad." He was simply who he was. I believe that our experience was positively affected by the fact that we had gotten information about cleft care prior to delivery. Instinctual concerns about his physical and emotional well-being were reduced because we knew there were resources and people who could help us care for him.

That didn't make our fears about surgery go away. After all, cleft repair is not minor surgery and the physical stress on the child should not be underestimated. A surgery to close the cleft lip generally will be offered at around 3 months and surgery to close the cleft palate will be offered at around one year of age. Any rush to repair a cleft lip in the immediate newborn period needs to be avoided. The most important thing that can be done to reduce physical risks is to wait until the baby is a little older and is more physically stable and robust. Waiting is not only in the best interest of the child but also the family. It would be a serious mistake to rush a child to surgery on the grounds that doing so would reduce the parents' anxiety.

I have suggested that it's important to recognize that, upon the birth of child with an anatomical difference, parents can experience confusion, sadness, anxiety, and shame. It's equally important to recognize, however, that in most cases parents stop thinking of their children as different. Because of this, when it comes time for the first surgery (lip closure) parents' clarity about how to balance the risks and benefits can dissipate. The cleft begins to become simply part of how your child looks. What initially seemed like a no-brainer can come to seem like a hard choice when the routine risks of anesthesia and surgery are reviewed. Parents can find themselves asking, "If I can come to accept my child as she looks without the surgery, then why can't others?" Although the risk of serious injury or death is rare, it is still present. It can feel wrong to have your baby undergo an operation, even if in the next moment it feels like the right thing.

In general, parents can easily imagine good reasons to give permission for their child to undergo surgery. Such good reasons might include things like broken legs or a burst appendix. In those cases there is physical pain and in some situations a life-threatening risk. But cleft surgery is not about preventing physical pain or a potential risk to life. As I mentioned above, it is primarily about protecting your child (and yourself?) from psychological pain. Preventing physical pain with the risk of physical pain seems to make sense. But trying to prevent psychological pain with even temporary physical pain just doesn't always seem to make sense to parents. So working toward a place where it makes sense to choose this trade-off (treating psychological pain with a treatment that involves physical pain) can seem wrong. Parents need time to work through their ambivalence. Again, making a conscious effort to explore these issues beginning in infancy can help to set the stage for future surgical and treatment discussions.

Once the long-anticipated day of the surgery comes, there is tremendous anxiety and worry. When you first see your child after the operation you must adjust to his new face. I often hear parents describe this moment as feeling bittersweet. The change in appearance feels like a fundamental change in who the child is. Parents often describe themselves as feeling confused. There is a sense of relief that it's over and that the defect has been fixed. But at the same time parents did not experience their children as unacceptable or unlovable before the surgery.

This is as close as parents can get to understanding the confusion their child may experience when she considers appearance-normalizing surgery in the future. Those children will be worried, as I have been, about why they are considering a change. They will question their sense of who they are and how those around them affect it. How worried should they be about what others think? And they will ask, "Is it okay to want to look better? Is that in any way a rejection or denial of who I am on the inside?"

Helping Children to Develop Their Identities

If we are lucky, as we grow up we are helped to figure out who we are and how our appearance is related to who we are. My parents, family, and friends helped me. The same is happening for my sons. Ultimately, only they can decide how important their appearance is. I watch this happening a little bit at a time along with all the other impressions they have about their individual characteristics. Which ones matter to them? Which ones matter to everyone else? And is what they think of themselves more important than what others think of them? In the end, I can only hope that all three of my children will develop positive perceptions of themselves, finding a balance between paying too little and too much attention to how they are perceived by others.

But my youngest son's journey is especially difficult. His differences are harder for him to understand by looking at those around him. His appearance varies in a somewhat rare and unusual way and finding comfort by finding someone else who is like him can sometimes seem impossible. I imagine that people who are culturally or racially different can experience similar difficulties. The question is: How much do we want to encourage children like my son to conform with what is normal to fit in and to avoid pain and suffering? How much pain is too much? Is all pain to be avoided? We no longer believe that those belonging to racial, ethnic, or sexual-preference minorities should conform to societal norms in order to fit in. Or do we? The truth is that the pressure for all minority groups to conform exists. The question is: What do we do with that pressure?

When it comes to bodily differences in children, the answer has often been that it is easier to offer children surgery to help them look more normal than it is to change the attitudes of those around them. But how can we be sure that a surgical treatment will really make a child's life better?

To start with, we can ask children and parents this simple question: Will changing what I or my child looks like make me or her feel better, or will it just make those around me or her more comfortable? Yes, of course, it's impossible to sharply distinguish between how comfortable people feel around us and how good we feel about ourselves. Those two things are complexly related. But asking the question allows everyone to slow down long enough to examine what is being done and why. Parents I work with often comment that they feel they are delivering mixed messages when they discuss appearance with their children. These parents are aware of the conflict within themselves when they simultaneously reassure their children that they are accepted for who they are—and prepare them for surgery.

Such conflicts can make parents feel that they've lost their moral compass. But there really is no way out of such ambivalence. Rather than seek a way out, the best parents can do is face it directly. In surgeries that involve older children, the children themselves need to be involved in a discussion that explores the child's own ambivalence. It's our job to help them say how they feel and what sort of treatment they think is in their own best interest.

Including children in open discussions about their health care can sometimes seem threatening to the authority of the parent or even to the integrity of the family. But this is not the intent. Making certain that children are included in their care does not mean that parents are excluded or undermined. And talking with parents does not mean excluding children. Parenting is neither a dictatorship nor a democracy and individuation is a process that cannot be planned nor does it happen in isolation from others.

Determining the Difference between What You Think and What Your Child Thinks

Let me give an example of how hard it can be to separate your own adult experience from your child's. I had arrived at the after-school daycare to pick up my two older boys, who at that time were ages 5 and 7. I had my youngest son (who has the one-sided cleft lip), age 3, in tow. An older boy (around 10) came up and looked at my oldest son and said, "Is that your little brother? He sure is ugly!" I felt my face turn red and it felt as if my heart was in my throat. My body was tense and I was ready to launch myself physically and verbally into the conversation. But I stopped myself. I took a breath and sensed that my reaction was just that: it was *my* reaction. I could see that neither my son with the cleft nor his older brothers knew what this older kid was talking about. The older boy's faced turned red as my oldest son looked at him blankly and said, "What do you mean he's ugly?" The older boy responded, "You know what I mean." But neither of my sons did. So they simply turned and walked away.

How was it that my reaction was so different from that of my son's older brothers? There are many differences in how we heard what this other boy said related to our ages and our life experiences. My older sons were still young enough to not have experienced (yet) the stigma attached to being related to someone who is different. And they weren't even old enough to realize that he *was* different. My response was related to the fact that I had grown to understand all of this and more. I could no longer go back and see my son through their eyes and not understand or interpret the comments to be anything but hurtful at worst and ignorant at best.

Had I expressed my rage, I would have risked putting emphasis on this other boy's interpretation of my son's difference. I could have made my rage their rage. But by waiting to see what the reaction was from my children, I could then take their lead before intervening. The comment that my youngest son was ugly was dismissed. I did check in with my boys later to make sure that I didn't miss something, and I hadn't. That they didn't share my feelings did not warrant further attention from me. I did use this as an opportunity to understand myself a little better.

I acknowledge that there will be (and have been) instances where my interpretation is the one that matters and leads me to step in to protect my children, even though they would prefer that I didn't. But it is important to remember that there are many ways to interpret the same set of circumstances. Your version may not be the most important one worth acting on.

Again, none of this is to say that parents should always defer to their children's interpretations or choices. The question is: Where do we draw the line? When is it morally justifiable to make decisions *for,* rather than *with,* children? Again, when change involves risk and uncertainty and the goal is primarily psychosocial, the importance of deciding *with* a child is greatly magnified. Acknowledging the incredible complexity of relationships, the intensity of social pressures, and how difficult it is for children to express their opinions means that time must be taken to do the right thing. The possibility of coercion cannot be ignored.

This issue came up for me during my youngest son's recent team visit at the Craniofacial Center where he is treated. He decided he didn't like the look of his nose and wanted to get rid of the scar on his upper lip. I told him that the surgeon could probably do something to make it look better and I encouraged him to ask him about it. He was a bit shy about bringing it up, but he was able to point out in the mirror what the problems with his lip and nose were. The surgeon described how he could change how his lip and nose looked. Then he described what the actual process would be. He explained that to make his nostrils look more symmetrical (one of them is somewhat flat) he would need to get some "soft bone" (cartilage) from his ear and put it inside the skin of his nostril to hold it up better.

Was it appropriate for my husband and me to let the surgeon give our son these details? We firmly believe we would have been remiss to do otherwise. As parents our assessment was that our son could ask questions to explore his hopes and fears about the surgery. We were confident that it was important to provide him with an open opportunity to consider on his own terms what the risks and benefits were from his perspective. Because we gave him this opportunity to explore the details, we felt comfortable when he decided he didn't want to have the surgery. He felt that the worry he had about his lip and nose was not "big enough" to go through the anxiety and pain that was described to him by the surgeon.

All families will make different decisions about how to play out this process. Our process worked well for us. There are many different ways to deliberate about surgical decisions. Taking the time to think through how you do this as a family and as a patient, and how you facilitate the process as a medical practitioner, is what is important.

Final Thoughts

When they are old enough to make it feasible, children should be involved in decisions that affect their health and well-being And it is the job of parents to try to improve their children's lives. Especially when children are too young to participate in the decision, parents may decide by themselves for elective surgery. While they grapple with that decision, they should consider questions such as: What is the problem that is being treated? Whose problem is it? and, Does this surgery have to be done now?

Without answers to questions like those, the decision-making process will be incomplete. Without a clear understanding of the motivations and goals behind pursuing a certain treatment plan, the child could be unintentionally harmed.

As a child grows into who she is, it is her right to have her parents help decide what she wants. It is also her parents' responsibility to talk with her as she becomes old enough to understand the potential costs and benefits of normalizing surgeries. We must not forsake this sacred trust and fall prey to any illusion that we can make children into something they *are not* or *do not want to be*. Parents need to consider what a child's appearance means to her: what it means for who she thinks she is and who she is becoming. It is from this vantage point that authentic decisions can be made.

CHAPTER THREE

My Shoe Size Stayed the Same

Maintaining a Positive Sense of Identity with Achondroplasia and Limb-Lengthening Surgeries

Emily Sullivan Sanford, B.A.

I was 11½ years old when I began my first limb-lengthening procedure, commencing a six-year-long process that would end with my gaining 11 inches of height; a proportionately sized body; two torn anterior tibialis tendons as surgical complications; and sixty scars. Several months before I began, I sat with an adolescent girl who had finished all three procedures, without complications, and listened as my parents and other adults inquired about her experience. Every time she was asked about her life before the surgeries, her expressions ranged from uncertain to indifferent. "I really don't remember . . . I'm just so glad I could have the surgeries cause life's easier now." This made me, the prepubescent child, very uneasy. How could she not remember? Although I could make no assumptions about her upbringing, I knew my own had left me very aware of my condition, so I considered it an essential and positive component of my identity.

Limb-lengthening surgeries cannot cure achondroplasia. All achondroplastic people will be affected by their condition throughout their lives. Doing limb-lengthening to erase the effect of achondroplasia on the child's sense of identity is dangerous, leaving the child ill-equipped to face the challenges posed both by the procedures and by the rest of her life.

All parents undoubtedly wish to expose their children to as little pain as possible. But everyone's life is indeed painful, and both having achondroplasia and undergoing limb-lengthening surgeries inflict pain on a child. However, an achondroplastic child is not stuck in a catch-22 scenario. On the contrary, she can transcend the suffering that goes with being designated as abnormal. A parent's responsibility is to recognize and then show his child how she can deal with pain and potential difficulties constructively. A strong sense of identity is what an achondroplastic child needs to grow to become an individual who is as, if not more, confident than her peers.

In this chapter I analyze how my personal experiences have brought me to this conclusion. Neither my achondroplastic condition nor my experience with limb-lengthening makes me an authority on any of the issues discussed in this book; however, I hope that my reflections on my experience will be helpful both to others who are contemplating particular surgeries like the ones I had and to those who are grappling with the more general questions posed by such surgeries. Like many others in this volume, I strongly recommend that parents delay decisions about limb-lengthening until the child is aware of her identity as a dwarf, and can voice an opinion and participate in the decision regarding this potential alteration of her body and thus her identity.

Achondroplastic Identity in Childhood

Georgia O'Keeffe once said, "When I was born and where and how I have lived is unimportant. It is what I have done with where I've been that should be of interest." Perhaps it is my artistic identity as a writer that compels me to quote a painter more readily than the president of Little People of America (LPA). As implied in O'Keeffe's words, not a single dwarf on this planet will experience her condition in the exact way I have because, while achondroplasia may be genetically caused, it is environmentally conditioned. The huge number of environmental variables across communities and homes help to shape very different experiences for different people. Although my experiences are different from the experiences of other people with achondroplasia, I know that I am not alone in concluding that achondroplasia has had a positive impact on my life.

From my upbringing in the face of achondroplasia, I have always considered myself different and fortunate because of that. Who can say her personality was shaped by her normality? Two days after I was born, the doctor explained to my parents that I had dwarfism. "No one has a normal body," he said to them, thank goodness. "Everyone is different, everyone has biological mistakes. One person has certain allergies, another has bad knees, another deals with chronic rashes. Her mistake is just more noticeable than other people's." A mistake? My mother says she saw the maturity necessary to understand the unreliability of life slowly being reflected in my 9-year-old eyes as she explained that my dwarfism was caused by a genetic mistake. I no longer accepted the adage "You can do anything if you put your mind to it," knowing full well that my chances of becoming an Olympic figure skater were not worth calculating, and that most people who used such a phrase were either gold-medal Olympians or individuals who had yet to face such words as *handicap* and *lifelong condition.* My mother and I had this conversation after I had been inquiring about exactly *how* this mistake had happened. Like the majority of achondroplastic people, I was born to average-sized parents and my family will never know from which parent I inherited the gene. This eternal mystery was helpful in teaching me that the events of the past were irrelevant to the present, which I had the option to either mourn or celebrate.

Apart from not being allowed on the trampoline with my friends due to my exceptionally fragile spinal cord, I saw very little to mourn about my condition throughout most of my childhood. Teachers were trained well in advance of my entry into primary school to have a stool under my feet and a backrest in my chair. Every year, from preschool to fifth grade, my teachers would introduce my condition to the class and read *Thinking Big* by Susan Kuklin, a biography of an 8-year-old girl with achondroplasia, to the entire class. I experienced this extra attention as positive. While strangers on the street and students from other classes would stare and sometimes poke fun, family and friends would quickly jump to my defense before I could open my mouth. When I was forced to react on my own, my parents' encouragement had taught me to respond flippantly to taunts. "More room for more brains!" I said to a student on the school bus who had gawked at my large head. As we learned in our schoolbooks about racism, I knew people who judged others' bodies were wrong and would be proven wrong.

The truths regarding my condition were never avoided but adapted so as to ensure that I could comprehend them and shrug off any stigmas peers might possibly attach to them. As I would recommend to parents of achondroplastic children, my parents used the term *dwarf* as early as I can remember, before I could understand its entire meaning. That helped me become comfortable with it by the time its full implications began to manifest themselves. The uses ranged from the serious to the silly; when I wore my sunbonnet my father affectionately called me "Little Dwarf on the Prairie." My mother recalls that she herself was uncomfortable in referring to her daughter solely as a "dwarf" and opted to say I was a "person/child/girl with dwarfism." I appreciated her distinction but never considered the term *dwarf* negatively; at worst it was burdensome to explain yet again to an ignorant playmate. The term *midget* was incorrect; it actually defines an individual who is proportionately small, but it is mostly seen as a colloquial, outdated, and derogatory term perhaps similar to the term *moron*. I have always told people this after it has been used in my presence. However, I also knew the difference between scolding the rude and informing the naïve; the difference was intention and if an adult affectionately referred to me as a "midget," I responded softly but firmly.

It would be dishonest of me to deny any substantial drawbacks in my childhood caused by achondroplasia. In spite of my general satisfaction with my own body, it being the only one I had ever known, I was often taken aback when I saw other achondroplastic people and realized that my body looked like theirs. Their round hands and high foreheads were familiar *and* they stood out harshly in the presence of average-sized people, reminding me how different my appearance was. It was an ambiguous feeling, a momentary reconsideration of identity, when I was reminded that I had company in my short stature with people outside of my family, neighborhood, and school. My two best friends in intermediate school were exceptionally tall girls, who treated me no differently from their other friends, except when enthusiastically helping me body-surf or complaining to a carnival worker who had said I was too short to join them on certain rides.

Although I considered most attention to my condition positive—to a point, becoming rather accustomed to if not spoiled by it—I also knew from an early age that my identity was not dominated by my achondroplasia. At age 10, when I saw an interview of an achondroplastic couple in a documentary and the woman said she had sought to have a partner who was also achondroplastic, I felt very uncomfortable and somewhat ashamed in realizing that many would think that this interviewee spoke for all achondroplastic people, including myself. I perceived her preference to be nothing but prejudice. As I grew older, I understood that many achondroplastic people of this particular woman's generation spent most of their lives out of contact with anyone slightly resembling them. Perhaps this experience made them think that it would be easier to build a community if people just looked more like they did. I was exposed to other individuals with achondroplasia from an early age; one of my closest playmates in early childhood was achondroplastic and my family attended regional LPA meetings, where I secretly enjoyed seeing my and other parents feel slightly out of place as they towered above everyone in the room. However, I knew adamantly that my friendships were based, as O'Keeffe asserted, on common interests rather than on genetics.

I believed achondroplasia did link me on some level to the LPA members and the actors seen in the movie *Willow*—for which I had been invited to audition by George Lucas when I was an infant—but it also linked me to all minorities, from the issues of race to gender. *Snow White and the Seven Dwarfs* was one of my favorite stories throughout my childhood, one that I often adapted into a play for my friends and me to put on in my living room. Although I would have been the only actor who didn't have to kneel to portray a dwarf, I played Snow White every time, feeling my female identity as a girl was automatically stronger than my short-statured identity, as important as it was.

Deciding about Limb-Lengthening and Identity Alteration

One evening when I was 10 years old, my parents announced that we needed to have a discussion. My parents showed me a *People* magazine article about Gillian Mueller, who had successfully completed all limb-lengthening procedures, and began to explain the opportunity of limb-lengthening to me as I played on the couch with my brother. As they spoke, I had vague recollections of my orthopedists mentioning limb-lengthening to my mother. My perceptions had been that it was very dangerous and painful, coming from far away in another culture where scientific experimentation was prioritized over self-acceptance. It had nothing to do with my life, and the news about Ms. Mueller did not change this. I was Emily Sullivan Sanford. I was born in December. I had strawberry-blonde hair. I had dwarfism. Why change any of this?

"No, no, no, and double no!" I smiled. My parents explained that they accepted my answer, that they were very proud of me, but why not research the surgeries a bit more together? An appointment was already scheduled with Dr. Paley in two months. He would examine me and determine whether my anatomy would respond well to the procedure. I spent the next two months asking every night in my prayers that Dr. Paley would discover that I was inoperable, deferring the decision from myself to a medical authority that would halt all discussion. I mentioned the news of the surgeries casually to my playmates, who loyally shrugged it off as no big deal. Dr. Paley, however, fell short of my expectations and said I was an excellent candidate for limb-lengthening. Contrary to my deepest hope, the discussion about surgery did not go away.

My friends remained neutral on the subject, which is what I wanted. Teachers and extended family, however, began expressing enthusiasm for my great opportunity. My parents' love for me assured me subconsciously that their intentions had to be good, but urgings from acquaintances—especially average-sized adults—tempted me to rebel. My instructor for modified physical education smiled, "*I'd* do it!" What did she know? I muttered to myself. In an autobiography written at age 14 during my arm-lengthening procedure, I wrote: "Everyone had told me I was perfect the way I was and now they wanted me to change." As far as I was concerned, no one with long legs could be qualified to decide for me based solely on the fact that they were older than I was. In fact, they were not allowed to have any opinion other than that which supported my own. What was my opinion? I wasn't sure.

To me, achondroplasia was *not* a disease; a disease could progress and cause harm, or it could be cured. My achondroplasia would never be cured and I was grateful for that. To do so would be to remove all physical evidence of an enormous piece of my identity and thus I was relieved that such a choice could never be presented to me. However, just as my parents' support of my achondroplastic body had nurtured my self-confidence about it, their support of limb-lengthening as an option suggested strongly to me that it was worth considering. Dr. Paley's staff photographed me and from the image produced a computer-generated portrait of me with 10 inches of height added to my legs. With that picture I happily imagined myself as an independent teenager traveling alone to France to visit my best friend's family, carrying my own luggage with no modifications for me. It was tempting, and I gradually began to realize that many of the activities from which I had always been excluded would no longer be off-limits. I had never known exactly what I was missing, but here was my chance to experience almost all of the world of average-sized people.

I was vaguely aware of the ethical controversy surrounding the surgeries, hearing that many achondroplastic people opposed the concept of physically blending in after so many efforts had been made to accept achondroplasia as a difference that should be celebrated, not erased. I remember being vehemently opposed to undergoing any sort of surgery and major body alteration for purely cosmetic reasons. For my own sense of morality and identity, I had to defend a decision to have limb-lengthening on the grounds of practicality, just as I had had fibular osteotomies at the age of 5 to curtail bowing. It took a very long time to comprehend not only how my present life would practically change but also what future obstacles would be eliminated. Consistent contact with many of Dr. Paley's patients who were my age gave me a strong sense of security and acceptance into the community of people who had similar experiences as well as this new one.

I cannot recall what potential benefit ultimately swayed me toward the procedures. I can recall, however, that an essential ingredient of the decision-making process was my sense that the decision was my own. I needed that sense of ownership both to reach a decision and to get through the procedures. Priscilla Alderson's reports of children's awareness are profoundly validating and nostalgic to me, reminding me that my memories of my own awareness are not sentimental figments of my imagination. As the surgeries approached, I began learning all the medical terms I overheard: from the parts of the fixators I wore to the drugs I was prescribed. By the age of 12, I insisted on being present at every instance in pre-op when the doctor read the long, detailed list of surgical risks before my parents signed a waiver. I felt brave and responsible in realizing what I had agreed to undergo. During one clinical check-up, I felt chills down my back and anger in my cheeks as I heard a mother confer with the surgeon about limb-lengthening for her 7-year-old daughter. "Children can't make the decision of course," she smiled, "they're too young." I pitied her daughter immediately because, although I was sitting in a wheelchair similar to the one to which she would also soon be confined, I had brought myself there. That was what mattered.

When I finished school three weeks early to embark on the first operation, I knew I had made the right decision and I had unwavering support from my family, friends, school, and the staff and patients at Dr. Paley's clinic. My fifth grade class threw me a goodbye party and sang a song they had crafted—"The Emily Song"—which put me in tears as it demonstrated an accurate understanding of my identity: "*You make us proud, you make us glad / Hate to see you leave our pad. The boys and girls at your school care / When you return, we'll all be here. In life you'll surely go real far / We think you're perfect as you are.*"

The Experience of Limb-Lengthening

With a few whacks of a surgical hammer, Dr. Paley not only began my six-year-long experience with limb-lengthening but also left my legs weaker than they had ever been. The day after that first surgery, I was made to stand for 60 seconds at the parallel bars in the physical therapy room to prevent blood clots. The pain was excruciating. My mother wept and I sobbed, and we both silently asked, What did we just get ourselves into?

The excruciating pain did subside once the immediate post-op effects wore off and I was taking heavy painkillers regularly. Creeping across the room like a turtle with a walker continued to hurt at different intensities over time, but the fact that I needed a walker at all was the initiation to the psychological impact of the procedure.

After having ridden a bike with training wheels and participated in modified gym class, I was suddenly unable to do either for one year during the first procedure (and for a collective five years in all). My parents received a Handicapped Parking sticker for our car. We purchased a wheelchair customized to my size. After being subconsciously aware of the world's practical preferences for people of average size, I was now acquainted with its intolerance for the nonambulatory. *Handicapped* was a term LPA bucked, but there was no question about my condition during the process that was to ironically bring me past all the limitations I had experienced by virtue of achondroplasia and was experiencing by virtue of my wheelchair.

Like physical pain, psychological pain can be dealt with passively or constructively. The painful fact that my legs could simply not race me across the room as they once had would leave me instantly frustrated and often depressed for various reasons at my different ages during each procedure. When I was younger, the desire to be physically active was greater and essential to my daily happiness. When I was older, I was more content to read or write on my laptop, but my self-consciousness from being so obviously handicapped was enormous.

However, at 16, while other girls my age had to overcome insecurity to wear the right bathing suit, I had to hold my head high (or at least down into a book) while being pushed through the mall by my friends or parents. There is no better test of one's loyalty to the maxim "I don't care what other people think"—which so many rebellious, body-altering adolescents profess—than being thrust into a bulky wheelchair with heavy apparatuses on both legs. My friends decorated my wheelchair with puffy-paint and named it after one of their cars that had recently died. One put my hair into fifty-odd braids as an excuse to avoid bed-head. To every classmate who boasted a piercing in some unconventional place, I would uncover a limb penetrated with four or more stainless steel pins. On bad days I wished that I could worry about what bathing suit to wear rather than about when I would walk again like I used to. On good days, I prided myself on the profundity of my mission in contrast to the petty worries of others.

Making friends in the hospital who shared my disability but little else was a disconcerting experience. I yearned to return home to those who might have no idea what I was going through—one of them accidentally sat on my foot fixed in place by pins—but who knew what books, films, and music could be good distractions as I had a muscle spasm. My younger brother—who certainly received less attention from our parents than I did and subtly expressed natural envy on occasion—became very familiar with my physical needs and volatile mood, and knew better than anyone in the hospital what could make me laugh. He and my friends, all of them average-sized and physically fit, were a confirmation that my identity expanded far beyond my physical condition.

One of the issues most debated by others who have not undergone limb-lengthening that makes me most uncomfortable is pain. Critics portray the procedures as torture, while surgeons emphasize that there really are hardly any difficulties at all. Both portrayals are inaccurate. As a patient who screamed, "I hate you!" to her surgeon until she was hoarse as he unscrewed pins from her thigh, I can attest that the procedures are indeed very painful. But I am not convinced by the argument that the pain associated with the surgeries outweighs the benefits. As I said before, many parents feel their duty is to expose their children to as little pain as possible. Although I risk sounding like an "in-my-day" conservative, I believe that too many parents fail to understand the nature and consequences of pain. Pain does not have to be traumatic. When dealt with constructively, it can reduce rather than increase the child's fears in life.

A college friend and I recently empathized about difficulties endured in childhood and adolescence. While coping with no major physical difficulties of his own, he had been forced into early independence and extra responsibility at a young age when one of his parents began to suffer on and off from an unknown mental illness. His entire family had naturally experienced tremendous stress but reacted with openness and solidarity. Both of us came to the conclusion that we would never erase the difficulties from our pasts were we to be presented with the option to do so. We both observed that, different from many of our classmates, when we face the challenges and pressures of college and the world beyond our homes, we tend to cope well—and perhaps even to be especially open to exploring new areas. When we face new challenges, we find assurance and strength in knowing that we have already successfully met others. For that we are grateful; we consider all of it to be essential components of our respective identities.

I differentiate here between embracing the lessons learned from having endured difficulty and stagnating in a victim complex. Although I may have become accustomed to the extra attention bestowed on me by my family, I am not defined by how much I have suffered, nor did I ever wish to be. In my experience, most individuals who become dependent on recognition for having suffered more than anyone else do not have a high threshold for any form of pain or were not raised with a strong sense of self-esteem. When parents instill in a child the confidence that she is every bit as valuable as her peers, that child learns to face challenges unfazed and to answer inquiries about her difference with pride or irony, depending on the nature of the inquiry. When a young person is unsure of her worth as a person, she may, in an effort to get positive attention, call attention to her anatomical difference. Alternatively, a person who does not have a strong sense of her worth as a person may desperately seek to camouflage her anatomical difference. I have encountered many young people who have adopted one of these strategies, especially in adolescence and postadolescence, and almost all of them did not have an "official" disability. Mild weight problems or weak joints were not significant enough to move their parents to assure these people that they were valuable and beautifully different, but they were significant enough to incite self-doubt and insecurity. Their self-doubt and insecurity moved them to try to construct a stronger sense of self, which too often seems to lapse into self-scrutinizing and hopelessly narcissistic monologues.

Whenever I went into a rage because I had come down with yet another burning pin-site infection or my muscles had tightened to the point that physical therapy was a scream fest, I did not blame anyone but myself. I certainly took my anger out on those around me—and my most constant companions were my parents—but I did not ever blame them for having encouraged me to undergo the surgeries. I knew I had made the choice and I never regretted my decision. On a few occasions, often at four in the morning as I wailed in pain, my tearful mother offered that we stop the lengthening process. I steadfastly refused. I had made a commitment to reach 6 inches of length on my tibias, 5 inches on my humeri, and 4 inches on my femurs, and quitting at any point short of the goal would render it all not worth it. This sense of conviction was the principal driving force throughout the six years.

However independent a child may be in the decision-making process, she is handicapped by her inability to fully comprehend all of the nuances and jargon of the health care establishment. Parents are thus responsible as interpreters when, for example, a child needs to understand that she must brace herself for upcoming pain. As with every trip to the doctor's office, parents of course should not scare their child with an overly honest emphasis on everything that could possibly cause pain because children are gifted with wild imaginations. I was no exception. Until I learned to catalogue all the different sorts of pain I had endured into a hierarchy ranging from wholly unpleasant to tolerable, I was terrified at the idea of the pre-op blood test and the intravenous needle. Downplaying the potential for pain should also be avoided; I felt betrayed and condescended toward every time the transparent lines "It will barely hurt for just a second; it's the smallest needle in the world" were fed to me. Children have reason to be suspicious and imaginative.

I no longer fear pain as I once did, because now I face it with the knowledge that I have endured far worse. This perhaps does not immediately calm all parents and the repercussions of pain in my life have not always been productive. I once impatiently told a 17-year-old classmate to shut up as she moaned from having mildly burned herself with a curling iron. I always win when peers compare hospital horror stories or reasons they were sent there. But, when I recently sprained my knee dancing, I found myself choosing: to wallow in frustration that my body that had required so much time and money once again demanded my attention, or to react casually since two weeks of using a cane, wearing an ace bandage, and doing odd exercises were nothing compared to what I had endured before. I easily chose the latter. My close friends and professors knew of my medical history and silently understood what this minor injury meant to me. As for the rest of the school, I didn't care what they thought of my cane or the scene of my two friends lifting me onto their shoulders off the dance floor. I had survived far more embarrassing situations and it required less than a moment's thought to know there was really nothing to be embarrassed about.

Every accomplishment during the procedures was magnificent. I crowed with joy the day I realized could stand up with my head well above water in the 4-foot-deep area of the hydrotherapy pool. I grinned when I successfully reached the top of my head with a brush in my hovering hand. I beamed as I felt along my back and could barely detect the once prominent curvature caused by lordosis and reduced in surgery by Dr. Paley as part of the procedure done to my femurs. I was elated when I took my

first steps for the second time at age 17 as a friend held his arms out to me like a father to a toddler. In my yearbook profile I listed that moment as one of my favorites
in all of high school. I did not list the joy I felt when I embraced my friends at their
shoulders for the very first time. Words would fall short of fully expressing that sensation.

And although I spent the entirety of all three limb-lengthening procedures saying,
"I can't wait to get these things off!" and felt genuine relief when the removal dates arrived, I kept every piece of each apparatus I was allowed to. The metal frames I had
named "cages" had accompanied me through some extremely difficult times—
granted, they had in fact caused them. I had never been truly embarrassed to have
them; I had chosen to have them. In a way I felt and sometimes continue to feel that
they were extensions of my identity, just as my achondroplasia has been. After all, the
night before my very first surgery I kissed my "old" shins goodbye, able to part with
them but kissing them nonetheless.

Now That the Procedures Are "behind" Me

The mundane advantages of limb-lengthening are important, and they are often
accompanied by reminders of my mundane but lingering disabilities. I can reach
more shelves in various public places than before. I do not need my car modified. I
can carry my own luggage for a year's worth of traveling across Europe. But I cannot
carry my computer, my mini-refrigerator, or my television set from my dorm room
to my car; whereas my peers do not need assistance with such tasks, I do. It is still rare
that I find a pair of pants that does not need to be hemmed. I do not dare participate
in full-contact games with my friends. I always need a hand when grappling over un-
even terrain and my friends have learned to automatically offer it, just as they have
learned to fall into my pace of walking and to find benches for me periodically when
we are out on our feet for more than an hour. Due to my ruptured tendons, I cannot
dismount from a bicycle without falling. Although I was wistfully envious of those
who could speedily bike around Berlin when I lived there, I knew that the surgeries
had increased my ability and endurance to live there at all. Furthermore, had I committed to another long stretch of tendon reconstruction and physical therapy, college
would have been interrupted and I wouldn't have been in Berlin at that time in the
first place.

Like anyone who has ever been labeled *handicapped,* I continue to derive joy from
physical achievements others take for granted. I am proud to see my endurance increase over the years that I have been working in a nursery school during college.
Whenever I trip in front of my friends as a result of my ruptured tendons, they help

me up and celebrate how long it has been since I last tripped. On a solely physical level, the effects of my achondroplasia and limb-lengthening are mundane but lingering. The effects on my identity have been anything but that.

I once thought a ridiculous percentage of the population was ignorant of the definition of achondroplasia, but joining the even more elite group of dwarfs who have undergone limb-lengthening has extended my explanatory monologue tenfold. However, it is never a monologue with people who become truly special to me. With such people, the event of explaining my condition is an interview if not a dialogue, always unique and interesting, including reactions and questions I have never heard before. With each new acquaintance, I gauge the relationship to tentatively plan the appropriate moment to discuss my achondroplasia and the procedures that have rendered it less obvious. (A gay friend and I once likened this planning to coming out of the closet.) Since many people notice my scars, hands, or gait, I prefer to bring up the topic as early as possible to put them at ease. However, since it is now more of an issue of the past influencing my present identity than anything else, I never intend to waste divulging such a thing to someone who would obviously not divulge such a complex side of his identity to me.

When I was an exchange student to France just over a year after I had let my last set of canes go, the profile my host saw described me as "lightly handicapped." She of course could not imagine what was implied by such a description, so I arrived with copies of medical articles in which I had appeared and I translated them to her until I was convinced she knew roughly how "handicapped" I am. At the daycare center in France where I volunteered, I was given an extra hour during my lunch break to relax in order to rest my back that had begun to hurt badly by the third day of following toddlers around and my supervisor noticed me trying to inconspicuously lie on the floormat. It was frustrating to continuously require more attention and care than those around me, but my needs were not obvious to everyone. It was my choice to mention it to anyone apart from those immediately concerned, and I realized that my newly evolved identity in the postsurgical context was very much concerned with choices rather than automatic judgments by others on my appearance.

At the end of my stay, I spotted a teenager with dwarfism across a platform in the Paris subway. She was flanked by friends who affectionately played with her dreadlocks and I sensed a smile creep across my face. After a minute, I suddenly realized not only how long I had been staring at her, but that, should she notice me watching her, she would have no reason to assume that I was connected to her in any way. She would most likely take me for an impolite, gawking person of average size. Did I want to shout to her what we shared? My priority was to look away before she noticed, and then I smiled more broadly to myself. What was my identity to her?

When my childhood friend with achondroplasia came to visit me for the first time after my first limb-lengthening surgery, she opened the door and her mouth hung open as her face traveled upward to meet mine. In attending the screening of Lisa Hedley's documentary *Dwarfs: Not a Fairy Tale*, I suddenly felt self-conscious—like my parents—as I towered above the other dwarfs featured in the film and felt my identity grow and shrink. One made the offhand comment, "She's not a dwarf! She cheated!" to which another responded by facing me, "I'm on your side, honey. No way did you cheat."

I have now described myself on occasion as a "dwarf," though this term seems inaccurate in light of the limb-lengthening procedures. I cannot name another of my traits that has had *more* of an effect on my individual identity than achondroplasia and limb-lengthening, yet achondroplasia does not define me. It is of equal significance to my gender, ethnicity, family, and personal passions. Am I a person with dwarfism? A young woman with dwarfism? A writer with dwarfism? An American with dwarfism? I am equally uncomfortable allowing any of these terms to summarize me, always preferring adjectives to nouns.

I was raised by a progressive family, and it was more likely my parents than my dwarfism that raised me to be accepting if not celebratory toward differences in ethnicity, sexual orientation, and physical conditions, yet having achondroplasia has sensitized me toward these issues by making them personal. For better or for worse, this contributed to what many of my friends and family have identified in me as righteous indignation over the world's many injustices. When a gay man was ostracized for the way he was born, I couldn't help but see our shared vulnerabilities. Who was to say a person prejudiced against certain skin colors would give me any more of a chance? Weren't dwarfs used in gruesome Nazi experiments along with twins and other genetic "deviants"? Three years ago on a language trip abroad, I found myself discussing the issue of having minority status with my three classmates and one cynically joked that all of us—a Catholic, a Jew, a lesbian, and a dwarf—could all have been shipped off on Hitler's trains.

I know many members of minorities take offense at emphasizing the universal experience of being different, arguing that this is a presumptuous generalization as dangerous as prejudice. The different qualities and forms of oppression we experience are what determine our very different identities. Yet how more automatically similar is my character supposed to be to that of another dwarf as opposed to a Catholic, Jewish, or lesbian person? One day I stumbled across a link to a religious group on the LPA website and was shocked to read the advertisement, "For dwarfs who just enjoy conservative chat." Didn't belonging to a minority automatically make it impossible to be conservative? Apparently not. They could not speak for me as I could not speak for them in spite of our anatomical similarities. Simply being able to literally put yourself in someone else's shoes does not guarantee that you will share perspectives.

As I mentioned before, every year, from preschool to fifth grade, my teachers would read *Thinking Big,* by Susan Kuklin. After fifth grade, I began my first limb-lengthening procedure and the book, geared toward younger children in any event, was no longer read as I moved on to middle school with a longer set of limbs. For five years, from eighth through twelfth grades, I used the book with several other resources to teach middle and high school health classes in two-day seminars about dwarfism and limb-lengthening at the urging of the instructor. The last time I saw the book was when I began working at the nursery school at Bard College. My scars triggered the conversation of my achondroplasia with my supervisor, who then jumped on the opportunity to purchase the book to enlighten the children. The book has been prevalent but not dominant in my life; it does not define me but it offers explanations to many parts of me. My identity as an achondroplastic, limb-lengthened dwarf serves to enlighten others, and to remind me that what I teach about it is what I have been learning from it. I endeavor to use what I have learned from my experiences with achondroplasia and limb-lengthening to the utmost advantage. These advantages are not always clear, but I am certain that my ambivalence is no deeper than anybody else's whose identity is in part rooted in how she is "different." I forge my identity in light of my difference with as much confidence as possible, hoping that I am making the right decisions for those who perceive me and for myself as the person I claim to be.

CHAPTER FOUR

The Seduction of the Surgical Fix

Lisa Abelow Hedley, J.D.

As the mother of a child born with the form of dwarfism called achondroplasia, I struggle to let her be who she is and recognize that there are two children growing up: the one I perceive and the one she is—and ultimately all that matters is the one she is. That means not letting my fantasies get in the way, which is harder than it sounds.

When our LilyClaire was born ten years ago, everything was confusion: how to react, how to proceed, what to *do*. As the frantic first days unfolded, it seemed that all we could focus on was how to repair the flaws, and we would listen to anyone from a faith healer to a surgeon if we thought there was a "fix" for her in it. I remember thinking: we can put men in space, surely we can fix this.

In our case, there was no immediate fix on offer, because the flaws are molecular, embedded in every cell of her body. So for us, the first order of business was to come to terms with a few central desires, not the least of which is that most troublesome one—the desire for normalcy. There are dangers both social and emotional in being different and a certain amount of safety in being normal. So as her guardian and protector, I am vulnerable to the enticing possibilities of a surgical fix that might bring her closer to that safety zone of normalcy.

When you are a parent busy adjusting to the loss of the idealized child and raising the one you do have, it takes time to come to terms with a couple of facts. First, flaws are an essential part of real, normal human lives. Second, the pursuit of some imagined, flawless life obscures the real parental work, which is to raise a resilient child who values her self. To do that you have to look closely at your own fantasies and balance them against the real medical and psychological needs of the child. This is the ongoing challenge and the best way to describe it is by example.

It is April 2002. LilyClaire is 7 years old and my husband and I are sitting in the office of a pediatric orthopedic surgeon whom we respect immensely, who has monitored LilyClaire since she was born and who has carefully evaluated the latest X-rays of her very bowed legs.

"If I was a betting man, I would say we will need to operate by Christmas," he says.

"So, strictly speaking, we don't *need* to correct her bowing right now," I say, trying to understand why we would opt for breaking both of her legs in two places to straighten them when she walks perfectly well. "I mean, right now there is no medical proof that she is wearing down cartilage, or even the *certainty* that she will?"

I am very much attached to the notion of certainty even though I know there is no such thing in the world of medicine. I am also very susceptible to authority figures in white lab coats. So I am worrying about the goals we would reasonably hope to achieve by operating now: medical repair or fantasy-fix or something in between?

"So, all we are saying for sure," I continue, "is that she will have straighter legs and that might stave off future problems."

"That is correct, but I believe she *will* need it." Our doctor repeats his view that we will probably eventually have to make the correction to avoid damaging misalignment and wear and tear on LilyClaire's cartilage.

My husband sighs and shifts. He hates it when I engage in the "on the one hand, on the other hand" thing I was trained to do as a lawyer. But I am no longer a frantic mother in search of solutions. I am not a maniac for the fix. Nor am I the clear and precise thinker I can be on other issues in my life. I am a mother seesawing between the nagging desire to alleviate some of my daughter's difference, to feel we are doing something—and the strong belief that I have to protect my daughter against those marauding, seductive, and unattainable notions of normalcy. I am a mother who needs to be sure in my own mind that we are doing the right thing.

At that moment, I am enticed by the idea of straighter legs, thinking it really is one of those things that matters in the real everyday world of being LilyClaire on the playground, in the face of staring, curious strangers. It seems just then that straight legs really would make things easier. And LilyClaire herself hates the way her legs are shaped. She complains about them regularly, sometimes telling us her knees hurt. But it is generally a fleeting complaint, more like fatigue, I always think hopefully, than a clinical finding. Or not, I always worry at 3:00 a.m. when I can't sleep and vulnerabilities swirl.

There in that antiseptic outpatient cubicle, my mind is a blur of statistics and likelihoods of arthritis, breakdowns, and damage done by leaving this severe bowing untreated, not to mention thoughts of my daughter's anger with me when as an adult she asks why we didn't fix the bowing way back when we had the chance. But the more I question, the more I realize the futility of my questions. There are only so many facts and statistics available, and no matter how I twist and turn and combine them, they will never yield any definitive answers.

I don't feel our doctor's impatience, but I am pressured by the awareness that my ambivalence is taking up a lot of his time and the waiting area is teeming with kids in multiple casts and my husband is definitely antsy. He knows from years of life together that it is time to force the decision.

I have one last gasp of reticence. I know how wrenching it is to hold your child as she goes limp under anesthesia. What if it is for a nonessential medical procedure that you are relinquishing your precious child to possible surgical errors, uncertain outcomes, and God knows what other unknowns? It is clear to me that if I am being driven by the insatiable desire for normalcy, I am lost in my attempt to do the right thing.

I finally wear myself out and am persuaded that now is the time to operate to forestall potential permanent damage and not disturb school schedules. I am still reluctant, however, to abandon the notion that if we wait, we might find that six months from now she doesn't need the surgery yet. I also give one more glancing thought to her choice—the idea that at some point, now or in the future, she should be part of the decision. But right now she is whining and fidgety and I know she is still too young. I will be very clear with her about what we are doing, but I will not yet consult her.

So finally, *finally* we feel we have to have faith in the "betting man" whom we have decided to trust, and we convert that trust into the belief that we are doing the right thing. So we sign all of those scary papers, which commit LilyClaire to a summer of full leg casts and videos and bedpans. And we read the fine print about the hazards of surgery and tremble.

After we have signed and the tension is eased by the satisfaction of a decision made, we are told that this surgery is procedurally the same as extended limb-lengthening (known as ELL). It's like this: we could prolong the procedure by six months, put on external fixators that open incrementally day by day, then get the cast we will have anyway for eight weeks and thereby gain a little height. If we really want to.

"What is a *little* height?" we ask.

"Two to four inches."

I know this doctor, this "betting man," and know that he does not like the odds of ELL. We know about the infections and potential neurological and tendon damage, we know that he thinks it is risky and the outlook down the road unknown, and we know that he particularly does not approve of the procedure for young kids not yet able to decide for themselves.

All I can process for a few seconds is the 4 inches. Quick calculations bring me to the fact that for LilyClaire that could mean as much as 4 feet, 7 inches as an adult. More seduction toward the norm. But I respect our doctor for making sure to present all of the options in as unbiased a way as possible, and then I am confused all over again.

The concept of ELL surgery is so supremely seductive because on the surface it strikes you as a magic pill capable of stretching someone out of the musty air at the level of belt buckles and into the fine air of reasonably normal stature. This particular surgical fix has even more power than most to overshadow instinct, sense, facts, statistics, and clear thinking, because it directly addresses concerns that matter so much to a social little girl like LilyClaire. At age 7 she is already self-conscious about going into rooms full of strangers, worried about using public bathrooms and needing the stool at school when other girls can reach.

For details about what it's like to have the procedure, you have to turn to those who have done ELL, and they are necessarily unreliable reporters. They have sublimated the awful, painful, frightening aspects and are confirmed in their belief, as they must be, that they did the right thing, the thing that has been their salvation. There is no going back from such a commitment, even, I find, for those who experienced complications and repeated surgeries to repair damage done by the ELL procedure itself.

So willing for a moment to suppress the risks, the question is: Can we take this shot and grab it before LilyClaire is old enough to have it affect her sense of self and psyche? I know fixing the bowing will do little to change the way people stare at her in airports, in supermarkets, on the street, and even that is appealing on some level, but height? Real height? That is something else again, even as I know it is no cure—just a measured amount of fix.

The lure of gaining a few inches on the sly, cloaked in medical necessity is achingly attractive. But then I know this is totally irrational—that is to say, it is a rationalization. It took years for my husband and me to know that we must never decide the ELL question for her, and here I am making room in my mind, preparing data space, for an elaborate rationale that will subvert all of my better judgment about the molecular reality, the *what is* reality, the identity-building reality of LilyClaire. But the lines are so blurry, where cosmetic meets psychosocial meets medical necessity.

I know that an experience this profound would not go unnoticed by 7-year-old LilyClaire's rapier mind. When I was 7, I fell down a flight of stairs and split open my chin. I have vivid memories of straining to hear the doctors confabbing at the foot of my emergency room cot. They were discussing something about a little more pain now, but I would be happy later and I can remember wanting to scream at them, Include me here! This is my chin! My face! My pain! No. I know that this is already an age of awareness and she would bloody well get the very message I know we must never send: we love you, you're perfect the way you are . . . now change.

I have always believed every parent must choose her own course, and have always thought that I have been respectful of decisions either way. I am disappointed in myself because now I can actually observe the process by which it would be possible to come around to a position I have already decided is untenable for us.

But then the danger passes. The charm, attraction, and seduction of the fantasy fix fall away. We will stick with the first step to straighten the bowing so there will be no cartilage degeneration or progressive misalignment. Our doctor reassures me that we will, in fact, gain a little in height anyway. A centimeter or two. I glom onto that absurdly small increment as a little icing on the cake, but even that comes at a price. Even when the surgery ordeal is over and it is September and I am bored watching the fiftieth hour of rehab, I feel cheated that after all that we didn't get just a little more satisfaction, just a little more esthetic upside. And what's worse, I am disappointed in myself for being seduced by their promise.

It is March 2003. I never hear complaints of achy knees, and the long scars on the front of LilyClaire's shins have faded to pale pink, like most of the pain, the terrors of the hospital, the long boring summer, and the rehab. My daughter and I are reading a book on the couch on a rainy afternoon. I have to start up one of those conversations that neither of us likes: one where we have to explore the way LilyClaire has responded to a playmate's questions the day before about why she is so small, why her head is big, why she had to have casts on both legs and stay in bed all summer, even if she did have a super cool bed that went up and down and unlimited television time.

LilyClaire is furious that I told the other girl the party line we tell every one of her classmates, teachers, parents who ask: that it is because LilyClaire was born different and is just smaller because that's the way she is made, like some people are fatter and some skinny, some wear glasses, and so on. She was spitting mad when the girl left, but would only say that I had no right to explain her to people. Door slammed.

She forgave me by dinner and did not mention it again.

So now that a day has passed and we are reading together and discussing the way that her hair has gotten so beautifully long, I have decided to explore her reaction. Nothing like a little psycho babble in the afternoon.

"LilyClaire," I begin, "when people ask about the way you look, what would you like to tell them?"

"Nothing." And she trains her knowing and intense brown eyes on mine in a way that says do not mess with me on this one.

"Well, we have to say something." I am as determined as she is. I am very aware that people with dwarfism say they get tired of explaining themselves, of being seen first as a person with dwarfism second to everything else about them as people, and I wonder if she really does have to say something or not. But now that these questions crop up pretty regularly, it does seem that she ought to have some direct, proud, and reasonable response at the ready. "Why not just say 'because I have achondroplasia and this is the way dwarfs are supposed to look'?" I suggest.

"No. I will say that I fell out of a tree and broke my legs and shrank." And now those eyes are full of foreboding . . . they are saying loud and clear that the conversation is over.

"But honey, you know you have dwarfism, right?" Now I need to be sure she is not slipping into a fantasy and somehow undermining that all-important sense of self, rooted in reality but ever optimistic, that we have been nurturing.

"Of course. But I like the tree idea."

I imagine that LilyClaire would rather say she fell from a tree because she does not want to feel that heavy hand of fate upon her, which separates her so decisively from her peers. I imagine this fantasy is one of her first assertions as an individual about how she wants to be perceived, and who am I to argue with a bit of fiction about which she is so resolute? It is her way of trying to fit in, and part of her process of sorting out her reality. For the most part I am in awe of how deftly she already handles the paradox that it is both uniquely formative to have challenges and hard on a daily basis to manage the reality of being the one who is different.

As she matures, she will, I hope, be able to distinguish between wanting not to be different and wanting to be normal. I hope she will make peace with herself and her difference and focus less on how others perceive her. The struggle to be herself as an individual, flawed and yet perfect in her own way, is how she will embrace her own reality, just as it is one way any of us comes to terms with ourselves.

Even as I hope this kind of peace for her, it is the daily realities of staring and quizzical glances, outright questions, and the practical difficulties of doing some things for herself that drive me to feel I might do almost anything to alleviate her pain and self-consciousness if a palatable fix came along. Proving of course that, for parents like me, when it comes to surgical fixes, all you can be sure of is doubt. Nothing is clear or irrefutable. It is just that at some point you get exhausted by statistics, possibilities, and probabilities and decide just to act and that is when the internal arguments end . . . and you go for it . . . whatever it is you have decided on.

The seductive promise of surgery as repair mingles with the realities of surgery as medical solution by way of psychosocial rationale. Providing clear, medically and psychologically appropriate guidance and reasonable goals are the surgeon's and physician's challenges. Sorting through it all, while remaining true to the best interests of the child and, finally, figuring out when it is time for the child to participate in decision making about her care, are the grand parental challenges.

PART II

TECHNOLOGY AND THE PURSUIT OF NORMALITY

Concepts of Technology and Their Role in Moral Reflection

James C. Edwards, Ph.D.

Most people think of technology as theoretical science's dull but dutiful companion: a sort of practical Doctor Watson plodding along after science's intellectually adventurous Sherlock Holmes. Science—so this standard story goes—tells us the odd and difficult truth about things; it exhibits the unexpected stuff out of which the universe is made. Technology, on the other hand, turns that shimmering weave into the solid things we crave; it figures out how to make theory's truth pay off. In its ideal at least, theoretical science is free of any requirement that it answer to human desires, save the thin but intense Desire to Know the World as It Truly Is. Technology, however, is the happy adjutant to desires of all sorts, some as thick as a Buffalo snowfall. It takes the world chastely undressed in laboratories and in journal articles and fashions it into light bulbs, napalm, soaring freeways, Viagra, television movies, Reece's Pieces, and much, much more, all of which answer to some desire, deep or adventitious, of some human being, representative or idiosyncratic.

Conceived in this standard way, technology is neither philosophically nor ethically interesting. Deep and persisting philosophical difficulties afflict the claims of theoretical science, of course, and ethical reflection on its practice and its social uses is increasingly recognized to be of great importance (Kitcher 2001). Naturally, one can raise all sorts of first-order ethical questions about the desires that motivate some particular pieces of technology. (What does one say about someone's desire for a weapon consisting of jellied gasoline, all the better to stick to the human flesh that it is, once ignited, designed to consume?) But technology itself is—in this common conception of it—both philosophically and ethically transparent. It claims neither objectivity nor virtue; it is merely the process of efficiently producing the things we want. It is the robotic servant of human knowledge and of human desire. Given what we know, and given what we want, technology neutrally (if ingeniously) matches means to ends: it is the colorless but essential instrument by means of which our wishes—good or bad, intelligent or silly, harmless or fatal—are fulfilled.

Such a commonsense view of technology is not false—how could it be?—but it may be simple-minded. There is, and here I follow Martin Heidegger, entirely another way to think about technology (Heidegger 1977a). In Heidegger's view, technology is itself *a particular way of revealing things, of letting something come to presence* before us. "Technology is therefore no mere means. Technology is a way of revealing. If we give heed to this, another whole realm for the essence of technology will open itself up to us. It is the realm of revealing, i.e., of truth" (12).

For Heidegger, truth is not fundamentally the correspondence of some representation (for example, a sentence) with the reality it represents; truth is the coming into presence of something in such a way that it can be seen as what it is (Heidegger 1977b). Truth is disclosure, uncovering, unconcealment. Technology, as a mode of such disclosure, brings things into presence—lets them be seen—in a particular way; it reveals them as having a particular character, a particular Being. Thus technology is not, for Heidegger, primarily the machines and the power tools we usually associate with the term: it is not just the hydroelectric plant on the banks of the Rhine or the superconducting supercollider half buried in the Texas plains. Technology is a way—according to Heidegger, it is now the *fundamental* way—in which the world of human beings is constituted and populated; it is an overarching set of linguistic and behavioral practices that allow our things to appear around us in a particular way, that give to the things that appear in our world a particular Being, a particular significance, a particular sense. The machines and procedures we think of as distinctively technological, such as power plants and particle accelerators, are just the most obvious instances of the Being of *all*—or at least *almost*[1] all—our things as they are constituted by our most basic social practices.

What is that characteristically technological Being of things?

> The revealing that rules throughout modern technology has the character of a setting-upon, in the sense of a challenging-forth. Such challenging happens in that the energy concealed in nature is unlocked, what is unlocked is transformed, what is transformed is stored up, what is stored up is in turn distributed, and what is distributed is switched about ever anew. Unlocking, transforming, storing, distributing, and switching about are ways of revealing. . . .
>
> What kind of unconcealment is it, then, that is peculiar to that which results from this setting-upon that challenges? Everywhere everything is ordered to stand by, to be immediately on hand, indeed to stand there just so that it may be on call for a further ordering. Whatever is ordered about in this way has its own standing. We call it the

standing-reserve [*Bestand*]. . . . [The word *Bestand*] designates nothing less than the way in which everything presences that is wrought upon by the challenging revealing. Whatever stands by in the sense of standing-reserve no longer stands over against us as object. (1977a, 16–17)

The characteristic kind of thing brought to light by the practices of technology is *Bestand*, "standing-reserve," "stock": that which in an orderly way awaits our use of it for the further ordering of things. When I walk into my study in the morning and glance at the computer on the desk, the computer, as the thing it is, is *Bestand*. It reveals itself to me as waiting patiently for me to turn it on, to "get its things in order," so I can use it to order and reorder those things and others. The data stored there— words, sentences, thoughts, digital photographs, recipes, bank balances—await my command so they can be transformed, distributed, and switched about: they too are *Bestand*. It's not just the glass-and-plastic machines that reveal themselves to me as standing-reserve. As I glance out the window at the leaves I have not yet raked, they too are *Bestand*: they patiently await my collection of them so they can be put on the compost heap ("stored up" so the energy in them can later be "unlocked") or bagged for the garbage collection ("switched about"). The very house I inhabit is, as we have famously been told, "a machine for living in," with the window out of which I gaze a device for the orderly collection of light (and the orderly retention of heat). The house patiently awaits its tenants for their use of it in ordering their lives; the land on which the house sits reveals itself through the window as garden and as landscape, waiting for the orderly touch that shapes and preserves and cultivates. The mugs on the kitchen shelf, the television in the loft, the cereal in the pantry, the toothbrush on the bathroom sink: all "stand by" (17) in the manner of "stock," as resources awaiting their call to orderly use in the ordering of things.

For us (almost) everything reveals itself as *Bestand*. Most of the time, of course, we are not explicitly aware that our things have that sort of Being. Our consciousness of them as "standing-reserve" shows itself not in anything we say or think about them; rather, it shows itself in how we comport ourselves to them in unselfconscious everyday action and reaction. How I "see" my television set or my coffee mug or my toothbrush shows itself in the way I carelessly handle them, in the way my eye passes over them without a pause, in the way I irritably react when they don't perform as expected, in the way I dispose of them when they are no longer useful, and so forth. When I press the remote-control button that turns on the television set, I don't punch it with the same delicacy of movement that a mother might use in playfully poking her child in the ribs to tickle him; when I pick up my mug at the breakfast table, there is no tactile attention to its surface in the way there might be when I am handling a piece of sculpture or stroking my cat's fur; when my toothbrush is worn out, I don't burn or bury it (as Scouts are taught to do with the country's flag)—I pitch it into the garbage and hurriedly rip another from its package. In all these unreflective ways (and others) I show what these things are for me: "standing-reserve."

And the things just named wonderfully conspire in our treatment of them as *Bestand*. The deftly shaped buttons on the television's remote control are made to be punched again and again (by anyone) with no delicacy or attention, just as the white ceramic coffee mug is intended to offer to my eye and hand (and to any eye and hand) no resistance or interest.[2] These things, like the toothbrush and innumerable others, are supposed to "disappear" into our use of them; they are supposed to be there for us only insofar as they are useful without impediment and without our careful scrutiny. "In themselves" they are, one wants to say, *anonymous and interchangeable;* they have no reality for us as *particular* things. My television set looks and performs much like every other one, and certainly my coffee mug and my toothbrush are virtually indistinguishable from an indefinitely large number of similar objects. Today's breakfast Grape Nuts taste exactly like yesterday's—and (this is the crucial point) *that's what makes them what they are.* That anonymous interchangeability is what makes all these things the kind of things they are; that's what gives them their Being as *Bestand*. Their nature, one might say, is to have only a *general* nature, a nature exhausted by their impersonal usefulness to us. All these things suppress their reality as *particular* things. Or, to put it more precisely (but in a way that will demand further exposition), all these things are things the Being of which covers over the manifold conditions of their coming to presence.

So the things that appear in a technological world appear as some kind of *Bestand*. But why should this be so? Why should technology reveal things in that particular way, as having that particular kind of Being? Here we are asking, says Heidegger, after the *essence* of technology. "We now name that challenging claim which gathers man thither to order the self-revealing as standing-reserve: *Gestell* [Enframing]" (19).

The appearance of things as *Bestand* is the inevitable result of those social practices that have as their nature and point what Heidegger calls *ordering*. In his highly wrought idiom (an idiom certainly *not* "anonymous and interchangeable"), technology is a "challenging-forth" (16), and "that challenging gathers man into ordering. This gathering concentrates man on ordering the real into standing-reserve" (19).

What is this ordering? The dominant social practices constituting our world are practices that "enframe": they are practices that put things in their proper places in such a way that they are readily available to be put to use by us with a maximum of efficiency and a minimum of attention to the conditions of their appearing. Such practices impose a "grid" (*Gestell*, "frame") on things so that within that grid—within the completely and immediately surveyable space created by that grid—those things are completely and immediately locatable and thus are completely and immediately available for whatever use we find it appropriate to put them to. In this way things are made *orderly*. They are located within a frame that transparently orients us to them and them to us; as a result of that perspicuous orientation within the frame they are ours to use and reuse easily and quickly and essentially thoughtlessly. And the point of our use of our orderly things is further ordering. Under the spell of technology, we come to order things primarily for the sake of ordering itself.

Of course, the "frames" Heidegger has in mind here are *conceptual* frames; following Rorty we might call them *vocabularies*. Technological practices are first of all practices of careful and precise linguistic categorization. They are practices that "enframe" by way of assigning clear senses to the things they constitute: the more clearly and completely we can say what kind of thing it is we are talking about, the more available that thing is for what we want to do with it. In the world of technology there should be no linguistic surplus value. Meaning and use should exactly coincide. That way of putting the matter is a bit misleading, however, because it makes it seem that (1) knowing what something is and means and (2) being able to do something with it are two different matters, and that the first is the best path to the second. In the world of technology, however, the two are precisely the same; they are simultaneously given in the notion of *Bestand*. Things are what they are only insofar as they patiently await our orderly use of them in our ordering of things.

Three techniques of erasure help secure the dominance of these technological practices. First, there is the erasure of the particular frame itself. Our dominant social practices seek—usually successfully—to obscure the fact that they are just our dominant social practices. They are practices that, through a shrewd combination of opportunistic rhetoric and institutional power, present themselves as not just the truth about things but as obvious common sense. Think how often one hears it said (or at least implied): "Only a fool would deny that. . . ." What replaces the ellipsis varies from platform to platform, but each such appeal to our "obvious common sense"—"Obviously that is a toothbrush"; "Obviously Yosemite Valley is there for us to enjoy"; "Obviously the spotted owl is not worth thousands of jobs"; "Obviously we must fix this genetic accident if we can"; "Obviously there are some moral absolutes"—is a way of disguising the particular conceptual and institutional "frames" that make the appeals effective (or not) in the first place. Each is a way—perhaps decisive in certain instances—of causing us to forget that our particular way of placing things in relation to one another and to ourselves is itself a particular historical construction. Technology is a frame that blinds us to itself as a frame. It is a way of revealing that makes us forget that it is *a* way of revealing.

Second, technological practices obscure not just their own character as particular ways of revealing things; they more generally blind us to the necessity of there being "ways of revealing" at all. Operating within such practices we forget not just that *this* particular account of things is contingent; we forget that such contingency is the condition of *any* account of what a thing is. "Thus the challenging Enframing . . . conceals revealing itself and with it that wherein unconcealment, i.e., truth, comes to pass" (27). Under the spell of characteristically technological practices we forget "revealing itself," that is, we forget history and ourselves as historical beings. We forget that—to use a Nietzschean image—perspective is not just an accident of this or that particular vocabulary or social practice; perspective is the necessary condition of any seeing at all. We are not gods, and our lack of a divine standpoint is not an unfortunate accident perhaps at some point to be remedied. All our seeing is, and always will be, a perspectival seeing; all our seeing will come as the result of a "revealing," that is, as the result of some contingent concatenation of opportunities and abilities, conceptual and otherwise. Engaged in certain practices—the ones Heidegger calls *technological*—we forget this necessary contingency, this necessary historical condition of all our thinking and acting.

Third, technological practices erase as inessential the particular conditions of the particular things they bring to presence. Here it is useful to think again about the defiantly mundane: coffee mugs, toothbrushes, and Post Grape Nuts. Specific instances of these things are, as I put it above, largely anonymous and interchangeable. This coffee mug looks and feels no different from that one; this bowl of Grape Nuts tastes just like the one I had yesterday; any Oral-B 60 is much the same as any other.[3] What is crucial to see is that this anonymity and this interchangeability are not just accidents, and not just unfortunate features of living in a society rich enough to mass-produce breakfast foods and implements of personal hygiene; they are essential to our need for these things readily to "disappear" into our use of them. In practices given over—as Heidegger thinks almost our whole life is—to ordering for the sake of ordering, the more easily and quickly an entity can be thoughtlessly taken up into its particular task of ordering, the better. Explicit attention to the tool one is using distracts one from the job the tool is being used to accomplish and in that way makes the successful completion of the job less likely. If I notice the texture of the handle of my coffee mug, and then begin to wonder how it was made, and maybe even to wonder who made it, and under what conditions, I may be led into a train of thought that disrupts my normal and efficient progress from breakfast to newspaper to car to classroom, thus introducing a bit of disorder into my quite ordinary life. And—to push the matter in a more sentimental and unlikely direction—if I become aware of the fact that my mug was made in China (as indeed it was), and then begin to think about the economic and political conditions of the workers who made it, and then am moved write a letter to my congressional representative protesting the continuance of most-favored-nation trade status for China in light of its atrocious disregard of human rights, and so on, my attention to my coffee mug might actually cause an even larger disorder. The more "unconditional" and "smoother" the appearance of the thing, the more readily it disappears into our use of it. The less we pay attention to particular things *qua* things, the more efficiently we carry on with the tasks we have inherited from the social practices that have constituted us.[4] An impetus to ordering for the sake of ordering—Heidegger's characterization of the essence of technology—will seek to efface anything that impedes such ordering. Thus it will seek to produce things that efface their own conditions of production. No wonder things like coffee mugs and television sets are so anonymous and interchangeable.

What is most frightening for Heidegger about technology is not that it turns consumer products such as coffee mugs or toothbrushes into anonymous and interchangeable markers in a great game of economic ordering; it is that *we ourselves* sooner or later come to see ourselves as *Bestand*. We too become raw material for human ingenuity to use in its attempt finally to order the world for the sake of order. You don't like the lay of the land on your shore property? Does it interfere with placing the house so that from the bedroom you can see the sun rise? Bring in the bulldozers and smooth out the contours. (And too bad about the Clapper Rails that will be displaced as your wetlands drain.) You don't like your sensitivity to criticism and the way it holds you back at work? You want that promotion this year rather than next? Here, pop a few of these pills that will leave a bit more serotonin in your synapses for a bit longer. You don't like the way your body looks? You don't like that spare tire of fat? You want more muscle to use in the NBA? Here's the knife or the hormone that will fix the situation. Nothing has to be left the way we find it. The world is *our* world; we own not only it, but ourselves. All of it, our bodies and minds included, is there to be shaped as we see fit, shaped into an order that answers to our own sense—what other?—of what order demands. We too aspire to be "anonymous and interchangeable." We wish to erase from ourselves anything that unfits us to fit in; we desire most of all that we be normal, that we in an orderly way be able to do our part in the ordering of things.

Does corrective surgery on children—some of which surgery was the focus of The Hastings Center working group that produced the essays in this volume—belong to what Heidegger would call the "essence" of technology? In particular, if we operate on an achondroplasic teenager to make her arms and legs a few inches longer, or on another child to repair her cleft palate, or on another to normalize her genital structures, are we falling into a way of revealing things that erases what, from Heidegger's own point of view, makes them most truly the things they are? Are we (with the best of intentions, of course) treating that child's body (and life) as *Bestand,* as raw material to be shaped so as to fit our (and presumably her) sense of what is natural, normal, and orderly? And if we are, is anything wrong with that?

It is clear that in Heidegger's mind a particular ethical valence attaches to *die Technik.* He hates (and I do not think the word is too strong) the world revealed purely as *Bestand* for human projects, and this hatred is connected to his more general hatred (or at least profound distrust) for the project of modernity in general. Heidegger is, as most of us probably are not, an old-fashioned reactionary. He harbors a romantic hankering for the preindustrial world of the Swabian small-hold farmer, a world from which the cosmopolitan city and its temptations of license and self-invention are far, far away. He despises, and fears, the idea that everything solid can melt into air at the touch of the human finger. For him, the "humanism" that goes hand in hand with *die Technik*—the idea that human beings should mold their world in accordance with their continuing discoveries of their own deepest desires, desires that may radically change as we continue to discover them—is a frightful and ugly degeneracy. We humans should, he thinks, be the dutiful shepherds of Being, not its willful shapers.

But, as I say, most of us do not share Heidegger's nostalgia for the premodern world, just as we do not share his philosophical anguish at our eagerness to reinvent ourselves in every generation. And so if his critique of technology is to have any resonance for us, it can't be because of its filiations to a larger project of turning back the clock. At least one feature of modernity has sedimented itself so deeply into our ethical consciousness that we cannot easily imagine ourselves without it: when Judith Shklar said that to be a liberal means to believe that "cruelty is the worst thing we do," she was speaking not just for liberalism but for what we have come to regard as common decency itself. That human suffering is the final touchstone of evil, and that nothing is worse than to cause or to collude in such suffering, strikes us as incontrovertible, especially when that suffering entails not only physical pain but humiliation. And is it not humiliation, or at least the threat of it, that most affects us when we think of the child with the cleft palate, or whose body is in some remediable way significantly different from the "norm"? How, we may exclaim, is it possible not to think that surgery is appropriate—assuming that the risks are fully understood and are acceptable to all the parties? Anyone who distrusts or opposes this sort of surgical technology, frankly call it "enhancement technology" if you like, can seem—notice I say "*can* seem"—a sort of monster.

And of course Heidegger seems exactly—and quite happily—that sort of monster, not because he would sadistically deny corrective surgery to a child (I have no idea what he'd do in the particular case of, say, achondroplasia), but because he truly doesn't take human suffering as the final court of appeal for our ethical practice: there is something worse for him than cruelty. It's not something for which he has a transparent name—he usually calls it *Seinsvergessenheit* ("the forgetfulness of Being")— but it's clear that it holds for him a kind of transcendent significance. In his devotion to something larger than our liberal humanism, he resembles the religious believer who says, "Human happiness is all very well, of course, but what really matters is the greater glory of God." And what can one say to that? Here one has reached a kind of impasse; one is making, and responding to, first-order ethical claims that cannot be finessed.

These reflections encourage one to recognize that it's a mistake to think that Heidegger's account of technology, however revelatory, can solve the incredibly difficult first-order ethical problems that come in the train of our increasing ability to order the world in accordance with our desires and our scruples. In spite of his animadversions on Platonism, Heidegger was still very much a metaphysician in a central respect: he still expected philosophical insights—insights at the meta-level, one might say—to settle first-order ethical quandaries.

Here's an example of what I mean, an example perhaps closer to home than Heidegger is. Hilde Lindemann Nelson has written a brilliant and moving essay that begins its reflection from her own childhood memories of her hydrocephalic younger sister Carla, who died of an uncontrollable fever at 3 years of age, having never spoken, nor sat up unaided, nor ever played with a toy (Nelson 2002). Lindemann Nelson is trying in the essay to construct what one might call a Wittgensteinian theory of personhood and to show how that category can be legitimately applied to human beings (such as Carla) who are unable to apply it to themselves. The result is stimulating and thoughtful, and my question to her will seem, perhaps, a naïve one: What do you want a theory of personhood *for*? For her answer is, I think, plain: she wants that theory because she thinks it will do some ethical work for her. She thinks it will show her what properly to say and to do about children like Carla, or about first-trimester fetuses, or about human beings in permanent vegetative states. Like other metaphysicians, Lindemann Nelson thinks that one can, so to speak, shove first-order ethical disputes upstairs and then solve them as metaphysical (though she might rather say "philosophical") problems. If we can just come up with a theory that will "establish the criteria of personhood," for example, then we'll know how to treat the ethically hard cases that drove us to philosophical reflection in the first place.

This is, I think, exactly the kind of move Heidegger is trying to make with his account of *die Technik*. Like lots of us he is frightened and baffled by our increasing ability (and willingness) to reshape the world—and ourselves—as we see fit. We are distressed by our inability to control ourselves; we seem unable to throttle back our rush to destitution. What can we say to stop the developers from draining all the wetlands to make room for yet more luxury second homes on the coast, or to stop the bioengineers from altering the genes of corn in such a way that the Monarch butterflies are endangered, or to stop the agribusiness conglomerates from driving the family farm out of existence, or . . . , or . . . , or . . . ? These are terribly hard questions to answer, and we'd like a way to cut the Gordian knot, to answer them all in a single pass. A philosopher like Heidegger says: all these matters involve the dominance of *die Technik* as a way of revealing the world; once you see that, you'll know what to think and to feel and to do about them.

But of course that's a naïve hope, as serious thinking about the surgical shaping of children quickly shows. In hard choices like those, the ethical questions aren't settled merely by fitting the cases into a Heideggerian template of "the essence of technology," any more than hard cases about what to say about killing fetuses are settled by fitting them into a Wittgensteinian template of "the essence of personhood" (even if there were such a thing, which I very much doubt). We expect too much of our philosophical ideas, if we expect them to settle first-order ethical quandaries. No parents would be satisfied if, faced with the possibility of limb-lengthening surgery for their child, we ethicists argued against that surgery on grounds that it treats the child as *Bestand.* In fact, I couldn't offer them such an argument with a straight face, much as I enjoy kicking around these ideas in class. At a certain point I realize that philosophy, no matter how compelling, can't be appealed to *itself* as *Bestand,* as raw material standing by for us to use in solving ethical problems. We don't get firm answers to such questions by kicking them upstairs into the airy realm of metaphysics. Yet that's very much what we'd like to do, whether we are philosophers like Heidegger and Lindemann Nelson or policy makers trying to draft ethical guidelines for a new surgical procedure for children.

This doesn't mean that Heidegger's account of technology has nothing to teach us as we struggle with such first-order problems. It's a mistake to think philosophy can solve our ethical quandaries, but even philosophical theories (such as Heidegger's or Lindemann Nelson's), if seen in the right light, can play a constructive role in our ethical reflection, a role connected to what Heidegger calls a more phenomenological understanding of truth. Once we understand that truth is disclosure, that seeking the truth is not about matching up our ideas with the reality they purport to represent but about letting our ideas call attention to aspects of what appears, aspects that we are likely otherwise to overlook, then it becomes possible to see the results of philosophical reflection not as theories of this or that, theories that will solve our problems of practice, but rather as *indicators of salience.* Philosophy can't tell us what to think (much as we would like it to); maybe in some cases, however, it can tell us what's worth thinking about, in relation to the case at issue. It can indicate resonances and saliences that, when folded into our first-order ethical reflections, may change their course in directions we find both useful and unexpected.

For example, Heidegger's emphasis on our desires for order and ordering, our need to shape our environment in accordance with patterns and practices that seem to us regular and proper, can let us see something relevant to some cases of surgically shaping children. It is especially relevant, I think, to those cases where surgery is argued (by surgeons, by parents, by ethicists) to be the proper response to infants born with (so-called) ambiguous genitalia. The different conditions comprised in such a description vary a great deal, of course, ranging from, on the one hand, those (such as male hypospadias) that don't necessarily involve a great deal of visibly unusual anatomy to, on the other, those anatomical formations (enlarged clitoris, for example) that don't allow an easy perception of "correct" gender at all. Such anatomically "ambiguous" infants are, for the parents and for the hospital personnel, shocking, since they seem to fall into no easily definable category, and the temptation is quickly to fix them. The temptation is, of course, understandable, and it will remain powerful even after the parents and the medical professionals fully appreciate the now clearly documented risks and difficulties of surgical intervention.[5]

Part of that temptation will be rooted in various kinds of fear: the parents' fear that their child will be stigmatized and humiliated; or the parents' fear that they will be seen by others (the doctors and nurses, the grandparents, and later, perhaps, even by the child) as insufficiently caring, or insufficiently aggressive in acting on that care; or the parents' fear that they themselves will become objects of derision or pity by the wider society; or the surgeons' fear of litigation or (at least) of criticism; and so on. Not all these fears are ethically of a piece, of course. Out of love for the child to fear the child's humiliation is not nearly the same as fearing one's own shame or fearing a nasty lawsuit. And the loving root of the temptation to surgery explains why that course of action won't easily be dismissed, or dismissible, by those who care about the child and her welfare. Nevertheless, to be tempted to operate is not necessarily to operate. The first-order ethical decision about surgery still has to be made, and perhaps it will be easier to make when one is aware of, and critical of, one's own impetus to and need for active ordering of what is perceived as disorderly.

The Heideggerian point—that the need to impose order on a world revealed to us as *Bestand* belongs essentially to the epoch we inhabit, and thus belongs inevitably to us in our deepest sensibilities—won't *make* that decision, but it may make it easier to identify one of the fears—the fear of disorder itself, especially when that disorder seems to attach to something so fundamental to us as gender identity, which shapes our response to this situation of emotional and ethical turmoil. Thinking about Heidegger's claims may, in this way, help us to *historicize* ourselves, help us to notice that our reactions to the child's ambiguous genitalia are not "the natural human reaction," since there's no such thing. Our reactions are *our own,* shaped not just by personal idiosyncrasy but also by large-scale cultural and philosophical formations ("the essence of technology," for example) that are likely to go unnoticed. But if our fears and hopes are our own, as I've insisted, they're not merely pieces of individual psychology. To treat those reactions as pieces of individual psychology, in hopes of altering them as the result of philosophical reflection, is just in another way unconsciously to assume the technological frame Heidegger abhors. Our fear of disorder, though powerfully *ours,* is not therefore a *given.* But in another way it *is* a given, given by our historical place in a long history of the reciprocal revelations of world and human being.

Notice that I say our fear of disorder is *one* of the fears in play here: it's important for us to realize, as Heidegger himself would not, that this hospital nursery we're imagining is a site of genuine contestation, and that what shapes one's fears and hopes for the child and her life is not a single or simple thing. It is not just "the essence of technology" that guides our thinking; our reflections are guided by a number of hopes and fears, some of which are rooted in—one may assume—a genuine love for the child and a genuine concern for her long-term good, combined with a perplexity as to how that love should best be expressed. To highlight our largely unexamined need for ordering, and our tendency to treat whatever we find—even the bodies of our beloved children—as raw material to be ordered, may help us to see something about the root of our distress in the situation and thus help us to discount that distress in a way we would otherwise not be able to. Heidegger's point won't (and shouldn't) carry the day, but it may add sufficient weight to others so as to tip the balance against the push to fix things.

Another way in which Heidegger's perspective may be useful in our first-order ethical deliberations about these matters has to do with a common refrain one hears in ethical discussions, usually voiced as a complaint, to the effect that "if we *can* do it, eventually we *will* do it." If the technology exists, even in a rudimentary and largely untested form, the strong impetus we feel is to use that technology. "If the problem can be fixed, why not fix it?" Of course, the question leaves much unexamined. Is this really a problem, and if so, whose problem is it to solve? Is it really so easy to fix it with the technology being touted, and what are the costs likely to be incurred? (And so on.) But even if these questions can be satisfactorily answered, there remains a more fundamental query: Why does the possibility of a fix seem to make almost inevitable our need to avail ourselves of it? Recently this theme has most visibly surfaced in connection with various pharmacological enhancement technologies: If I can be more energetic/more focused/more self-confident by taking this (safe, effective, affordable) pill, then what's to stop me? Why should I deny myself the benefits of pharmaceutical technology? Why shouldn't I be as satisfied with myself as I can?

Substantial philosophers have worried these questions, sometimes to very good effect (Elliott 2003). They have articulated and questioned the ethic of authenticity, the identification of happiness with self-fulfillment, that underlies our easy slide from pill-as-therapy to pill-as-enhancement, and no doubt these more obviously ethical considerations—our conception of the good life as authentic self-satisfaction, to put it crudely—play a large role in our cultural moment. But I think Heidegger is correct in suggesting that something deeper than the patently ethical may be determinative in these matters. For what so much as gives us the idea that our lives are, in every aspect, our own to shape in accordance with whatever we take to be normative? What gives us the idea that our lives are our own raw material to fashion into an order we desire? Here Heidegger's account of *die Technik* is helpful. Our ruling ethical conceptions (a conception of happiness as authentic self-satisfaction, say) didn't emerge from thin air; they belong to a way of thinking about what there is as a whole. (Ethics is always a reflection of metaphysics, to put it bluntly.) And Heidegger is right, I think, in maintaining that so long as that metaphysics remains in place, our first-order ethical reflection will, one way or another, map its outlines rather than challenge them. If we see our world, and ourselves in it, as *Bestand* waiting patiently to be shaped into an order not otherwise given, then is it any wonder that we feel impelled to impose that order when its imposition is possible? Is it any surprise that we instinctively are puzzled why anyone would *not* use some available technological means to fix an infant's ambiguous genitalia, a condition that is likely to strike even the most sophisticated of us as disorderly, because it flouts a pattern of difference so obvious and culturally significant to us all?

These questions bring me to a third way in which Heidegger's reflections on technology may be of use to ethicists trying to aid those who have to make the hard decisions about surgically shaping children. I'll begin with a story. After a trip to The Hastings Center, I was visiting my 87-year-old mother, a former schoolteacher now living alone on a South Carolina farm, filling her in on what I'd been doing. She was fascinated by my account of our discussions, clearly moved by the distress and perplexity of the children and parents we had been talking about, and at one point she said, "Well, if I were in that situation, I don't really know what I'd do, but God would have had some reason for sending me the child he did, and I would need to love that child as a gift from Him."

Now—trust me—this is not something I would ever have said, or even thought about saying. Partly that's because I'm not religious, and partly it's because as a philosopher I've been taught to substitute an ethical discourse for a religious one. From the point of view I typically inhabit, Mama's remark is, however heartfelt, naïve and out of place (if not actually obscurantist and dangerous). But then it struck me: in none of our Hastings Center discussions did I ever hear a distinctly religious perspective brought to bear on the hard cases we were considering. Nobody like my mother was sitting around the big brown tables in the library; or, if they were, they didn't speak up. As nurses, physicians, and ethicists we don't think in Mama's terms; we must set aside whatever religious views we personally hold (if any) and pursue ethical issues on a ground undetermined by traditional faith. And we do this in spite of our knowing, if my own experience is a reliable guide, that a great many of the patients and families we deal with in situations of crisis—though not all of them, certainly—*do* appeal to religious stories and conceptions to sort out their confusions and to guide their actions.

I am not—certainly not—arguing that we should revert to theology to tell us when surgery is appropriate, nor am I suggesting that there's something wrong with our culture's long (and politically productive) attempt to separate ethics from faith. I'm only suggesting that a religious perspective like my mother's reveals a perhaps unnoticed aspect of our own preconceptions. Our whole ethical perspective is one that takes nothing as finally given. For us, life appears as a problem and a challenge, not as a gift. Whatever uncomfortable facts we confront—an infant with ambiguous genitalia, a marriage gone stale and comfortless, a cruel dictator in Iraq, famine raging on the Indian subcontinent—we confront them as *our own to order.* If we do not like them, we can fix them. The world is *our* world, and we are responsible for it.[6] We may, of course, decide to leave things as they are, because we don't (yet) have a cheap and effective way to alter them as we wish we could; but even so, it's our decision. We have solved the problem of evil in the world by becoming ourselves fully responsible for it.[7] Ideally, nothing must be left as we find it; to do so is a sort of criminal negligence. "Why not the best?" We must improve even the shining hour; the dark and dangerous ones must be changed beyond all recognition.

There is much that is noble in such a perspective. Who would wish merely to stand by and let people starve? And maybe there is something necessary in our finally becoming gods, in taking upon ourselves the responsibility for ordering the world as we see fit. I would not say no. But I would want to remind us of two things. First, it's important to attend to how our ordinary ethical perspective merely *assumes* that transition to divinity, and assumes it invisibly. Of course, human life is about remaking the world, we think; about making it, for the first time, truly a home for us. Ethical reflection seeks the necessary standards we need to direct and constrain that remaking. For we want (this time) to do it *right*. God is dead (justifiably assassinated, perhaps, given his mismanagement), and we ourselves must now set in order the run-down estate we've inherited.

Heidegger and my mother have in common an attitude—in her case rooted in theological conviction, in his not—that there are some facts that face us not as problems to be solved but as realities to which we must, joyfully or sadly, with resistance or with acceptance, accommodate. And the difference marked here is not the obvious difference between those facts we can presently alter and those we cannot. (We know how effectively to cure certain common infections with antibiotics; we don't know how to cure last-stage cancer metastasized to the bones.) The difference marks some things we see as *proper* to alter, as *our own* to remake, and those that are not. (If on our wedding day my partner gives me a silver cup to carry on my birding hikes ["Water always tastes better from silver, even in the woods."], but I know of another cup shape I'd like better, would I blithely go to the jeweler and swap it out?) Usually we demand that the facts answer to us, to our needs that the world be ordered as we see fit; some facts, however, have the demand on their side: it is we who must answer to them. One can hear in my mother's talk of God's gifts or in Heidegger's contempt for the conversion of the world into *Bestand* something that one also hears in a thinker like Thoreau: "If you stand right fronting and face to face to a fact, you will see the sun glimmer on both its surfaces, as if it were a cimeter, and feel its sweet edge dividing you through the heart and marrow, and so you will happily conclude your mortal career" (Thoreau 1985, 400). For him, it's what the fact does to you that is important; not what you do to the fact. Such a fact, were one able to front it directly, might, as he puts it, "end one's mortal career." That, I take it, is for Thoreau a good thing: the end of one's careering back and forth between one thing and the next; the end of the mortal life of rush and inattention most of us live; the happy conclusion of ordinary existence for something better; finding oneself part of something *to* which one is responsible but *for* which one isn't. "Be it life or death, we crave only reality. If we are really dying, let us hear the rattle in our throats and feel cold in the extremities; if we are alive, let us go about our business" (ibid.). This is not reality understood as *Bestand*, craved for its plasticity and patience; it is reality as a power to which we can and may accommodate, reality given as an important gift is given, with no happy possibility of exchange.

My point here is not that we should agree with Thoreau, Heidegger, and my mother in this attitude. I very much doubt that we can, or that we should. In the hospital we have another role to play: we are, given the grace of a chance, advisors to action in difficult, distressing, and confusing circumstances, and some of us actually carry out those actions with sharp knives and steady hands. Professionally and (I suspect) personally most of us are happy to be charged with responsibility for the world; we are glad to take on its evils and, if we can, turn them into goods. We are glad to be agents, not Thoreavean witnesses and recorders. As I say, my point is not to assert we should try to be something we are not; my point is just that, with Heidegger's (or Thoreau's or Emily Edwards's) help we might be reminded that our stance toward the world is not the only serious one, and that some of those we encounter (some of our patients, our clients, our friends) might not fully share our particular way of dealing with the world's evils by becoming the gods who vanquish them.

It's a mistake to think of our ethical lives as a branch of philosophy, even as a branch of moral philosophy.[8] Most philosophers, and maybe most intellectuals, would surely resist my counsel in that assertion, I know; since they would see it as promoting, if not despair, then at least the surrender of any hope of reasonable agreement about how to live in relation to our hard cases. I disagree. I suspect Wittgenstein was finally right in his famous remark (section 127) in the *Philosophical Investigations:* all philosophy can do is to assemble reminders in service of some purpose or other (Wittgenstein 1953). It cannot offer a map of Reality, or of The Good Life for Human Beings; all it can offer are "sketches of landscapes" that may, in a particular situation, help us to orient ourselves as we slog through the countryside (ibid., preface). But such sketches are not useless. They can, after all, help us to pay attention and thus to see what we need to see in order to get on. Heidegger's account of "the essence of technology" is such a landscape-sketch, even though he of course thinks it's (part of) a (or in fact part of *the*) Map. Will it be a sketch, a reminder, that will help us to see our way more clearly, or will it—as it certainly could—distract us from our proper path of thinking? It would be nice to know in advance, but in this, as in so much else, the proof of the pudding will be in the eating.

NOTES

1. The qualification will become important later on.

2. Here there is no necessary implication that anyone in particular consciously said or thought: "Let's make the mug this way."

3. Of course, there are differences at the margins. The point is that those differences, to the extent they can't be suppressed, are not supposed to matter.

4. The connection to what he says in *Being and Time* about *Zeug* is obvious.

5. It is impossible to overstate the contribution made by Cheryl Chase and her colleagues in the Intersex Society of North America to educating and sensitizing medical professionals, ethicists, and others in relation to these matters.

6. Here I am relying on Susan Neiman's wonderful book *Evil in Modern Thought.*. In the context of this discussion, evil is just whatever we say "This ought not to be" about when we confront it.

7. Hegel thought so, of course. See Neiman (2002, chap. 1).

8. To the attentive reader it may seem there's an inconsistency between this sentence and what I say above about ethical conceptions reflecting metaphysical commitments (perhaps unconsciously held). I don't think so. I think there's an important difference between recognizing the influence of metaphysics on ethics and in thinking that the true solution to our ethical quandaries can be found in a better metaphysical conception.

REFERENCES

Elliott, C. 2003. *Better than Well: American Medicine Meets the American Dream.* New York: W. W. Norton.

Heidegger, M. 1977a. The question concerning technology. In *The Question Concerning Technology and Other Essays,* translated by William Lovitt. New York: Harper & Row.

———. 1977b. On the essence of truth. Reprinted in Martin Heidegger, *Basic Writings,* edited by David F. Krell. New York: Harper & Row.

Kitcher, P. 2001. *Science, Truth, and Democracy.* New York: Oxford University Press.

Neiman, Susan. 2002. *Evil in Modern Thought: An Alternative History of Philosophy.* Princeton: Princeton University Press.

Nelson, H. L. 2002. What child is this? *The Hastings Center Report* 32 (6):29–38.

Thoreau, H. D. 1985. *Walden.* New York: The Library of America.

Wittgenstein, L. 1953. *Philosophical Investigations,* translated by G.E.M. Anscombe. Oxford: Basil Blackwell.

CHAPTER SIX

Emily's Scars

Surgical Shapings, Technoluxe, and Bioethics

Arthur W. Frank, Ph.D.

> The limits are unknown between the possible and the impossible, what
> is just and what is unjust, legitimate claims and hopes and those which
> are immoderate.
>
> *Emile Durkheim, Suicide* (1896)

Any illusion that The Hastings Center's Surgically Shaping Children (SSC) project
was about *other* people—people with rare conditions, including achondroplasia (genetic dwarfism), anomalous genitalia, and craniofacial deformities—was lost one day
as I went for a walk. I passed a person with a physical characteristic that was normal
enough but still precipitated my thinking, "I'm glad my body's not like that." And then
without discernable pause: "But if it were, I could get that sort of thing fixed." At that
point, moral and sociological sense returned and I noted that my judgmental reaction to another's body was shaped by my coincidental assessment that surgeons work
on conditions like that. Judgment conflates the body itself with the quality of work
done on that body or the potential to have that work done. The possibility of fixing
renders inescapable the question of whether or not to fix—a problem affecting far
more people than the groups studied during the SSC project.

My unworthy but useful reaction to my fellow walker led me to realize how uneasy
my sense of boundaries is between what I consider fixable about my body and what
I believe I am called on to live not only *with* but *as*. I wash, groom, exercise, and reflect on my diet; I convince myself—or am I convinced by an increasingly undiffer-
entiated mixture of commercial advertisements and health promotion campaigns—
that these actions have not only practical benefits but moral implications: caring for
myself in these ways enhances the person I am. It is a short step along the continuum

to seeking medical advice on matters not only potentially critical but also mundane: physiotherapy and wart removal. These consultations seem to raise no ethical issues. But my fix-it reaction to my fellow walker raises the question of where to draw limits of self-fixing. My initial modernist reaction is to phrase the issue in individualist terms: Is there some core of me that I should work with, not work on, or are some body parts no more than unwanted contingencies, like warts, that temporarily intrude on my life? If the latter, is the decision to fix determined only by a comparatively simple cost- and risk-benefit assessment? Need I ask only whether the promised improvement will be worth the time, trouble, and pain to me that the fixing involves?

The bioethics appropriate to such cost-benefit questions is a kind of consumer protectionism; it insists, for example, on full disclosure of risks, preferably based on follow-up studies of how such fixings have worked, or not, in past interventions. *Protectionist bioethics* takes for granted the presuppositions of consumerism; thus it wants people to know exactly what is being delivered at what cost and with what risk. The ethical standards are liberal, requiring medical professionals to be responsible salespeople and then leaving the choice to patient-consumers. One (of many) problems with this project is the difficulty of accurately specifying the potential benefits, costs, and risks. On a less functional level, this kind of bioethics has trouble taking seriously how one individual's choice—not only what is chosen, but also being in a position to choose—affects others.

Of course, there has always been another kind of bioethics, which can be called *Socratic*. Socratic bioethics questions what protectionist bioethics takes for granted; it asks disconcerting questions about the good life and what kind of *health* is part of this good life. These questions widen the scope of concerned parties whose needs ought to count in any individual's health-related decisions. No one lives a good life alone. In this Socratic mode, whether my fix-it reaction is conducive to the kind of person I want to be depends on whether my reaction is conducive to my participation in the communities that support my good life. I then have to specify which parts I play in which communities, and how those parts need to be played for those communities to be good—as I understand "good." My understanding of *good* is not fixed but remains perpetually open to questioning from all sides, with specific decisions responding to that questioning.

This essay follows the Socratic approach to bioethics, but unlike the Platonic Socrates, I am more concerned with practices and experiences than with the logic of arguments. I start with the social context in which surgical modification makes sense as a solution to bodily conditions that are perceived as troubles. I then consider what people say about decisions for surgical modification. My objective is not to offer guidelines for practice; it seems more useful to open up the discourses in which people—both professionals and potential patients—are able to think about how their actions affect themselves and their communities.

Socratic bioethics seeks to offer alternative courses of action as real possibilities for people who face decisions. If consumer-protection bioethics can be beneficial to people's physical, emotional, and economic welfare, Socratic bioethics can be liberating, in the sense of helping people to realize they have more options for how they live than they had imagined.

The Context in which Children Are Surgically Shaped

Only at a certain historical and cultural moment do the surgeries considered by the SSC project—limb-lengthening, intersex surgery, and craniofacial surgery—make sense. The technologies of medical intervention presuppose the willingness to use these technologies in certain ways. The problem of who is willing to do what in order to achieve what end is endemic to the culture of high modernity. The sociologist Emile Durkheim, writing in 1896 about the relation of suicide to modernity, raised the question, "how [to] determine the quantity of well-being, comfort and luxury legitimately to be craved by a human being?" (Durkheim 1951, 247). The SSC project could be understood as yet another attempt to wrestle with Durkheim's question, which we have now learned will not and cannot be answered. What Durkheim understood clearly, more than a century ago, is that the energy of modernity is always toward *more:* the cultural impetus is to expand what it is legitimate to crave. In reacting as I did to my fellow walker, I was being no less than modern.

Three aspects of the contemporary context of the SSC surgeries can be singled out to suggest why these surgeries make sense to people: neoliberal medicine, the idea of the body as project, and the moral language of personal authenticity.

Neoliberal medicine denotes the political-economic ideology that considers it proper for the for-profit, corporate sphere to set the agenda for professional medicine (Smart 2003). This corporate agenda makes it increasingly commonsensical to understand medical services as *products.* Health maintenance organizations refer to the "product lines" that they sell, and that language diffuses into the way people think of delivering and receiving services. Recently I heard a radio interview with a physician who used the words *patient* and *client* interchangeably, so far as I could tell, with no apparent awareness of a distinction between them. Patients become consumers of medical products—a status that empowers those with sufficient resources and disenfranchises others who lack these resources (Henderson and Peterson 2002).

Within neoliberal medicine, the boundaries of professional medicine increasingly blur. During the past century these boundaries were fairly clear, but in the nineteenth century they were less clear (Starr 1982), so there is no reason to suppose that professional boundaries will remain as they have been. In the century we have now entered, physicians, especially but not exclusively American physicians, become the delivery agents of corporate products, and corporate entities deliver these physicians' time as a product. Physicians remain *privileged* delivery agents—privileged in what they can do and in how much they are paid for doing it—but they take their place as one category of *providers*, with increasing overlaps between what different providers can offer patients, who are also known as clients and customers (Special Issue on Consumers and Collaborative Care 2002, among many other examples). Neoliberal medicine can be recognized by this breakdown of traditional labels for who people are: physicians become providers; patients become consumers. As new interests assert themselves, different sorts of actors have to be identified in ways that suggest their new roles and entitlements.

Neoliberal medicine happens at the same time that an increasing number of people regard their bodies as *projects* (Shilling 1993). The flesh as God-given reality—for better or worse, this is how I am—gives way to the flesh as stuff to be worked with by various sorts of body workers—among whom physicians are but one, albeit privileged, type. Cosmetic surgery websites feature the image of the surgeon as "flesh artist" (Atkinson 2003). At the interventionist extreme of the continuum of body projects is the French performance artist Orlan, who incites reflection on body modification by orchestrating surgeries to reshape herself. Orlan's reshaping has proceeded through a series of cosmetic surgeries that she directs while under local anesthetic. Her art is both her face itself and the videos of her surgeries. She treats surgeons as instruments of her art and speaks of *using* them, as a traditional artist would use a brush to paint or a chisel to sculpt. Orlan is sculpting herself, using surgery as her artistic medium (Pitts 2003; K. Davis 2003).

Neither most middle-class consumers of traditional cosmetic surgeries nor younger body modifiers among whom tattooing and discrete piercing are popular have ever heard of Orlan, but she affects the milieu that eventually, through layers of diffusion, makes a navel ring seem like a moderate choice for a suburban housewife. Orlan pushes to new extremes both the material use of her body as a project and the self as inextricably tied to how that project is realized. What she does with her body becomes as real a moral responsibility for her, in the twenty-first century, as what people did with their souls was real in earlier centuries.

The body as project extends the trajectory that Charles Taylor argues emerged in the late eighteenth century, when for the first time in history each individual life became something new, a *self*. Life became a project of finding each self's unique point; as Taylor writes, it became possible to miss the point of your life (Taylor 1991). In other words, one's life became something—raw material—that people expected themselves to *do something* with. The contemporary twist on the modern project of the self is that many of us moderns—most observers agree the number is increasing—include doing things with our bodies among the ways to seek the unique point of our lives. At the extreme, the point of one's life can be the modification of one's body (Elliott 2003).

Here lies the crucial difference between contemporary body projects and various forms of body modification that have been practiced in traditional societies since the beginning of humanity. Traditional body modification, including initiation ceremonies, marks the body's membership in a group; particular markings indicate a prescribed status in that group. Undergoing these modifications is not something that individuals decide on or negotiate. Markings express, but they are not *expressive,* which is a modern concept requiring a post-Romantic self. Markings are a non-negotiable expectation, expressing such matters as a member's gender, family status, and age group (such as having attained puberty) (Frank 2003a).[1] Those who elect contemporary body projects speak of these projects in a language of *personal* decision making and *individual* choice. At least in the eyes of the modifier, although not necessarily as perceived by others, tattoos and piercings (not to mention more extreme modifications like branding and scarification) are marks of *unique* individuality. When body modifications do express membership—such as when members of sports teams get a common tattoo at the end of the season—those affiliations are individually chosen and often competed for (ibid.). The tattoo or more extreme modification is understood to say something about the individual, because the affiliations are expressive of who the individual is. Contemporary individualism includes memberships, but the marks of membership are elective, not prescribed expectations.

To illustrate how these contextual elements of neoliberal medicine, body projects, and moral claims conjoin, and to complicate the question of what ought to be fixed by surgery, I offer a single example: feet. Looking at what people are doing with their feet, or more specifically, the cultural threshold of what it now makes sense to do with one's feet, is a provocative way to suggest the uses of surgery that already make sense to people when they find themselves confronted with decisions about surgically shaping children.

Surgically Shaping Feet

In March 2003, *Vogue* ran a story in its "beauty, health & fitness" section—a concatenation of topics typical of neoliberal medicine—titled "the flawless foot" (Lamont 2003, 442). The story interviewed several New York podiatrists whose surgical practice includes shaping women's feet so that they can fit into and can look good wearing designer shoes. These shoes "require designer feet" (ibid.). As *Vogue* told the story, surgical practice is being pushed by patient-consumers, who in turn are being pushed by shoe designs. Thus *Vogue* quoted a "Manhattan-based podiatrist and podiatric surgeon" who said: "Until recently, my patients would have surgery only to relieve painful foot deformities like ingrown toenails and plantar warts. Now they come in for a consultation, pull a strappy stiletto out of their bag, and say, 'I want to wear this shoe'" (ibid.). This scene is certainly not typical of twenty-first-century medicine, but the description instigates a cultural expectation among *Vogue*'s many readers. Whether or not these readers actually have their feet reshaped, *Vogue* presents a potent lesson in what patients are entitled to expect from their physicians, as well as what people should expect of their bodies.

The cultural resonance of *Vogue*'s story is suggested by the appearance of a similar—the unkind adjective would be *clone*—story that appeared in June 2003 in the "style" section of Toronto's *Globe & Mail,* one of Canada's two national newspapers (Pearce 2003). The *Globe*'s story focuses on Suzanne Levine, the same New York podiatrist who is quoted extensively in *Vogue*'s story. Her statement expresses the taken-for-granted values of neoliberal medicine: "The shoes out there right now are like looking at jewelry. I just saw these sandals, with stones and gems . . . they're gorgeous. You want to be able to wear them. If your foot is unsightly, it detracts from the shoe." This statement lends a new twist to Martin Heidegger's critique of modern technology. In two of Heidegger's examples, technology causes the river to be seen as a source of hydroelectric power and the forest to be seen as a source of lumber. The water becomes "standing-reserve" for the power plant and the trees standing reserve for the sawmill (Heidegger 1993). Levine presents the foot as standing-reserve for surgery, which is how Heidegger describes patients in clinics.[2] But she then broadens the frame as she presents the practice of surgery as standing reserve for fashion. What comes first is the shoe, which then dictates the shape of feet. If the shoe does not fit, then perform surgery on the foot.

The moral justification of this ordering of priorities lies in what *Vogue* called "a woman's confidence." "I got tired of burying my toes in the sand when I went to the beach. It was humiliating," says a woman who had surgery to shorten several toes. Cinderella stories are ancient and culturally diffuse; this woman's description of the effect of surgery sounds like Peter Kramer's biotech version of the Cinderella plot, told in his best-selling *Listening to Prozac* (Chambers and Elliott 2004). Kramer describes patients who experience Prozac as a transformation of self. "At first I thought I was just being nit-picky," the podiatric patient says. "But the transformation is amazing. And I was back in high-heels in less than two months" (Lamont 2003, 442). "It changed my life," says another woman, speaking not about medical podiatry but about the effect of treatments from those medical adjuncts whom *Vogue* describes as "expert pedi-curists at Buff Spa in Manhattan's Bergdorf Goodman" (ibid., 446). I note these *expert* pedicurists as an example of the point made earlier, that physicians practice as delivery agents of services within an array of agents offering complementary services. But my main point is the Prozac-like language of transformation and life change as a justification for surgery. These patients and *Vogue*'s writer may well have read Kramer, but whether they have or not, the diffusion of Kramer's language sets their rhetorical expectations, and they perpetuate the diffusion of this language.

Vogue refers to this form of podiatric practice as "technoluxe," a useful description of what neoliberal medicine brings about.[3] Technoluxe comprises both product lines and conditions of delivery. Neither discretionary medical services nor high-end de-livery is new; when I was a boy, one floor in the local hospital was referred to as the gold coast. But in those days, the gold coast could offer little more—though no less—than more comfortable surroundings in which to receive the same medicine. What is new is the profusion—the sheer quantity and accessibility at different income levels, in different sites—of medical product lines. Technoluxe depends, first, on the in-creasing public and professional acceptance of the body as something to shape and life as a project of shaping. It depends equally on the idea that projects are realized through acts of consumption. Those who are disturbed by technoluxe have to ask a question that specifies the problem of modernity that Durkheim and Heidegger brooded over: What exactly is wrong with the aspiration to have, and to use medicine to produce, designer feet?

One objection is functional. *Vogue* quotes one sole medical dissenter, a podiatrist from Moline, Illinois, and the rhetoric of locating dissent there is interesting, since the other prosurgical podiatrists quoted in the article are all New Yorkers. "When I oper-ate, my goal is to alleviate pain," says the Midwestern medical traditionalist. "The risk with all podiatric surgery, no matter how minor, is that it fundamentally alters the structure of the foot and the way you walk, which may cause new calluses and pain you didn't have to begin with" (ibid., 446). Especially in the world of technoluxe med-icine, caveat emptor applies. As the patient becomes more of a consumer—a buyer—the need to beware intensifies. But I do not regard the functional objection, impor-tant as it is, to be the most provocative, since it relegates the moral question of *should we?* to the level of whether it works.

If the only objection were functional, then it could be argued that the rich do the rest of us a favor by acting as guinea pigs for new medical technologies (Baldi 2001, 217n. 13). The objection I consider more significant for more people, more of the time, is that technoluxe medicine distorts the allocation of medical services and distracts medicine from its original and still-predominant purpose. This purpose is clearly stated by the dissident podiatrist: "to alleviate pain." But pain is not what it used to be, and here I return to the moral justification of the satisfied medical consumer who says going to the beach pretreatment was "humiliating." I react to this statement as an inflation of the language of pain: if having unfashionable toes counts as humiliation, in what words can we describe the lives of people living with massive facial deformities? But as troubling as I find the usage of *humiliating* in this instance, it is important to hear the very real problem that this woman is working to express.

This woman exists, like all of us, in what Pierre Bourdieu calls a field (Bourdieu 1990, 1998). What counts most about fields for the present argument is that positions within them are hierarchical, and one's place depends on possessing capital. Bourdieu delineates different forms of capital, including physical capital, and calls attention to how different forms of capital count in some fields but not others, and how some forms of capital hold their value between fields (Crossley 2001). This woman's capital, in at least one of the multiple fields of her life, includes being able to go barefoot or wear scandals and have her feet look a certain way. The field determines what this *certain way* is. Fields set the terms of *what counts* as capital, and fields are also sites of perpetual *contest* between rival forms of capital. This woman, in her field, is doing with her feet what all members of any society, including bioethicists, do with our bodies and with our talents: we shape and allocate them in order to make them count as capital. Feet can be a form of capital not only in dating and marriage markets, but in job markets as well.

What counts as capital goes well beyond the feet themselves. Reshaped feet *display the willingness to reshape one's body* to conform to the demands of the field. The woman's feet mark her *ability to read properly* what counts as capital and to endure what has to be endured to accrue that capital. This interpretive skill and the complementary endurance are the woman's real capital. Any self-reshaping, whether of body, language (as in Shaw's *Pygmalion,* a resonant plot later adapted to become *My Fair Lady*), or skills (in education, certification and recertification) is properly brought off when and because it demonstrates the person's *attunement* to the demands of a specific field. In modernity, attunement is no longer an automatic corollary of membership. Members of traditional societies accepted being told when and how to reshape their bodies. Their decision was binary: either participate or leave the group. In contemporary society, each individual is responsible for choosing and effecting her *own* reshaping, thus demonstrating her fitness for membership within a given field. Hierarchical position depends on displaying attunement to the field, and what counts as capital changes; people have to anticipate shifts. Bourdieu emphasizes throughout his writing that playing in any field requires the correct assessment of what counts as capital *there,* and *then,* including what kind of body counts as *right.* The right body demonstrates having made the right assessment of capital, and thus becomes a potent display of rights to participation and position.

If Bourdieu's argument stopped here, it would be a neoliberal defense of anyone doing anything that enhances his market position. This defense would effectively end ethical discourse, since our capacity to claim that some actions are good and others are not so good would be determined only by what counts as capital in specific fields. Nothing could be further from Bourdieu's point, which is to oppose neoliberalism. I lack space to pursue this argument, however. I use Bourdieu's ideas not to make technoluxe surgery legitimate, but only to show that it is plausible.

Recognizing the demands of capital and fields allows us to take a generous view of the podiatry patient who seeks designer feet, and it complicates the question of what's wrong with these feet. Unless this woman leads a charmed life, she will have other experiences that will shift her scale of what counts as humiliation. But for now she is doing what we all do: she is *trying to hold her own*. And so is her podiatrist. The website of Suzanne Levine, the podiatrist who wants to shape feet to fit designer shoes, tells us that only 8 percent of podiatrists are women, and Levine's success is singular for a woman in this field (www.footfacial.com). Although she may not be a feminist hero, she too, in her field, is working to hold her own.

To suggest what may be troublesome about how they are holding their own, I turn to the SSC surgeries.

In the Gravitational Field of Technoluxe

The SSC surgeries are not shaping children so that they can wear designer shoes, but the same basic equation applies: if the body does not fit, reshape it. The problem of how to respond to these surgeries is tied to this equation. The SSC surgeries—most evidently, limb-lengthening surgery—can be presented as the leading edge of a slippery slope that relegates all medicine to technoluxe market values: those who have the most resources to put into their bodies can produce bodies that accrue the most capital in the most rewarding fields. The body is called forth as a site of investment and accrual, and in neoliberal society, those who have the most to invest have the first call on services. Alternatively, these surgeries can be defended as medicine in the cause of democratic humanism: they offer the best chance for people who have been allocated low physical capital to get back onto as level a playing field as possible. And who can say they should not have that chance?[4] Both perspectives have some merit, which is what makes bioethical response so difficult. A beginning is to consider the moral justifications people offer for each type of surgery.

The language of moral justification for limb-lengthening surgery is individualistic.[5] The following statement is taken from a long article posted on the website of the Little People of America (LPA). The author is a Little Person named Gillian Mueller, whose experience of limb-lengthening was the subject of a 1992 article in *People* magazine. Her updated story is posted on the LPA website, dated September 2002 (Mueller 2003). Mueller describes her near-total satisfaction with how limb-lengthening has affected her life. She concludes:

> Undergoing limb-lengthening was clearly the right decision for me. That is not to say it is the answer for everyone, or even a majority. It is a personal decision that every individual whose lives [*sic*] can be functionally improved by the procedure should be allowed to make for him/herself, without being judged by anyone for that decision.

This dual emphasis—that only the individual can decide for herself, and that no one else can judge that decision—is repeated in Internet chat groups of people who are planning or considering limb-lengthening surgery (Frank 2003a). Moreover, Mueller's statement is entirely consistent with the language of people who practice both conventional and extreme body modification (Atkinson 2003).

Mueller's rationale for undergoing surgery appeals to mundane matters of convenience—she writes of driving an unmodified car and reaching objects on supermarket shelves. She downplays issues of identity, writing that before her surgery, "I knew I really was no different from anyone else, and I knew if I set my mind to it I could do anything any average person could do, if not more . . . My mother made sure I came home to a place where I knew I was loved for who I was, even though I was small." But the "even though" qualification is inescapable, and the decision to have surgery reinforces how much "even though" counts. By asserting how much better her life is since she made herself less small, she makes "even though" count for others as well. She necessarily poses a choice whether or not to make it count less. When being small is presented as a choice, the "even though" becomes a heavier weight.

That her choice affects others does not impugn the validity of what she chooses. When, as a young teenager, she is sent to a medical presentation on limb-lengthening, she too *cannot avoid* choosing. Some people's discovery of choices that they find liberating will force others to confront choices they would rather not have recognized in the first place; this chaining of possibilities seems inevitable. But Mueller should be aware that her choices affect other Little People's ability to choose, and she should take responsibility for how she frames the choices that do affect others. The recognition that none of us chooses anything consequential "for herself" seems fundamental to moral participation in society. That means only that we must choose carefully, because as we choose for ourselves, we also confront others with choice.

The choice of limb-lengthening surgery is a form of normalization—fitting the body to the demands of society rather than calling on society to create accommodations for different bodies—and normalization has a bad name in an age of disability rights (L. Davis 1995). Yet who among us of normal height wants to tell Gillian Mueller that she has no right to a technology allowing her the advantages she claims? What, then, needs to be offered to those who are affected by the expectations that her decision generates in their lives? These questions are typical of modernity, a defining characteristic of which is the dislocation of people's lives by technologies. These dislocations have always brought benefits and losses, often to the same people. At this stage in modernity, bioethics can offer those who must choose the reflective observation that practices reinforce each other's acceptability; bioethics can heighten people's awareness of how their practices affect their sense of connection with other people.

Simply the reporting of technoluxe podiatry in *Vogue*, followed by various clone stories, regardless of how many feet are actually reshaped—even in Manhattan—affects the acceptability of surgically reshaping limbs. In a technoluxe context, achondroplasia is readily understood as another individual problem that requires medical fixing. Surgical intervention is one of a series of available choices for fixing some part of one's life—choices from pharmacology to promises of gene therapy.

In this framework of choice, living with achondroplasia becomes understood as *a choice of body projects*. This understanding can be either liberating or constraining, or both. What constitutes liberation and what constitutes constraint depends on values and politics and will remain contested. Participation in disability rights—claiming one's disability as a cultural difference, even as a positive value—is one available body project. Another project is to minimize disability through surgery. Many people—probably an increasing number—will mix both projects, since the projects are mutually exclusive in theory more than in practice. Decisions of which project to pursue—when to pursue it, how far to go, and to what extent that pursuit excludes other projects—depend on expectations that are constantly being conditioned. The conditioning of expectations is not unidirectional from technoluxe to disability; it cuts the other way as well: once limb-lengthening becomes known as a standard of surgical body modification in the cause of convenience, cosmetic podiatric surgeries like bunionectomies will seem like pedicures.

The consequences of normalization darken when we move from the legs to the genitals. Limb-lengthening surgery is performed on teenagers who participate in the decision for surgery, as Mueller carefully specifies she did. Intersex surgery is usually decided between parents and surgeons, excluding the child from the decision. Children are often considered too young to be informed—infants clearly are too young, but age of consent becomes contested as children grow older (Alderson 1993)—or, in some of the most disturbing stories we heard in this project, older children are intentionally misinformed as to what surgery will do to their bodies. The stories of those who have been subjected to this surgery are filled with expressions of shame and recriminations for familial secrecy. Both academic research and the website of the Intersex Society of North America (ISNA) present stories of people who feel mutilated by surgeries that sought to correct differences in genitalia (Dreger 1999). What we have been lacking are the stories of the decision makers. (See, however, Ellen Feder's chapter in this volume, which considers some parents' stories, as well as the narratives in Part I.)

The observations of the SSC group, while falling short of formal ethnographic research, suggest that surgeons present a threefold justification for their intersex-related interventions. First, surgeons believe that they carry out the wishes of the parents, who are the child's surrogate decision makers. When pressed as to why they operate on infants so soon after their birth, surgeons appeal to the level of parental distress and their responsibility to relieve it, a responsibility that is equated with intervening as fast as possible. Second, they claim to achieve the surgical outcome of normal-appearing genitalia and support that claim by showing numerous before-and-after slides. Third, their descriptions of their patients' lives foreground the risk of social humiliations—in locker rooms and other change rooms and in public bathrooms—that could make embarrassment over one's toes seem trivial. If patient stories are about shame and loss as the effects of surgery, surgeons' stories are about how surgery can prevent teasing, and they claim the moral responsibility to do so.

In intersex surgery as in technoluxe podiatry, it is no surprise that the need to reinforce self-esteem or confidence—whatever words are used—is presented as a moral trump. Self-esteem is a crucial resource for the modern self precisely because this self's uniqueness entails being out there by itself, on its own, responsible for itself. Surgeons have good reason to believe that medicine must use its resources to protect this self-esteem (Taylor 1991).

Again, there is a functional objection, this time expressed in personal accounts of loss of genital sensation as a result of surgery, as well as the trauma of repeated operations for more complex conditions. Too often professional surgery chooses not to hear these stories. One such refusal to listen—an angry response to a video produced by the ISNA, in which several people described not only their sense of physical loss but also their sense of violation—was perhaps the most dramatic, confrontational moment in the SSC meetings. What is at stake is crucial for medicine: Whose opinion trumps in the determination of surgical success? And, based on that question, whose opinion ought to count in decisions about future interventions? But again, surgeons have considerable justification for believing that they are doing what those around the intersexed person—if not that person himself—wants to have done.

In contrast to Mueller's story of limb-lengthening, people who have had surgery for intersex conditions believe that their families and society at large find them acceptable *only if* their anomaly is fixed. Many believe that the attempted fixing created only a crude simulacrum of normality. They remain marginalized from the society of normal genitalia, and they are alienated from the bodies they had been born with.

We can only speculate about why parents elect surgical correction for their children's intersex conditions. Those stories would be difficult to elicit.[6] The SSC project meetings left us with grave reservations about the quality of medical information on which parents base their consent for surgery. As important as standards of practice for patient information are, the use of any information confronts an inherent limitation. Information always requires interpretation in order to be acted on, and even the most accurate, appropriate information will be interpreted within dominant cultural paradigms. Thus, any advice concerning surgery risks being understood within the same equation that applies to feet: failing to fit the fashion is humiliating, and surgery provides a fix. Most of these parents undoubtedly would feel they had failed to be responsible if they did not offer their children the more approximately normal future that surgery promises.

This same hope for a normal future pervades decisions around craniofacial surgeries. It may be easy to regard intersex surgery as medicine acting to police physiologies that threaten the conventional binaries of gender normality—and more threatening still, physiologies that people claim to take pleasure in—but this critique of surgical normalization is difficult to apply to the craniofacial surgeries that our project group saw. Our seeing again took place through the conventional medical rhetoric of before-and-after slides, and these slides, like the word *deformity,* depend on normative visual convention, and those conventions need to be contested. Yet it would challenge most observers to see these pictures and not feel the appropriateness of this language of deformity. Faced with such faces, it is difficult not to affirm the value of surgery as at least an improvement in what are readily (perhaps too readily) perceived as life-impairing conditions. Moreover, there is no craniofacial group equivalent to ISNA: no survivors of craniofacial surgery protest what has been inflicted on them and claim they would have better lives if they had been left alone. The problem craniofacial surgery presents is not understanding why surgery is first undertaken. The question is deciding when, after years of operations, surgery ought to end.

Jeffrey Marsh, a craniofacial surgeon and a member of our project group, crystallized the issue when he said that after what is often more than a decade of operations, the current surgery is being undertaken to ameliorate the effects of earlier surgery. Candidates for continuing surgery eventually have to ask when is *enough.* Is the next surgical revision going to effect any improvement in appearance, or will it only rearrange past damage? Perhaps more to the point, the potential patient, much of whose life has been invested in undergoing surgery, eventually has to ask whether she *needs* that promised improvement (even if surgery achieves it) to get on with the life she needs to get on with. This life may not be the one that the person would prefer, and the difficulty lies in reconciling the difference between what has been hoped for with what now seems to be the reality.

Medicine, in a variety of contemporary forms that the SSC surgeries represent, becomes the business of rewriting what counts as reality. In response to any patient's condition, some surgeon somewhere will probably offer the possibility—which from another perspective is a fantasy—that the face and the life that goes with it could be a great deal better if only that last surgical revision is agreed to. When we asked why both craniofacial and intersex surgical interventions continued past a point when it seemed to our group, as detached observers, that little could be gained and harm was being risked, the best answer we found was that the momentum of previous decisions made stopping difficult to consider as an option. Momentum reinforces the quality that intersex and craniofacial surgeries share with technoluxe: the promise of a better life—more particularly, a better self—if *one more* medical step is taken.

Craniofacial surgery, like limb-lengthening and intersex surgery, takes place in the gravitational orbit of technoluxe. Many of the surgeons operating on what might be agreed on as facial deformity are or have been engaged in cosmetic surgery as well, and assumptions, like language, diffuse between activities. Yet craniofacial surgery differs from limb-lengthening and intersex surgery because among human body parts faces have a unique place.[7] Potential patients of cosmetic podiatry can choose to wear other shoes, even on the beach. In our intersex meeting we heard stories of young people who managed to keep their genitals out of public view. Living with a face that will attract horrified stares from strangers is where the word *humiliation* seems to find its most uninflated and unavoidable usage.[8] The public visibility of the face and the symbolic importance that links faces to character—exemplified by the aphorism attributed to Lincoln that after a certain age a person is responsible for his or her own face—make facial deformity a problem of a different magnitude, and that difference commands our respect.

Here we reach the crux of what makes responding to these surgeries difficult. How far do we expand the sphere of persons to whom we offer that respect? I believe that trying to compare forms of suffering—comparing the woman humiliated by her toes with a young person deformed by a facial hemangioma—is not useful. The attraction of such a comparison is that it promises apparently clear-cut medical guidelines for practice. Unfortunately, practice will have to confront a reality that is not clearly divisible into categories. The issue may be better thought of not in terms of *what suffer-*

ing we allow as legitimately in need of fixing, but rather *what form of decision making* we respect.

What Is a Bioethical Response to Surgical Shapings?

I suggested earlier that there are two forms of bioethics. Bioethics as consumer protection responds by recommending procedures that seek to protect those subject to surgical shaping; those protections include but are hardly limited to more fully informed consent. The need for whatever protection bioethics can instigate is most pressing in intersex surgery. What I have called Socratic bioethics poses questions about what sort of people we become by choosing to act as we do. My sociological Socraticism broadens the scope of those who are involved when questioning who we are becoming. It calls attention to connections: connections between practices, so that people recognize how one practice reinforces another, and also connections between people, breaking down the idea that any decision can be strictly *individual,* insofar as that word suggests that one person's decision does not affect how another person chooses. In conclusion, I want to suggest another dimension of Socratic bioethics: the significance of dialogue. In Socratic dialogues, people are having a good deal more than a pleasant chat.

Dialogue takes on a distinctive significance as a response to two features of neoliberal society and the medical practices that seem natural within it. One defining characteristic of neoliberalism is the absence of any alternative political-economic discourse that challenges it; the old Marxist-socialist alternative is effectively dead as any kind of opposition. The resulting fatalism is relieved by the glitz of consumerism, including technoluxe, and diverse panics, including epidemiological panics. Second, the pervasive myth of the market privileges an assumption that personal choice trumps in all matters. I suggested this language of personal choice in the discussion of rationales for limb-lengthening surgery as the individual's private decision. The personal is equated with the private. In this neoliberal context, *dialogue* means opening an oppositional space that is too often closed, and it means recognizing that the personal is communal. A Socratic bioethics can instigate dialogue that informs people's sense of how their particular trouble relates to others' troubles, and how their proposed solutions might cause others more trouble.

The technoluxe podiatry patient who is humiliated by her toes is, as I wrote, trying to hold her own, and such efforts are worth a certain respect. The limit of this respect depends on whether this person thinks about how her strategies for holding her own affect others' capacity to hold their own. If I am reluctant to call the woman's sense of humiliation trivial, I am willing to say she is not looking around very far or talking to a sufficient range of people. She is responding to her field, but only to *her* field and *her* need to position herself in this field. To paraphrase Michel Foucault, she knows what she is doing, but she seems to have little awareness or interest in what her doing does (Dreyfus and Rabinow 1983). In a world in which medicine has more work than it can do alleviating pain, how far anyone is entitled to plead ignorance of the needs of others is questionable. It is questionable whether surgeons who operate on anomalous genitalia can ignore the testimony of those who have had these surgeries; this testimony may not take the form of controlled trials, but as organized by ISNA, it is a compelling aggregation. Technoluxe patients and overly aggressive surgeons both lack sufficient participation in dialogue as a process of testing their needs and assumptions against others' realities.

Lisa Hedley, another SSC project group member, provides a specific illustration of dialogue as a kind of talk (Hedley 1997). She writes about what it meant when her daughter, LilyClaire, was born with achondroplasia, an unknown condition in their family. One day soon after LilyClaire was born, Hedley saw a Little Person, approached him, and told him—as a stranger—that her daughter was also a Little Person. I imagine him looking at her as people do when they are not sure on what basis strangers have approached them. He replied, "Right, well, is she healthy?" That simple question shifted Hedley's sense of her daughter's having achondroplasia. The question *repositioned* Hedley: her daughter's condition was no longer a problem, though problems might certainly occur related to that condition. Socratic bioethics recognizes that bodies and diseases are not there to be solved, but how one lives with them depends on how one positions oneself with respect to them. Of course, Hedley was already open to dialogue. The bioethical problem is to lead those not yet open to dialogue toward that openness.

Hedley's story suggests that Socratic bioethics often proceeds best through questions that are not especially clever; in that sense, my allusion to the philosophical Socrates is misplaced.[9] But Socrates remains a founding figure for this form of bioethics for several other reasons: he worked in the public square, where he talked to people about their everyday problems; he forced people to account for why they held the opinions they believed to be true; despite his cleverness, he operated in ordinary, accessible language; he did not make it the measure of his success to disturb people, but his questions did disturb; and, most important, he kept people focused on ideals of truth and the good while keeping the content of these ideals unfixed.[10] Truth and the good seem to have more to do with sustaining the *process* of dialogue than with being *outcomes* of dialogue.

Yet medicine, especially surgery, is about acting and producing an outcome; dialogical surgery can seem a contradiction in terms. A hard lesson of the SSC project is that surgery must be dialogical in order to be ethical: focused, mutual inquiry about what surgery can do must be open to multiple voices, and decisions need to be held open longer; these are recommendations for practice, though they are hard to wrestle into formal guidelines. In stories about surgical outcomes that most of the SSC group felt were bad—though our feelings could be contested—the trouble began when not enough people were involved in the conversation over a long enough time. The fullest range of possible outcomes, and their fullest range of consequences, were not considered; nor was the fullest range of alternatives explored. These alternatives include that posed implicitly by the Little Person who responds to Lisa Hedley by asking, in effect, why she thinks she has a problem.

Another distinction now cuts across my initial one between consumer-protection bioethics and Socratic bioethics. There are problems that arise *in the course of* medical practice—such as consent issues—and there are problems that arise *as a result of* the possibility of medical practice. Consumer-protection bioethics is more useful responding to the former sort of problems, since these problems seem amenable to solution. Socratic bioethics presents very different kinds of responses to the latter problems because these problems are ones that we cannot solve but instead must learn to live with. Medical technologies and science, almost instantaneously transformed into marketed commodities, will continue to present problems that require individuals and communities to rethink who they want to be, just as my reaction to the person I passed while walking—the story that begins this chapter—required me to rethink who I was becoming and whether I wanted to be that person (Frank 2003b).

Limb-lengthening, intersex, and craniofacial surgeries all pose problems about what constitutes a good life, and about when medicine should be used and when refused in pursuit of the good life. In a neoliberal age it is difficult to convince people that they cannot lead good lives by themselves. The neoliberal subjectivity does not readily accept that "personal" decisions implicate others, because any person's good life depends on others also leading good lives.[11] At this point neoliberal economic thinking converges with a postmodern philosophical recognition—which probably finds its earliest, most explicit statement in Nietzsche—that there is no gold standard of the good. Carl Elliott ends his recent consideration of issues complementary to SSC by observing: "Our problem, of course, is that most of us don't have Aristotle's confidence about the purpose of human life" (Elliott 2003, 199). I especially like Elliott's "of course." It is no longer news that old certainties are gone. The question is how to live after.

Sociologist Alan Wolfe puts an optimistic spin on this lack of confidence, calling it "moral freedom" (Wolfe 2001). The people whom Wolfe interviewed about what they understood as moral problems demonstrate their will to do the right thing alongside their distrust of canonical standards of what is right. They seem to be using the interviews as occasions to engage in dialogue, testing their sense of what is right in some specific situation against the interviewer's reaction to their stories of moral action. That perpetual process of testing one's views against the reactions of others seems to be the dialogue that Charles Taylor, among many others, believes is fundamental to moral life.

It seems both politically and culturally naïve to believe that bioethics can respond to the SSC cases by drawing lines between types of surgeries and giving some but not others an ethical seal of approval. We cannot adjudicate either what forms of suffering are sufficiently authentic to warrant medical intervention or what medical interventions are sufficiently effective to be ethical responses to that suffering. What seems useful is to show how decision making can proceed in ways that command respect.

Coda

Our meeting on limb-lengthening was attended by Emily Sullivan Sanford, a young woman who had this surgery several years earlier[12]—and who has written a narrative for this volume. She wore a sleeveless top, and on her upper arms were prominent rectangular scars where, during surgery, the bone had been broken and pins inserted, so that the bone's length could be increased by continually pulling the two fragments apart, preventing healing and generating new bone growth over several months. The scars were not neat, surgical scars. The skin looked well healed, but the past trauma was visible.

Emily talked about her scars at some point in our discussion. She said she had been encouraged to have a skin graft to remove them, but she refused. They were an emblem of the ordeal she had gone through. She was clear about her choice of word, *ordeal*. Her scars reminded me of an interview in *Habits of the Heart*, a major study of American values by Robert Bellah and his colleagues. They quote a woman whom they call Ruth Levy, who tells this story:

> The woman who took care of my daughter when she was little was a Greek Jew. She was very young, nine, ten, eleven, when the war broke out, and was lying at the crematorium door when the American troops came through. So that she has a number tattooed on her arm. And it was always like being hit in the stomach with a brick when she would take my baby and sit and circle her with her arm, and there was the number. (Bellah et al.1996, 138)

Scars do hit us like a brick, as they connect immediate persons to imagined forms of suffering and thus render that suffering tangible.

Bellah and his colleagues use Ruth Levy's story as an example of what they call communities of memory (ibid., 152), a term that does not quite fit Emily's situation. Memory is one issue for Emily, but her scars also look forward to the person she is becoming; they hold her surgery as partial foundation of that becoming. What kind of community Emily and her scars will figure in remains unknown. We do not yet know what to call a community of those who will define themselves as sharing some aspect of Emily's experience, or what aspects of her experiences will be shared within different communities.

Emily is normalized in height; when I first saw her across a room I did not identify her as a Little Person. But to suggest that Emily underwent surgery to trade a disability identity for a normal identity—that her limb-lengthening is a form of "passing"—would underestimate both Emily's moral awareness and the complexity of surgical shaping. Emily negotiates multiple resources, including medicine, to live in multiple fields. She is aware that she does not act for herself alone; like our other SSC guests who had had the surgeries we were discussing, she came to our meeting to talk about what limb-lengthening means for others. Her moral freedom is embodied in her scars and her self-conscious decision not to fix them. Her scars keep open both her identity and the dialogue about disability and difference. That openness is good, for us all.

ACKNOWLEDGMENTS

My thanks to my colleagues on the SSC project, especially to Erik Parens and Jim Edwards for specific advice on this essay, to Alice Dreger for her research on intersex surgeries, and to Lisa Hedley, Paul Miller, and Tom Shakespeare for help on limb-lengthening. Research materials on feet were generously provided by Rachael Meziere. A much shorter version of this essay was presented at the "Vital Politics" conference, London School of Economics, September 2003; particular thanks to Monica Greco. The SSC project is funded by the National Endowment for the Humanities. Additional research support for my work is from the Social Sciences and Humanities Research Council of Canada. Perhaps most of all, thanks to Emily Sullivan Sanford for the quality of embodied witness that she, along with Cheryl Chase and Cassandra Aspinall, brought to the SSC meetings.

NOTES

1. Nelson Mandela's autobiography uses such a language of external determination: "When I was sixteen, the regent decided that it was time that I became a man," which required ritual

circumcision. "An uncircumcised Xhosa man is a contradiction in terms," Mandela continues, "for he is not considered a man at all, but a boy. For the Xhosa people, circumcision represents the formal incorporation of males into society" (1995, 30). Compare Mandela's account to the language of those interviewed in contemporary studies like Atkinson (2003) and Pitts (2003).

2. In Heidegger's terms, Dr. Levine presents medicine as a technology with which fashion *sets upon* the body; medicine legitimates the capacity of fashion to *challenge* the body. The contested issue is whether and how this subordination of medicine to fashion affects the moral standing of medicine as a social enterprise. Part of what is contested is how much moral standing medicine has anyway, and what sort of moral standing it ought to have.

3. The complementary term is *boutique medicine.* See, for example, Cascardo (2003).

4. Kathy Davis makes this argument by reviewing the career of the pioneering French cosmetic surgeon, "Madame Noel," who wrote eloquently about her women patients' fear "of losing their jobs as their faces begin to show the first signs of aging" (2003, 27). Madame Noel considered her surgical practice an expression of her feminism—a self-image for which Davis provides considerable justification.

5. Disability rights activists certainly express objections to limb-lengthening, but in my search of publicly available materials—quick web hits—those voices are comparatively hidden behind issues of function that ask whether it will work, at what cost, and with what risk.

6. Another surgical rationale for quick, early intervention is that infants will be too young to remember the experience. Family secrecy begins in the parental hope that the intervention can effectively disappear, the child growing up as if she had been born with the genitals that surgery has recreated. Groups like ISNA never hear from those people for whom this strategy is effective.

7. These surgeons are acting in accordance with moral norms deeply ingrained in modernity that privilege the face. With reference to diffuse social usage, Goffman made the face his trope for that which members of a social group have a responsibility to protect: both their own face and the faces of other people. See Goffman (1967a, b).

8. Erving Goffman defines stigma as that which spoils identity. Stigmas allow various kinds of management of the effects of this spoiling; at the extreme, "passing" as normal allows the condition to remain unnoticed. Goffman presents facial deformity as the exemplar of stigmatizing conditions that do not allow "passing." See Goffman (1963).

9. Perhaps I should call it Parzival bioethics, in honor of the wise simpleton who, alone among the Arthurian knights, has the moral sense to ask the wounded Fisher King the obvious but previously unasked question of what's wrong with him. This simple but profound question breaks the spell and relieves the King's suffering. See Eschenbach (1980).

10. Socrates also sought the sort of universal attributes that my line of argument rejects. For an especially useful discussion, see Flyvbjerg (2001, esp. 67–71). Flyvbjerg argues for an Aristotelian *phronesis* as the basis of social science. Bioethics can choose what it needs from both philosophers.

11. Thus Lisa Hedley (1997) writes: "Early on I learned that the way other people respond to a child of difference becomes integral to your experience of the world." If this statement falls at the personal end of a continuum, at the global end is the theological ideal, emphasized in but not exclusive to Buddhism, that no person's suffering can be fully relieved until everyone's suffering is relieved.

12. Emily's surgery is depicted in Lisa Abelow Hedley's film, *Dwarfs: Not a Fairy Tale.* A project of the Children of Difference Foundation. Emily's name is used in this essay with her permission.

REFERENCES

Alderson, P. 1993. *Children's Consent to Surgery.* Buckingham: Open University Press.

Atkinson, M. 2003. *Tattooed: The Sociogenesis of a Body Art.* Toronto: University of Toronto Press.

Baldi, P. 2001. *The Shattered Self: The End of Natural Evolution.* Cambridge, Mass.: MIT Press.

Bellah, R. N., et al. 1996. *Habits of the Heart: Individualism and Commitment in American Life.* Updated ed. Berkeley: University of California Press, 138, 152.

Bourdieu, P. 1990. *The Logic of Practice.* Translated by Richard Nice. Stanford: Stanford University Press.

————. *Practical Reason: On the Theory of Action.* Stanford: Stanford University Press, 1998.

Cascardo, D. C. 2003. Boutique medicine: A new concept based on traditional ideals. *Medscape Medicine* 4 (2), at www.medscape.com, accessed September 17, 2003.

Chambers, T., and C. Elliott, eds. 2004. *Prozac as a Way of Life.* Chapel Hill: University of North Carolina Press.

Crossley, N. 2001. *The Social Body: Habit, Identity, and Desire.* London: Sage.

Davis, K. 2003a. Cosmetic surgery in a different voice. In *Dubious Equalities and Embodied Differences.* Lanham, MD: Rowman & Littlefield, 19–39.

Davis, K. 2003b. My body is my art: Cosmetic surgery as feminist utopia? In *Dubious Equalities and Embodied Differences.* Lanham, MD: Rowman & Littlefield, 105–16.

Davis, L. 1995. *Enforcing Normalcy: Disability, Deafness, and Body.* London: Verso.

Dreger, A. D., ed. 1999. *Intersex in the Age of Ethics.* Hagerstown, MD: University Publishing Group.

Dreyfus, H. L., and P. Rabinow. 1983. *Michel Foucault: Beyond Structuralism and Hermeneutics.* 2d ed. Chicago: University of Chicago Press, 187.

Durkheim, E. 1951. *Suicide.* Translated by J. A. Spaulding and G. Simpson. New York: The Free Press.

Elliott, C. 2003. *Better than Well: American Medicine Meets the American Dream.* New York: W. W. Norton.

Eschenbach, Wolfram von. *Parzival.* Translated by A. T. Hatto. London: Penguin.

Flyvbjerg, B. 2001. *Making Social Science Matter: Why Social Inquiry Fails and How It Can Succeed Again.* Translated by S. Sampson. Cambridge: Cambridge University Press.

Frank, A. W. 2003a. Surgical body modification and altruistic individualism: A case for cyborg ethics and methods. *Qualitative Health Research* 13 (10):1407–18.

————2003b. The bioethics of biotechnologies: Alternative claims of posthuman futures. In *Debating Biology: Sociological Reflections on Health, Medicine, and Society,* edited by S. J. Williams, L. Birke, and G. Bendelow, 261–70. London: Routledge.

Goffman, E. *Stigma: Notes on the Management of Spoiled Identity.* Englewood Cliffs, NJ: Prentice Hall.

————. 1967a. Embarrassment and social organization. In *Interaction Ritual: Essays in Face-to-Face Behavior*. Garden City, NY: Anchor, 97–112.

————. 1967b. On face work. In *Interaction Ritual: Essays in Face-to-Face Behavior*. Garden City, NY: Anchor, 5–45.

Hedley, L. A. 1997. A child of difference. *New York Times Magazine,* October 12; available at www.home.earthlink.net/~dkennedy56/dwarfism_nytmag.html, accessed September 21, 2003.

Heidegger, M. 1993. The question concerning technology. In *Basic Writings,* edited by D. F. Krell, 311–41. Revised and expanded ed. New York: HarperCollins.

Henderson, S., and A. Petersen, eds. 2002. *Consuming Health: The Commodification of Health-Care*. London: Routledge, including A. W. Frank, What's wrong with medical consumerism? 13–30.

Lamont, E. 2003. The flawless foot. *Vogue,* March: 437, 422, 444.

Levine, Suzanne. www.footfacial.com, accessed August 2003.

Mandela, N. 1995. *Long Walk to Freedom*. London: Abacus.

Mueller, G. 2003. Extended limb-lengthening: Setting the record straight. Revised posting, 09–27/02. http://www.lpaonline.org/library_ellmueller.html, accessed August 31.

Pearce, T. 2003. The new T & A. *The Globe & Mail,* June 24.

Pitts, V. 2003. *In the Flesh: The Cultural Politics of Body Modification*. New York: Palgrave.

Shilling, C. 1993. *The Body and Social Theory*. London: Sage.

Smart, B. 2003. *Economy, Culture and Society: A Sociological Critique of Neo-Liberalism*. Buckingham: Open University Press.

Special Issue on Consumers and Collaborative Care. 2000. *Families, Systems & Health* 18 (2) (Summer).

Starr, P. 1982. *The Social Transformation of American Medicine*. New York: Basic Books.

Taylor, C. 1991. *The Malaise of Modernity*. Concord, ON: Anansi (published in the United States as *The Ethics of Authenticity*).

Wolfe, A. 2001. *Moral Freedom: The Search for Virtue in a World of Choice*. New York: W. W. Norton.

CHAPTER SEVEN

Thoughts on the Desire for Normality

Eva Feder Kittay, Ph.D.

The desire for normality—not what normality *is,* but our desire for it—is the subject of this chapter. The various procedures for surgically shaping children that are discussed in this volume all appear to presume that what is normal is desirable, what is not normal is to be avoided. The price of normalcy and the cost of avoiding what is not normal are high, especially when surgical procedures, often repeated, are intrusive, painful, time-consuming, emotionally wrenching, minimally helpful in improving the body's functionality (and sometimes, as in the case of genital surgery, impede function), and expensive. Against all these material and emotional costs are placed the advantages of normalcy, or at least the appearance of normalcy. In this chapter, I will not try to assess whether the desire for normalcy weighs heavily enough rationally and morally to justify the efforts to achieve (the semblance of) normalcy. Instead, I will explore what the desire is, and from whence it comes. As I contend that the desire for the normal is a powerful one, not easily swayed by a rational weighing of costs and benefits, I believe it is important to consider what means there are to satisfy that desire without necessarily acquiescing to the norm implied in the standard of the normal. This is especially important when the attempt to meet that norm is potentially destructive for the individual, the family, and, arguably, the larger society.

To begin, it is helpful to evoke the desire for normality in order to fix on what such a desire is. The evocation is easy enough, *especially* when one feels that one's life is not normal, or not normal now. At such a time, one often finds oneself yearning for what one supposes is the safety, the comfort, the uncomplicated nature of what one supposes is the normal. Or one evokes a time of stability or order, or a time when expectations and predictions were less tenuous than in times we think of as other than normal.

Who among us would claim to have a *normal* life? For my part, I'm not sure that my life has ever been normal—and that is, in fact, the reason I consented to write a chapter about something about which I hold no pretensions of expertise. Doubtless most of us can claim features of ourselves or our history that fall outside the norm taken in either the descriptive or prescriptive sense, and I, at least, can point to features of my own life that are genuine outliers. As a child of two Holocaust survivors and an immigrant at the age of 6, my life as a child was marked by a singularity and a silence. In the late 1940s, 1950s, and even well into the 1960s, the Holocaust was rarely a subject of discussion in the general culture of the United States. If it was spoken of outside my home and our close circle of friends and relatives, it was in hushed tones. The experiences of the war and the pain and horror of Nazi crimes were too difficult to be assimilated into the cultural fabric of everyday life; the war, directly experienced here only by the returning GIs, was at once remote and frighteningly close, for soldiers who had been in the war were found in most all families. In the decade that followed, the 1950s, normality was deeply sought and deeply desired. Young men and women had had an early adulthood interrupted by a devastating war. War never is normal—it disrupts normality. After a war, people desperately want a return to stability and normality. I suggest that if the 1950s was a socially conservative, even socially repressive period in that the range of the normal was highly constricted, that if it was a time marked by conformity and concerns about conformity, it was because all that was regarded to be outside the normal—be it a revolutionary philosophy, an atypical sexuality, a deviant body, an unruly mind, a history of brutality, and surely grandparents, aunts, uncles, and cousins sent to gas chambers—all these were banished from sight and from memory so that life could assume a predictability and stability that contrasted with war conditions. The uneventful and unexceptional were celebrated. Racial and ethnic differences were assimilated, erased, or made invisible, only whiteness and normal bodies were visible in national representations. I grew up with the difference of being an immigrant, the difference of being a Jew, the difference of having no living grandparents, and, worst of all, the difference of having parents who had endured unspeakable horrors. I desired above all to be normal—to be like everyone else, to hide the pain of abnormality.

At the same time, there was a quiet pride, quite unbidden, in not being like everyone else, in having my own secrets, terrible as they were. Like Joy in Flannery O'Connor's "Good Country People," who had one leg and renamed herself "Hulga" because it was "the ugliest name in any language" (O'Connor 1996, 310), I took the deviance as a point of pride. I, however, attempted to conceal my scorn—and my envy—for those who lead normal lives. Thus I had, even as a child, tasted the ambivalence of normality—the desire as well as the disdain for what is common, what is routine, what is normal.

But a preoccupation with normality, especially human normality, was not the exclusive obsession of the post–World War II years. A wide political swathe—before the war—endorsed social programs aimed at producing "more normal" or "perfect" human beings. These programs shared an effort to rid humanity of human impairments—physical, intellectual, and psychological.

The source of my anomaly while a child was a heritage, a history, a cultural wound. My anomaly was invisible, but the source of the disabilities that are under investigation in this book is their visibility: manifest in the case of facial disfiguration and dwarfism, more intimate in genital cases. While the phenomenon of "passing" is available to those with invisible anomalies (physical or cultural) and not so when the outlier status is marked on the body, the difference that comes to be enmeshed in one's own self-understanding is, I venture, not so different. I venture this because the non-normal in the form of disability has also become an important part of my life.

I have a daughter, now grown, who meets few of the standard norms of 34-year-old women. She is profoundly dependent, having very significant cognitive impairments, seizure disorders, and cerebral palsy. When she was first born, many well-meaning persons urged us to put her in an institution so that my husband and I could live "normal lives." But we had immediately fallen deeply in love with our sweet, beautiful Sesha and I felt very much like a normal mother—one who would not consider giving up her child, discarding a child because she didn't meet someone's expectations of what a child should be. In this, my normality as a mother normalized my child. We wanted to live normal lives and be a normal family, not by excluding my non-normal daughter, but by creating our own sense of normal. But can one ever create one's own sense of the normal. And why would we want to?

In what follows I want to explore the conceptual relationship between what is normal and what is desired—a relationship filled with ambivalence. To do this, we need to spend some time thinking about what the concept of the normal means, for it is a concept with much ambiguity. I argue that in the very understanding of the concept of normalcy sits the concept of desirability. I then argue that normality, bound as it is to norms, is intrinsically a social concept, in much the same way that language is, and like language, norms cannot be private. This will suggest that those who stand outside the normal, stand outside what is desirable and have to be judged as abnormal and with it undesirable. This unpleasant conclusion is, I argue, not conclusive. It is possible to establish new norms, to alter existing norms, just as language itself can break into dialects, or can alter by the addition of new terms and new concepts. In this possibility resides the hope to retain what is desirable about the normal. For thinking of ourself and being seen by others as normal has important effects first, on our own self-regard, second, on others' willingness to recognize our worth, and third, on our acceptance within the community of which we are a part. If this is so, establishing a norm that allows us within "the normal" is not only desirable, but urgent for those who are excluded. At a still deeper level, I conclude, the desire for normalcy is the desire to be loved, a desire realizable through the background of norms that establish and are established by self-regard, recognition, and community.

Normality and Ambiguity

When I quipped "who among us would claim to have a *normal* life?" the tone of irony hints at a (subversive) pride we share with Flannery O'Connor's character, Hulga, in evading the stamp of normality. Claiming normality also is admitting to a certain banality, a lack of distinctiveness and so distinction. While being recognized by our own community and our peers as belonging, as fitting in, as being "one of the gang" gives a positive valence to normality, there is a negative valence attached to being merely normal, when we understand normality as an average, a mean, or a statistical norm. Being just like everyone else can be felt to be undesirable when it effaces what we take to be distinctive in ourselves, and what we take as the identifying features of ourselves, characteristics that make us who we are. This ambivalence derives from a sense of normal as descriptive of how things are for the most part. Sometimes we want to be exceptional while sometimes we want to be as others are.

The ambivalence may also derive from an acknowledgment of the deficits that mar the lives of almost everyone—the interruptions and disruptions, the failings and sufferings. In this latter sense, the desire for normality is the desire for the perfect realization of the life we think we should have, or the selves we think we should be—in this sense it is prescriptive and indicates how things ought to be. Yet while we may rue falling short of the prescriptive norm, we also recognize that life rarely admits of the perfections we seek. We understand that often the best we can do is to accept the failings and forgo meeting the standard of normality. At times, we may go on to question the very norm or ideal on which the normal is based and reject it in favor of a norm more in conformity with the conditions of our lives.

What Is Normal?

Normal, as the discussion above suggests, has both an objective sense and a subjective sense. It has both a descriptive sense and a prescriptive sense. While the objective is generally taken to be what is descriptive and what is subjective is thought to be what is prescriptive, I want to say that both the objective and subjective senses of normal have descriptive and prescriptive senses. Furthermore, much of the ambiguity surrounding the term *normal* derives from the fact that the descriptive and objective senses of the term are in fact infused with prescriptive and subjective elements—that the notion of the normal is, in short, value-laden through and through.

Lennard Davis (1995), in a historical analysis, locates the origin of the term *normal* in the nineteenth century and argues that it acquired its ascendance with the development of statistics and the introduction of a precise way of speaking of the *typical,* or the *average,* or the *mean.*[1] This gives to normal a descriptive and objective aspect. The statistical norm provides a representation of what *is*—as in the *typical,* or the *average,* or the *mean.* While average and averaging seem to be distant from the idea of an ideal, the average can itself become an ideal. So recent theories of the understanding of human beauty have maintained that the face that is ranked as most beautiful is the one that contains features that are averages of the different variants of human faces (Baudouin and Tiberghien 2004). Still the statistical norm as captured by the bell or "normal distribution curve" (Figure 1) epitomizes a statistical understanding of "normal" (and, as Davis notes, "is a symbol of the tyranny of the norm" [ibid., 29]), whereby the most numerous instances of something are those that constitute the norm of that thing. What was desirable, claims Davis, shifted from what was "ideal" to what was "normal," giving to the presumably descriptive norm of normal, a prescriptive force. In fact, argues Davis, a new kind of ideal emerges. The idea of a statistical norm is captured by the bell curve. The center of the bell curve is simply the statistical mean between two quantitatively uncommon, but qualitatively neutral, extremes. But when one extreme is viewed as less desirable than the midpoint and the other extreme as more desirable a new curve emerges, along with a new ideal. This is the ogive curve (Figure 2).

Thus, we see that there is an ambiguity in the notion of the normal, even when understood as a statistical norm. We may be offering merely a description of the statistical midpoint in a bell curve, or we may be invoking the prescriptive ideal conveyed by the ogive curve.

Another way to state this ambiguity of the term *normal* is to say that, while the term appears to be an objective "judgment of reality," it is in fact a subjective "judgment of value." These are terms employed by the French historian of science George Canguilhem, who, in his study *The Normal and the Pathological,* speaks of the normal as involving both a judgment of reality and a judgment of values. Using his work, we can introduce a layer of complexity beyond that found in Davis's account. Canguilhem notes that the etymology of normal is *norma,* a T-square that "bends neither to the right or left, hence that which remains in a happy medium" (Canguilhem 1991). (The bell curve is just an elaboration of the *norma.*) But if we take the way things are to be a realization of an ideal of how things ought to be, as we do when we take what

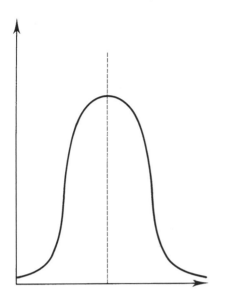

Figure 1. The normal distribution curve.
Source: Davis, 1995, p. 34.

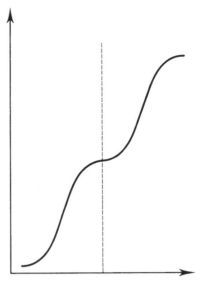

Figure 2. The ogive curve.
Source: David, 1995, p. 34.

is common as at once indicative of how things ought to be, then again the descriptive sense of normality takes on a prescriptive force.

The idea that the way things are is pretty much the way they ought to be, in part, accounts for what has been referred to as the moral model of disability (Silvers and Francis 2000). This model of disability seeks an explanation of abnormality in someone's moral failing and as a retribution for moral wrongdoing. Thus what is not normal not only fails to conform to what *is* (for the most part), but is also indicative of someone's moral lapse. In Ursula Hegi's (1994) riveting novel about Trudi Montag, a young girl born a dwarf during World War I in Germany, Trudi's mother is certain (and is driven insane by the thought) that her daughter's abnormality is actually her punishment for a marital indiscretion committed when her husband was off to war. As Silvers and Francis (2000) point out, the moral model precedes the medical model of disability that is currently the focus of critique by disability scholars.

The prescriptive sense of normal, as found in medicine, is also not necessarily objective in the sense that it is given by eternal and universal criteria. What is healthy or what is normal is first something valued, and valued by someone, as given by that individual's maximum capacity. The long-distance swimmer Lynne Cox (2004) was able to train her body to endure temperatures near freezing for durations that almost always send others into life-threatening hypothermia. Yet her endurance was normal for her. (A subsequent failure to withstand these temperatures would not have been normal *for her*—they would have indicated a failing of some sort *for her*.)

The judgment of value that is normalcy can also be seen in the normal from the patient's point of view, so returning to normal means returning to some previous state, even when the previous state to which we return is not itself optimal, perhaps even subnormal for another. This is a notion of normality that is sensed only in the breach, in the way in which sickness is only understood in the absence of a previous state of health, and it too is not a judgment of reality, but of value.

Normality as a Judgment of Value and the Desire for Normality

If we ask about the *desire* for normalcy when we understand normal as a judgment of value (of what is desirable), not of reality, the statement that we desire normality becomes a near tautology—for to be normal is to be something desirable. Conversely, the stigma that attaches to the abnormal is again analytically entailed by this notion of normalcy, for that which is not normal is precisely that which is not valued and so not desirable. Those who inhabit the space of the non-normal do not merely occupy value-neutral positions that deviate from a norm. They occupy positions marked as not valued, not desirable, stigmatized.

But what of the merely descriptive sense of the statistical norm? In this case, it is far more puzzling why we should desire what is simply more frequently found. Indeed, as I already pointed out there is good reason to be ambivalent about being normal in this sense. Lynne Cox's ability to swim in near-freezing temperatures was surely not normal in this sense, nor is it a normality to which she aspired. Two opposing terms to *normal* capture the ambiguity and the value relations in that ambiguity: the *anomalous* (or variation) and the *abnormal* (or pathological). Cox's capacity is an anomaly, but it is not an abnormality. It is not pathological because it enhances and does not diminish what we take to be useful functioning. Canguilhem writes, "As long as the anomaly has no functional repercussions experienced consciously by the individual . . . the anomaly is either ignored . . . or constitutes an indifferent variety, a variation on a specific theme" (1991, 135). This distinction is of crucial importance in many discussions among persons with disabilities because what is at stake is whether the condition in question is a mere anomaly that becomes a disability only because the built or social environment renders it so or because it is a pathological (abnormal) condition of the individual herself that requires a "fix."

We might say that there is not a two-part, but a three-part distinction. Among anomalies there are those that are "simple variations" and then there are those that are more significant, or obvious, or questionable. Variations that, given a bell-shaped curve, are at the limits of the demarcation of normal and abnormal may have functional repercussions sufficient to render them pathologies. These I am calling "questionable variations."

The distinction between a "simple variation," and a "questionable variation" seems at first to be a mere statistical fact, namely, a function of the distance from the norm. But it is also a function of what is often a socially construed and constructed conception of functional adequacy, both because what may be considered a suitable functional capacity is subject to social negotiation, and because social institutions either promote or inhibit functional capacity by the ways in which they are constructed. That is, what resolves the question in favor of pathology or of variation is a not a simple fact but a social valuation, and, at times, even that fact may have been socially constructed. The claim that some variations are considered pathologies not because they necessarily entail functional limitations, but because social practices and institutions lead to functional constraints is one frequently made with respect to disability. A similar point can be made with respect to phenomena such as homosexuality. Homosexuality is not statistically the human norm, at least within most societies. Whether homosexuality is a variation of human sexuality or a pathology has formally been resolved by no longer including homosexuality in the catalogue of psychological diseases. Because there are fewer homosexuals than heterosexuals does not render homosexuality an abnormality, only a variation.

Yet being homosexual in many parts of the world, including most parts of our own nation, still has functional repercussions—ones that are strictly social, but nonetheless effectively render homosexuality pathological. Being and having families is normally set within the structure of marriage (although that norm is itself breaking down). To be excluded from marriage has socially induced functional repercussions that are entirely a product of social restrictions. Once an anomalous condition comes to have functional repercussions by virtue of a social intolerance of the anomaly, then the desire for the normal may be seen to be simply the desire for functional capacity, a desire that is hardly puzzling.

This insight has important implications for understanding the desire for normality. The desire to normalize gay and lesbian unions by making marriage an option is not the desire to fit homosexuality into a value-neutral statistical norm—a desire that in itself is puzzling. It is instead a desire on the part of gays and lesbians to be included in a set of *functionally relevant and valued* social norms and institutions and this desire is perfectly comprehensible.[2]

In this discussion, the question of the desirability of normality comes to be: Why is difference so devalued that what is statistically normal comes to be precisely that which is desired? One answer to this revised question is that the statistical norm becomes the basis of social norms and institutions, exclusion from which has important functional repercussions and reflects on the extent to which we feel valued—or endangered—by the community of which we are a part.

Each of the conditions examined in this volume is, at least in large measure, an anomaly that is experienced as a functional limitation, largely because of the social intolerance of difference. The negative functional consequences of being little or having ambiguous genitalia or having facial deformities are often themselves a result of the intolerance of the difference. Even when there are functional aspects to the anomaly, the surgical fix is rarely directed at these consequences of the condition, and so the question of *if* and *when* to engage in surgery is more directed at the functional consequences that result from the lack of social value, in other words, social stigma.

This social stigma is a source not only of exclusion but also of danger. In this volume, Lisa Hedley writes about her thoughts for limb-lengthening surgery for her daughter who has achondroplasia, "There are dangers both social and emotional in being different and a certain amount of safety in being normal. So as her guardian and protector I am vulnerable to the enticing possibilities of a surgical fix that might bring her closer to that safety zone of normalcy." Where nonpathological anomalies are concerned and where difference is not tolerated, the desire for normalcy is at least in part a desire to reside in the safety zone it is seen to establish.

I have spoken of the value-laden nature of even the statistical norm, in that some variations come to be constructed as pathologies rather than mere anomalies. But there is a still deeper sense in which the apparently value-neutral understanding of a statistical norm (for example, a mean height or average height) is in fact value-laden. Canguilhem argues that "the norm is not deduced from, but rather expressed in the average." Consider longevity. In one sense the normal lifespan of a human being could be said to be approximately 100 years, for earlier death is due not to old age itself but to some disturbance or dysfunction: accident, disease, a wearing down of the organism that is in fact avoidable with better care and living conditions and the like. But whether or not these factors—hygiene, negligence, fatigue, inadequate or poor nutrition—receive attention depends on social values.[3] Again Canguilhem: "A human trait would not be normal because frequent but frequent because normal, that is, normative in one given kind of life" (Canguilhem 1991, 160).

If Canguilhem is right on this last point, then even the desire for normalcy taken in the sense of the most clearly descriptive and objective statistical norm may be less puzzling and, instead, akin to the desire for normalcy taken in the sense of an ideal. If the frequency of a human trait is not a raw fact but expresses a value (especially as values are generated by structures that are unquestioned and shared by a community that demands adherence to these values), then to wish to be among the many who exhibit the feature is once again nearly an analytic entailment: the frequency itself expresses a value.[4] To be normal is to be included within the scope of what is of value and hence what is desirable and desired. By this reasoning, it is in fact difficult to see how we could wish to be anything other than normal!

If the normal is what is desirable and what is desirable is what people either do or should desire, then the intolerance to difference begins to reveal itself as less baffling. To confirm that something deemed desirable is actually desirable, people must, in fact, desire it, or come to believe that they should desire it. If we have judged something to be desirable and someone fails to desire it, then we can say that it is irrational or evil or in some way bad for them not to desire it. In other words, we say they *ought to* desire it. We may have stumbled on an answer to the question of why difference per se should be so threatening to others that they place in jeopardy the one who exhibits difference. The stigma, the danger, attached to the anomaly, the insistence that those exhibiting the anomaly either try to conform or feel shame at their inability to do so, are all ways to *affirm* the value attached to that which is expressed in the frequency of the phenomenon that comes to be the statistical norm, and so to ward off the possibility of a challenge to the value ascribed to the norm.[5]

The negative responses to statistical difference in the form of shaming, threat, exclusion, and demand for conformity offer us compelling reasons to desire normality. For as long as adherence to certain norms is demanded of persons if they are to be included in the zone of safety or the zone of the valued, the desire for normality is transparent. How could we not desire that which makes us safe and which is deemed desirable—except perhaps if we reject that which is deemed desirable, establish values that are contrary to those prized by those who demand our adherence to their norms, and do what we can to establish new and individual norms for ourselves and provide for our own zone of safety, our own zone of value? After all, we saw before that at least one understanding of normality is what is normal *for a given individual.* But how do we do this?

We cannot establish values by ourselves, outside a social world and in opposition to conditions of existence that pose certain external necessities to us. Value, like language, is not a purely private matter. We can no more establish a private value system than we can (as Wittgenstein demonstrates) create a private language. He wrote: "One forgets that a great deal of stagesetting in the language is presupposed if the mere act of naming is to make sense." I suggest that one can substitute "value" for "name," "culture" for "language" to make of Wittgenstein's remarks a perfectly sensible argument against a private system of values.[6] We set values within a grammar of cultural valuations, a product of what French sociologist Pierre Bourdieu called *habitus,* which Ellen Feder (this volume) in turn speaks of as the "realm of the taken for granted, . . .

a kind of implicit normative order—a normative order that nowhere spells out the rules, that nowhere commands obedience to rules, but works, at the same time, to regulate practices in conformity with a prevailing social order." The *habitus* generates preferences, as well as practices. Structures of a determinate mode of life—for instance, the sexual division of labor, household objects, and modes of consumption—are the stagesetting and produce the grammar ("the basis of the perception and appreciation of all subsequent experience") from which are generated values. Thus, we cannot conceive of the formation of values outside a social existence, and these values cannot be merely privately constructed if they, like language, are to be meaningful to ourselves and intelligible to others. The *habitus*, then, is the set of dispositions, constraints, implicit rules, practices, and structures from which we derive our understanding of what is normal, which, as I have argued, is at once that which is deemed valuable and desirable. Our desire for the normal is tethered to valuations generated by structures that emerge from conditions of a social existence.

Normalizing the Anomalous and Dealing with the Ambivalence

I want to maintain that we can reject those values and the normalcy from which they derive. We can normalize the anomalous, even the pathological, and we must do so if we are to proceed with our varied lives in a satisfactory and satisfying manner. A way out is suggested by the thought that there is a flavor of the sophistical in the reasoning that has us conclude that the normal entails, virtually analytically, the desirable—not only where the normal is an ideal but even when the normal is merely a statistical norm. Perhaps the desire in the desire for the normal is simply an expression of a not very admirable feature of humans that Nietzsche called the *herd instinct*—a need to obey, to follow commands, to acquiesce to authority.[7] If desiring normality, understood as a prescriptive norm, implies a rule of how we ought to be or behave, then this desire may be nothing but such a herd instinct that has become a need to conform and follow authority. Nietzsche, of course, excoriated those who are herd humans, along with their morality of leveling, of obedience, of conformity. Still, to explain the need or desire to be normal, it will not do to use Nietzsche's invocation of an instinct to explain herdlike behavior. Herdlike behavior itself requires a better explanation, and appealing to instinct is too often a way not to explain anything but only name it. If the arguments above are right, then the ways in which normality, even when it seems purely descriptive, is enmeshed in judgments of value, provide reason enough to fear abnormality, if not to directly desire normality.

Furthermore, those reading Nietzsche with a commitment to democratic ideals and social justice inevitably feel a great deal of ambivalence concerning his remarks, for he derides the values of democracy, of equality, and of social welfare as deriving from the herd instinct.

Yet reading Nietzsche reminds us of what is undesirable about normality, revealing that, contrary to the conclusions we reached above, the desire for normality cannot be reduced to a desire for the desirable. That we desire normality cannot be merely tautological or analytically given. The conformity to a given standard carries with it a revulsion to and exclusion of any variation. It gives rise to a blandness for those who remain within the norm and it results in isolation—even immiseration—for those excluded.

Not only can we say that excessive conformity is morally repugnant, but we find that at the level of biology the persistence of life, evolution itself, depends on variation and anomaly. That there are deviations from a norm allows a species to persist through adverse environmental changes. Even anomaly that appears pathological in one circumstance can prove to be beneficial in another. It is safe to say that the persistence of a species and the possibility of its evolving depends on both its simple variations and its distinct outliers.[8]

At the same time, without some standards of normality, we risk outrageous behaviors that can be massively and disastrously destructive. Without some norms—such as norms of well-being, for instance—it is too easy to acquiesce in the suffering of others. Without some norms of health or proper nourishment, for instance, the fact of illness or malnutrition can go unacknowledged and consequently untreated. Norms and conceptions of normal health are frequently preconditions for treatments and interventions.

Resolving the Ambivalence

I hinted earlier that only by constructing new norms, different normals, can we avoid the tyranny of normalcy. But we also saw that these norms are socially established and cannot be merely individual. Yet we know that we do sometimes establish our own sense of normal—of what is normal for us. How do we do it?

During my childhood, my family created their own sense of normality by confining their social circle to those who had shared their own trauma and their immigrant status. In this environment, the members of their circle were not outliers, but normal. While they would poke fun of themselves as "*green,*" and as yet unassimilated, they also felt very much at ease in their own circle and viewed many of the features of their own lives as not only the true normal, but also as more desirable or more real or more savvy than those of Americans. After all, as painful as their experiences had been, it had made them tough and able to withstand what others cannot even imagine. In these and other respects, their survival, when recognized and shared, garnered them a sense of self-regard, even a sense of superiority of sorts. As in the case of biological populations, the anomaly that could result in dysfunction under some conditions can serve as an advantage in others. But to effect this result, one requires first a community to make intelligible the distinctive norm and a set of conditions that allow for the variation to function positively.

In a not dissimilar fashion, once my spouse and I had digested the difficult understanding that our daughter was never to have a normal life, we closed ranks and associated primarily with those who shared our valuing of our daughter, if not the experience of having a child with a serious impairment. By the time of her birth, the late 1960s, the *habitus,* as Bourdieu would call it, or background cultural understandings were in flux and the sense of normalcy that dominated the period after World War II was getting a bad name, at least in some circles.

Yet even as my spouse and I rejected the social imposition of what a normal family was like, we didn't entirely reject normality. In wanting a child, we desired a family and we never could nor would we want to entirely reinvent the concept. Families exist within a *habitus.* Such a *habitus* gives rise to expectations that need to be met if confirmation and approval by and inclusion into the community are sought. There are expectations of parents and parenting that are inescapable and not undesirable. For example, that a parent tries to do the best for her child is part of the norm. Abusive relations, even if common, stand outside it (and for this reason are concealed as much as possible when they do occur).

When parents of a disabled child insist on the normalcy of their special position as parents, they affirm the desirability of normalcy. But what they affirm is an altered conception of the norm. The new norms are generated out of a newly constituted *habitus*—one that emerges under changed conditions of existence and through the formation of a different community. The new community is not distinct from the old, nor are its conditions of existence entirely different. There are continuities and discontinuities. Again, the analogy with language is useful. A language will be modified as conditions of existence alter and as the community of speakers changes. It need not become a new language, but novel words, unfamiliar meanings, and different grammatical forms are generated. Values and norms are subject to these sorts of alterations as well and while we cannot have a private language we can have many dialects and variations on an established language. Furthermore, new dialects can, although they do not necessarily, reform the dominant language. What was first comprehensible only to a few becomes recognizable and intelligible to many. Similarly, what is normal for a few only can challenge dominant conceptions of what is viewed as normal for the larger group. The new understandings can open a space for political change, for challenges and struggles over the meaning of normal.

Why, one might ask, does one want the recognition as being of a certain kind? Why did my family wish to be confirmed/recognized *as a family?* Implicit in the desire for a family that is normal is the desire for confirmation that one is a family. One's family must be recognizable as such to others as well as to oneself. To be a family is to be a part of a social configuration, to share in the lives of others not as an individual but as one with ties and responsibilities. As a family, you would want to be included in discussions about the future of your children, about the responsibilities of parenthood, the responsibilities of society to parents and children, and so forth. You want people to ask about your children. You want to be able to speak of their accomplishments, share their delights, enjoy their friends. You want people to empathize, and when appropriate, help with pains, hardships, and heartbreaks recognizable as those of life in a family. And you want others to understand the degree to which your own well-being is tied up with that of those who are your family.

When recognition that one is a family is denied, the acceptance and inclusion of such attitudes, understanding, and gestures are not forthcoming and one feels isolated, undermined, and not valued. A terrible hurt is inflicted, for example, if grandparents reject a grandchild because of an impairment and try to insist that the parents institutionalize and abandon that child. The failure to confirm the group as a family constitutes a serious wound. But that confirmation requires a recognition and such a recognition depends on the meeting of expectations, which in turn is generated by a norm, the norm of normal.

What I have posited with respect to one's desire for the recognition, acceptance, and inclusion as a family can be generalized to other deeply held features of one's self-understanding or identity. When we conceive of ourselves as (or we aspire to be of) a certain kind, we want others to recognize us *as* such. For with that recognition we come to be treated by others in ways that involve us in networks of relationships of which we want to be part, and which give our lives meaning. That recognition requires we meet and act in accordance with expectations and norms determined by what is normal for that category.

Furthermore, these norms are not merely imposed from the outside; they are internalized as our own understanding of what it means to be of that sort. My own understanding of what it was to be a young American girl was to be a child without the burdensome history I carried with me. All the families I had known configured my own expectation of what it is like to have a child, build a family, and watch babies grow up—and having my daughter did not meet many of these expectations. And yet, of course, in both experiences, not all traditional norms were unmet. I was a young girl living in the United States, speaking English, going to school, dressing like an American child, and generally sharing the childhood of an American child. Similarly, I had gone through pregnancy and childbirth just as most mothers and had an infant to nurture and love. That is, where a situation or person does not fit the image of the normal, it is not because there is no match between the norms and the situation or person in question. Instead, some expectations are met while others are not. There are few matters that are necessary and sufficient for an identity. Those who are anomalous in certain regards, but meet some other conditions, can then work to redefine the normal, to create their own sense of normality, and so to find a way to live with the anomaly in a way that is more or less satisfying. But they will be successful only if there is enough of a community that can recognize the new normal as normal.

That is what my spouse and I did as a family. We created our own sense of normality. We found those friends who accepted our family as a family. We worked through the larger familial discomfort with our child and our situation. We figured out what was normal for our daughter, in terms of her health, well-being, and development. We learned to appreciate the small steps in development she did make. We refused the pity of those who could not understand, and we refused the attempts of others to sanctify us, to call us "remarkable" or "saintly," insisting instead that we were only doing what we assumed parents normally would do—care for, love, protect, and foster the growth of their child. We tried to extend the sense of normality to our other child, and he likewise found his way to normalizing his family by his choice of friends, his understanding of his role in the family, and his understanding of what a sister can be.

As the author of *A Difference in the Family* (Featherstone 1980) wrote, the greatest difficulty is at times when you are caught off guard and suddenly see your child as a stranger does. Until the new normality that we have developed together with others offers a vigorous challenge to the standard one, the important things that rest on our own revision of the norms remain tenuous. Our sense of normality falls apart when we view our child through the stranger's gaze—if only for a moment—and it needs to be recovered. It is worth noting what exactly falls apart at these times. What falls apart is the vision of your child as the individual he or she is and not as just someone with the impairment he or she has. What falls apart is seeing yourself first as a parent and not first as a parent of a disabled child. It is holding on to the connection you have with this singular person and not allowing the hateful attitudes of others to stand between you and the love you have for your child.

When we think of what it is to recover *that* sense of normality, I believe we see most deeply what the desire for normality is about. True, we want normality for the safety it promises, for the stability it entails, for the functionality it provides. But still more profoundly the desire for normality is about a self-regard that arises from being recognized as who we wish to be recognized as, and as the distinct individual we know ourselves to be. It is about an acceptance into a community and a sharing of one's life with others, either the community into which we have been "thrown" by birth or circumstance or a community that we have chosen to embrace. And lastly, but perhaps most urgently, it is about love, that is, about being able to give and receive love.

I have already made a number of remarks about community. Community is crucial because without some community norms themselves cannot be established as they arise through a shared life. But it is also important because without norms the recognition needed for self-regard or self-respect (which John Rawls took to be the most important of primary goods, the goods we need for all other goods) is not possible. While the importance of self-regard needs little comment, and the importance of social interactions in the establishment of self-regard has been widely discussed, what the present discussion adds is that situating oneself within some set of norms—some sort of normal—is crucial for that self-regard to be possible.

The desire for normality and love was revealed when I spoke of what falls apart when you see your anomalous child through the eyes of those who see her disability and not her. When I normalize my situation, seeing my child and myself as a parent through the formation of a norm that diverges from those of standard families (that is, when I see myself simply as a parent and my child as my child), my love for my child is as intense as that of any mother for her child. The distancing that comes from assuming the stranger's gaze is one in which I no longer see her as the distinctive person she is, but as the oddity she is for the stranger. That vision threatens to disrupt the bond that love is, that appreciation of her individuality, her own spirit. There is a paradox since what's normal is what commonly is, yet when someone is abnormal you can't see past the abnormality to the individuality of that person. The abnormality obliterates the individuality. Why should seeing someone as not normal be an inhibition to love?

The Desire for the Normal—What Does Love Have to Do with It?

I have been speaking of the desire for the normal and I have largely talked about the normal and focused little on the nature of desire. There is a great deal of literature on the nature of desire, especially in literature characterized by a term preceded by *post*—postmodernism, poststructuralism, and so on. In these contexts, desire is eroticized, or rather it is erotic desire that is explored. The desire for the normal seems to be far less sexy—far more pedestrian and far less chic.

Yet I have also come to appreciate how the desire for the normal is not as far from the erotic desire with which I just contrasted it—that, in fact, the desire for the normal is intimately tied to our desire for love, for sexual satisfaction, for affiliation, and for affective relations. "Good Country People," O'Connor's story to which I referred earlier, highlights the ambivalence, the ambiguity, and the erotic in our relation to the normal. O'Connor's heroine wanted to be loved, not in spite of her difference, but because of it. Did she transcend the desire for the normal? I want to suggest that she didn't. She had studiously avoided desires that made her vulnerable because of her difference. By her choice of name and her refusal to comply with the norms of feminine beauty, norms that she felt unable to meet because of her deformity, she guarded herself against the defeat of being a failed pretty woman. Yet vulnerable she was. She fell for a man who conned her into believing that he loved her for her uniqueness. He claimed to love her for her distinctiveness, appreciating and loving the fact that she had just one leg. But in the desire to be loved for her singularity, she turned out to be fatally normal. As a consequence, she was all too easily vanquished by this con artist who instead turned her into a freak, and in so doing exposed the vulnerability of her difference.

In O'Connor's story, in my love for my daughter, in my love for my parents, and in the decisions of the parents who consider the surgical procedures under discussion in this project, I believe we can discover a dialectical relation to the normal—a dialectics imbued with desire, with eros, with love.

I have already argued that the desire for normality is importantly tied to the desire to be recognized as who we are and what we want ourselves to be recognized as. When we fall outside the norm, we fall outside the set of categories and concepts by which we can be understood and be made intelligible to others. But, as I suggested earlier, we do not fall outside all norms, only some. Yet to the extent that we come to be identified with the anomaly, we simply are identified as someone who lacks value and even intelligibility. That is all of what is seen. So oddly enough, what is distinctive about us—but distinctive within the values and concepts that are accepted and intelligible—can be seen only when we fall within the bounds of normal—the norm that expresses what is desirable. When we fall outside that norm we are outside what is desirable, and so fear that we cannot be the object of desire, the object of love itself. But to be loved is to be loved for what is not merely typical or shared by everyone else, but for what distinguishes us.

This is a paradox that goes beyond the ambivalence. Lennard Davis suggested that the ancient conception of the ideal is less coercive than the modern conception of the normal. And this coerciveness is especially evident in the case of love. If, for example, the ideal of perfect feminine beauty is embodied only in a goddess, then a mortal woman might desire to approximate the ideal. But to the extent that a lover desires actual women, a woman who falls short of the ideal is not shut out of the possibility of love. But if every woman portrayed in magazine after magazine, image after image, embodies the ideal, then it appears to be the way a woman—any woman—ought to look. To the extent that a woman falls short, she experiences herself as failing to be what she should be—-failing to be the woman that other women in fact are and what a woman must be if she is to be the object of desire. Failing to have a normal-looking nose, for instance, then appears to jeopardize even the prospect of being desirable at all.

Locating the emergence of the normal at the historical moment that Davis does engages a rather interesting question—for the historical moment is also one that coincides with the emergence of individualism. Nietzsche contrasts the modern European's herd instinct to the nobility of hierarchical societies that eschewed the norms and values of the herd. And yet it is modernity that brings with it the valorization of individualism. Perhaps no nation partakes more of the values Nietzsche so scorned when he spoke of the herd human being than our own, but no nation so extols the individual. Individualism is the norm to which the herd human being aspires—impossible as that seems. Even as our young female students preen themselves with mass-marketed cosmetics, aiming to attain the perfect beauty modeled in magazines and on television, they want ardently to be loved for who they are as individuals—just as ardently as did Flannery O'Connor's Hulga. And in this desire for individuality and normality, they too are as vulnerable as Hulga. How is it that these two seeming opposing desires sit in the same breast? How is it that parents who will insist that they love their children for who they are in their uniqueness, so ardently want the same children to be no different than other children, that is, normal?

It is because, as I argued earlier, the contention that the normal is what is desired follows from the very conception and construction of normality. And while every parent, every family, adopts a set of norms with respect to their child, and it is against that backdrop that they see their child as valuable and unique, a parent also recognizes that this set of norms is not always the one against which the child will be viewed, and fears that the child they see as lovable will not be seen by others who see the child against the backdrop of norms that diminish the child's value and uniqueness.

To accept the view that what is normal is fixed and cannot be altered is itself problematic. If we can love and accept our children, if our norms are malleable, then why should we suppose that others cannot? The qualities that are valuable and intelligible can break through the rigidity of the normal and refashion it. The community we forge with our child can be enlarged and love need not be out of her reach. With the love we give to those of our children who deviate from standard norms, we exhibit that they are, in fact, valuable, valued, and desirable. In so doing, we already challenge the norm of normality insofar as that norm carries within it the supposition of its desirability. In that challenge lies the start of political and social struggles to alter pernicious norms, norms that exclude the children we love.

Trudie Montag (from Ursula Hegi's *Stones in the River*) first decided that her father lied to her when, as she expressed her burning desire to grow as tall as others, he told her that she was perfect as she was. She did not yet understand that he did not see her against the backdrop of people with typical height, but against the norms of parenthood. Viewed against this norm, she was perfect. She had to encounter another dwarf, a circus performer who told her of a wonderful world in which there were only dwarfs and how, when the performer felt sad, she retreated to that special world. Trudie had to envision a new norm, one in which she was valued, in order to give up the desire for the norm that surrounded her. With that vision and the love she secured through her father, and even her sadly deranged mother, she could find the self-regard she needed to handle the dangers and difficulties of dealing with those who saw her only as "a dwarf," not as Trudie Montag. She could forge a community with those who devised their own norms, revising the morally corrupt norms of Nazi Germany, and she could seek romantic attachments—she could find love and give love. And it was only when she joined in resisting the Nazi imposition of one standard of normality that she secured the sense of herself that sustained her.

Normality, then, is the backdrop against which our individuality, that individuality for which we desire to be loved, becomes foregrounded. We fear that without normality we move outside of the recognizable and so the cognizable. When we move beyond or outside the normal we fear the loss of intelligibility, intelligibility that at once serves as a condition for our own self-regard and as a precondition for another's love and desire—even as love and desire necessarily move beyond the intelligible. But normality becomes a tyrant when it becomes immutable, rigid, impervious to the fact of its own construction, and blind to the subjectivity with which it is infused. Love and care enacted in community that views us both as singular and "normal" enable us to gain the self-regard needed to struggle against and refashion a *habitus* that would place us outside the norm (and who is *always* within?) and render us undesirable.

NOTES

1. In a classic article, Edmond Murphy (1972) elucidated seven meanings of the word *normal*. These are (1) the Gaussian normal distribution curve; (2) most representative of its class, that is, the average or median; (3) commonly encountered in its class or the typical; (4) most suited to survival and reproduction or optimal or fittest; (5) carrying no penalty or innocuous or harmless; (6) most commonly aspired to or conventional; and (7) most perfect of its class or an ideal. I group the first three under the category of *descriptive* or *statistical norms,* and the last four under the heading *prescriptive norms.*

2. The above can also, interestingly, serve as an argument for those gay and lesbians who refuse to join the chorus of supporters of gay and lesbian marriage. To argue for gay and lesbian marriage works to confer on the institution of marriage the distinctive, perhaps even the exclusive, power to confer on intimate ties a status of normality, of valued and valuable bonds. Those who want to resist yielding such power to marriage, and not only those who wish to deny the rights of marriage to gays and lesbians, may wish to oppose homosexual marriage. But the controversy indicates that marriage possesses this power now and that gays and lesbians are barred from a certain form of normality because of the ban.

3. Canguilhem writes: "The number of dead and their distribution into different age groups express[es] . . . the importance which the society does or does not give to the protraction of life" (Canguilhem 1991, 161).

4. The large population of deaf people on Martha's Vineyard that was a consequence of hereditary deafness (see Groce 1985) expresses not only the presence of that hereditary trait, but also a tolerance of deafness as other than the pathology it is viewed as today in our own society. At that historical moment and place, deafness was normalized, a fact that is not only a consequence of, but also an effect of a certain valuing of deafness.

5. If, for example, deaf couples insist that they prefer to have a deaf child, that preference throws into question the unquestioned assumption that living a life as a hearing person is *superior* to living life as a deaf person. Allowing people who are deaf to propagate and have deaf children—actually select for deaf offspring—presents the possibility of more and more deaf persons in the community. This shifting of the population can either give rise to a community such as the one Groce describes or be experienced as a threat to the hearing community who have a stake in maintaining the importance of hearing. See note 4.

6. I believe that one can use the very same argument to establish that there are no private value systems that Wittgenstein used to establish the impossibility of a private language making the appropriate substitutions in the (Investigations, §258 and onward). The same problems of confirmation exist as do the questions about the intelligibility of the private denotations of meaning or value.

7. He wrote: "At all times, as long as there have been human beings, there have been human herds . . . and very many who obeyed compared with very few who were in command; [obedience] was the trait best and longest exercised and cultivated among men . . . It has become an innate need" (Nietzsche 1995, 107).

8. See Robert Wachbroit, who cites Elliot Sober's contention that Darwinian theory rejects the idea that "a biological system can be decomposed into an unperturbed state (. . . the normal . . .) and perturbations (deviations from the normal state or abnormalities)" and states that, "with variation the rule, the aim of evolutionary explanations is to explain the *constraints on* variation rather than the *presence* of variation" (Wachbroit 1994, 589–90). Also see Lloyd (1994).

REFERENCES

Baudouin, J. Y., and G. Tiberghien. 2004. Symmetry, averageness, and feature size in facial attractiveness of women. *Acta Psychologica* 117(3):313–32.
Bourdieu, P. 1990. *The Logic of Practice.* Stanford: Stanford University Press.

Canguilhem, G. 1991. *The Normal and the Pathological.* New York: Zone.

Cox, L. 2004. *Swimming to Antarctica: Tales of a Long-Distance Swimmer.* New York: Knopf.

Davis, L. J. 1995. *Enforcing Normalcy: Disability, Deafness, and the Body.* New York: Verso.

Davis, P. V., and J. G. Bradley. 1996. The meaning of normal. *Perspectives in Biology and Medicine* 40(1):68–76.

Ellison, R. 1952. *Invisible Man.* New York: Random House.

Featherstone, H. 1980. *A Difference in the Family: Life with a Disabled Child.* New York: Basic.

Groce, N. E. 1985. *Everyone Spoke Sign Language Here: Hereditary Deafness on Martha's Vineyard.* Cambridge, MA: Harvard University Press.

Hegi, U. 1994. *Stones from the River.* New York: Simon & Schuster.

Lloyd, E. 1994. Normality and variation: The Human Genome Project and the ideal human type. In *Are Genes Us? The Social Consequences of the New Genetics,* edited by C. F. Cranor, 99–112. New Brunswick: Rutgers University Press. Reprinted in *The Philosophy of Biology,* edited by D. L. Hull and M. Ruse. New York: Oxford University Press, 1998.

Minkowski, E. 1938. A la recherche de la norme en psychopathologie. *Èvolution de psychiatrique* 1.

Murphy, E. A. 1972. The normal and the perils of the sylleptic argument. *Perspectives in Biology and Medicine* Summer:566–82.

Nietzsche, F. 1995. *Beyond Good and Evil.* Chicago: Gateway.

O'Connor, F. 1996. Good country people. In *The Tyranny of the Normal: An Anthology,* edited by C. Donley and S. Buckley, 307. Kent, OH: Kent State University Press: 307–26.

Riesman, D., R. Denney, and N. Glazer. 1950. *The Lonely Crowd: A Study of the Changing American Character.* New Haven: Yale University Press.

Silvers, A., and L. P. Francis. 2000. Introduction. In *Americans with Disabilities,* by L. P. Francis and A. Silvers. New York: Routledge.

Wachbroit, R. 1994. Normality as a biological concept. *Philosophy of Science* 61:579–91.

PART III

THE SURGICAL CONTEXT

CHAPTER EIGHT

To Cut or Not to Cut?

A Surgeon's Perspective on Surgically Shaping Children

Jeffrey L. Marsh, M.D.

I have been privileged to participate in The Hasting Center's Surgically Shaping Children project in two roles: narrowly, as the surgical expert for the specific discussion of congenital craniofacial anomalies (that is, birth defects of the skull and/or face), and, more generally, as a representative of surgeons and surgery at the working group's final summation meeting. This chapter has developed out of my presentation at that final meeting, but necessarily includes some of the material from my earlier presentation to provide a richer context. My initial presentation as an "expert witness" was much simpler for me, since I was introducing to an intelligent (if untutored) audience information about what I have been doing for the past twenty-five years. My second presentation was much more challenging, in that it was a novel topic for me and it required me to speak at once about all three clinical conditions considered by the working group: short limbs, ambiguous genitalia, and craniofacial deformity.

Furthermore, the response of some members of our working group to a fundamental principle of contemporary care for congenital craniofacial deformities caused me to examine why I do what I do and whether the assumptions that my professional behavior rest on are valid. This principle is that the goal of treatment is to minimize the stigmata of the deformity so that the individual can enter adult life as if the deformity had not happened. Before the group discussion of my presentation, I had not appreciated the tension between the goal of making a child look more normal and the goal of affirming a wide variety of human appearance.

At the meetings I noticed that at least three positions were articulated: (1) we should use surgery to normalize individuals, that is, to make their anatomy more closely resemble that of the very large majority of the population; (2) we should change the opinions of others to affirm diversity and defer surgical alteration until the affected individual is old enough to give informed assent/consent; (3) we should find some combination of (1) and (2). Over the past nine months, I have reflected on these positions and those reflections stimulated this chapter.

Comparing Surgeries for Cleft Lip and Palate, Ambiguous Genitalia, and Short Limbs

American society has become increasingly aware of and sensitive to consequences, both unintentional and intended, of labels—so much so, that a novel abbreviation, "pc" ("politically correct"), has become commonplace in conversation, media, and litigation. In my opinion, based on discussions with health care professionals and laypersons, there is a fundamental difference between the linguistic formulation *craniofacial deformity* and that of *short limbs* and *ambiguous genitalia.* In *craniofacial deformity,* the noun (*deformity*) is a pejorative term, which is modified by a neutral anatomic designator adjective (*craniofacial*). Alternative nomenclature in current usage for such a condition—for example, craniofacial disorder, craniofacial anomaly, craniofacial birth defect—does not avoid the pejorative connotation. Deformity, disorder, anomaly, and birth defect evoke a set of responses that includes a need for correction, repair, fixing as well as undesired negativity. In contrast, *limbs* and *genitalia* are nonpejorative anatomic nouns. Their descriptive adjectives, *short* and *ambiguous,* respectively, may have pejorative connotations but they are not necessarily pejorative. *Short* usually did not evoke a set of responses that includes a need for correction, repair, fixing as well as undesired negativity among the people I spoke with, though *ambiguous* sometimes did.

English does not have a *neutral* descriptor for the type of craniofacial conditions that I evaluate and provide care for. Nor does it have an unmodified noun or single adjective that includes the condition such as *dwarf* for people with short limbs or the recent neologism *intersexed* for people with ambiguous genitalia. These comments are not meant to imply that *short* and *ambiguous* cannot negatively affect perception of a condition, but rather to note that there seems to be a difference in degree and consistency of response when the noun is necessarily pejorative. That is, whereas the label *craniofacial deformity* includes a necessarily pejorative noun, the labels *short limbs* and *ambiguous genitalia* include adjectives that can be—but are not necessarily—pejorative.

The discrepancy in terminology between *craniofacial deformity* and *short limbs* or *ambiguous genitalia* may reflect the fact that a facial difference is evident at birth and, if concealed through nonsurgical means, can be magnified in its significance by the very act of concealment. Short limbs might not be so apparent to others before the individual is ambulatory and outgrown by peers; ambiguous genitalia rarely have to become apparent to strangers. That a craniofacial difference is apparent early and cannot be concealed without added stigma makes it different from the other two cases— and makes it an especially compelling target for surgical intervention.

Beyond the questions concerning how the conditions are labeled and when the conditions become apparent to outsiders is the question concerning the effect of the condition on biological function. The critical element here is vital functions. Vital functions are those necessary for physical existence: breathing, eating, excreting waste, and maintaining homeostasis (keeping the inside of the body in and the outside world out). Of the three conditions examined, craniofacial deformities can impair the ability of the neonate to breathe or to eat, and ambiguous genitalia can be associated with impairment of excretion of waste. In such cases, there is no argument about the appropriateness of surgical intervention when required for preserving life. However, most neonates with craniofacial deformities or ambiguous genitalia do not have life-threatening impairments and so in that aspect resemble neonates with short limbs.

In trying to understand how the three conditions are similar and different, a final question regards the effect of the condition on psychosocial function. My colleagues and I have observed, in our experiences in the less-industrialized world, that individuals with the most common craniofacial deformities, cleft lip and cleft palate, who do not have surgical repair, have very limited options for socialization and employment. Surgical repair usually reverses that overt discrimination. Whereas short stature may limit some vocational opportunities, most individuals with short limbs integrate well into their society. Furthermore, it has not been demonstrated that limb-lengthening, the surgical alteration examined by The Hastings Center working group, facilitates social integration. Ambiguous genitalia, surgically altered or not, do not affect employment, with the possible exception of those few jobs that are performed nude.

Having considered the differences and similarities among the three conditions examined by the working group, I can formulate a set of questions regarding surgical alteration of the children who have them:

1. Is surgery needed to reduce physical or psychosocial risk?
2. If surgery is necessary to reduce physical or psychosocial risk, when should it be performed?
3. If surgery is necessary to reduce physical or psychosocial risk, how much surgery should be performed?
4. What is the evidence that the benefits of surgical intervention are likely to outweigh the liabilities?
5. What, if any, is the role of the affected individual and that person's legal guardian in determining the necessity for, technique of, and extent of surgery?

The Initial Consultation with a Surgeon

Before addressing the issue of need, I explore why parents might seek surgical consultation for their child with short limbs, ambiguous genitalia, or a craniofacial deformity. (*Legal guardian* is a more inclusive term than *parents;* recognizing that, I have chosen to use *parents* throughout this chapter as a shorthand for *parents or legal guardians.*) Most new parents expect their baby to be normal, that is, to have body parts and configuration that match that of most of the other individuals in their awareness. When the condition is inherited, as for some of the craniofacial deformities and some of the conditions associated with short stature, or it has been identified *in utero* by ultrasonography, the parents will have been relatively more informed before their child's birth and have the opportunity of becoming educated about the condition and its possible managements well before having to make decisions about management. In either case, the discrepancy between what was expected and what is leads to consultations that do not occur following the birth of an infant without such a discrepancy.

Surgeons are not considered primary care givers. This has at least three implications. First, people do not visit a surgeon for well-care. Second, one usually does not choose one's surgeon, but is referred to the surgeon by another, primary or specialist, health care provider. Further, patients and families expect the surgeon not only to diagnose but also to manage a specific problem. As a consequence, the potential patient, or her parent, expects that the consultation will focus on surgery—the act of physically altering the body, using techniques of physical penetration and often entailing the removal of a body part. While those seeking a surgeon's advice may not know anything about the specifics of surgical management prior to the consultation, they know that surgery is a possible management strategy.

Based on twenty-five years of focusing on the evaluation and management of children with birth defects of the skull and face, I have observed that parents consistently ask three questions: "Why did this happen? What does it mean? Can it be fixed?" It is only after these questions have been addressed that the discussion moves to surgery per se as a means of management. These questions should have been addressed by at least one, and hopefully several, health care providers before the family presents to the surgeon. Nonetheless, it is an iterative process that requires addressing, readdressing, and readdressing yet again until the family comprehends what is and is not known about their child's condition.

That many parents use the verb *to fix* during the initial surgical consultation reflects back on the tension between surgical normalization and diversity affirmation. Do parents innately perceive the difference of their infant as an abnormality that needs to be fixed? Or, has that concept been instilled in them by society and by the health care professionals with whom they first had contact after becoming aware of their child's difference? I am unaware of any literature that addresses this critical distinction.

Surgical Decision Making

The process of surgical decision making proceeds through a set of superficially simplistic binary choices. An individual with a potentially surgically manageable condition has a consultation with a surgeon. Surgery is either recommended by the surgeon or not. If the surgeon recommends surgery, the parent (with the child's assent if she is old enough to participate in decision making) either gives or refuses permission to do the surgery.

What motivates a surgeon to recommend surgery for a condition? I personally use a hierarchy of four indicants for surgical management: (1) to postpone death; (2) to prevent irrevocable consequences; (3) to alleviate pain and suffering; and (4) to improve the quality of life.

There is no argument that a newborn who cannot breathe, or eat, or excrete waste will die without intervention. In some cases, the initial life-preserving intervention is nonsurgical—for example, the insertion of a tube into the trachea to allow mechanical ventilation or a tube into a vein to allow intravenous feeding. Such temporizing methods may be sufficient in themselves and obviate surgery or may temporize until a definitive surgical solution can be implemented. In other cases, there is no option other than a temporizing or definitive operation such as drainage of a blocked bladder or rectum. Surgery is necessary in such cases to postpone death. (I use the verb *postpone* rather than the more common usage *prevent* because the institution of medicine does not have the ability to prevent death.)

When it is clear that an untreated condition will lead to irrevocable consequences and there is an operation that can prevent that downward spiral, surgery is also necessary. For example, an infant with a cleft palate (split in the roof of the mouth) cannot develop intelligible speech without surgical repair of the palate. However, when surgery purports to avoid irrevocable consequences, surgeons don't always know with certainty that the consequences are irrevocable or that surgery can forestall whatever unwanted consequences could occur. The surgeon must recognize and distinguish between consequences that are well documented in peer-reviewed literature and accepted by the medical profession in general and those that are speculative. This distinction should temper the authority with which the surgeon advocates surgical management.

The alleviation of pain and suffering, both physical and mental, is a fundamental objective of the profession of medicine. While some holistic assessments of the outcome of specific surgical interventions have been published, most outcome assessments are very focal, being concerned with specific anatomic configuration, function, or physiologic parameters. A further complicating factor is that some birth defects are almost always operated upon in infancy or early childhood in industrialized nations, making it difficult if not impossible to compare the holistic outcome of individuals with and without surgical intervention. Finally, there is no direct correlation between the magnitude of the difference and the magnitude of the pain and suffering. In the world of facial differences, where I have expertise, it is well documented that a minor blemish may cause far more psychological impairment than a major deformity. The surgeon must recognize the difficulty of knowing, for any individual patient, how much pain and suffering a condition will induce and to what degree it can be alleviated by an operation. If one deformity is exchanged for another, have pain and suffering been alleviated?

To improve the quality of life through surgery is the reconstructive surgeon's goal. Yet we lack consensus on the definition of "quality of life." We debate who should define it. (See Mouradian et al., this volume.) Quantification of "quality of life" remains elusive. Nonetheless, the justification for much surgical alteration of children is improvement in the affected individual's quality of life. This objective seems to be met for those facial deformities that surgery can reconstruct with minimal residual difference (for example, cleft lip and cleft palate). It is questionable whether it has been achieved for severe craniofacial deformities, for short limbs, or for ambiguous genitalia.

Before any operation, there should be a mutually respectful exchange between the surgeon and those seeking her help, rather than a paternalistic surgeon's monologue delivered to the family. For the patient and parents to process the information provided by the health care expert and then to make an informed decision about whether to intervene and, if so, with which type of intervention, first requires answers to a specific set of questions. The educated patient's (and parent's) consultation with a surgeon should address all of the following:

1. Why is surgery an appropriate management for this particular problem and what nonsurgical alternatives are available? (That is, what are the indications for surgery?)
2. What kind of surgery is appropriate? (That is, what surgical techniques are available?)
3. What are the benefits of surgical versus nonsurgical management?

4. What are the risks of surgery and how do they compare to nonsurgical management?
5. What is the cost-benefit ratio for surgery and how does it compare to nonsurgical management? ("Cost" is the composite of direct economic cost [for example, fees for the surgeon, the operating room, consumable supplies], indirect economic costs [for example, lost income for missed work, extra cost for childcare], physical costs [for example, removed body parts and other physiological losses from the surgery], and psychosocial costs [for example, missed school, missed vacation, and psychological distress]).

The responses to the first three questions are condition-specific and are beyond the scope of the current discussion. I can, however, make some general comments about risks and benefits of surgery. Clearly, if there are no good data or reasons to suggest that a given surgery can produce a benefit, then it should not be performed. As long as risks are low and potential benefits range from modest to significant, surgery is usually recommended; the intensity of the recommendation is directly related to the magnitude of the benefit. A more difficult situation arises when the potential benefits are significant but the risks are high. Such would be the case for an experimental procedure in a life-threatening situation.

Curiously, in the usual risk-benefit formulation, risks are thought of as short-term, while benefits include those in the short and long terms. The risks enumerated to the parents and assenting/consenting patient are those of any operation (reaction to anesthesia, excessive blood loss, infection, tissue loss, and permanent deformity) plus the specific risks of the operation in question. I have never heard "dissatisfaction with the results of the operation" or simply "regret about having been operated on in infancy or childhood when the affected individual becomes an adolescent or adult" voiced as a risk of surgery. In contrast, improvement of psychosocial adjustment and integration into society as an adolescent and adult is often voiced as a major benefit of elective surgery for anatomic differences in infants and children. Similarly in the cost-benefit analysis, the cost of psychological support services in the future is discussed as a negative aspect of nonsurgical management while the cost of the psychological services associated with nonsurgical management is not credited against the cost of surgery. Also, there is also an unfounded assumption that surgery will obviate the need for future psychological support services. The absence of any hard data regarding true costs of surgical versus nonsurgical management for short limbs, ambiguous genitalia, or craniofacial deformities precludes such comparisons, even if one were motivated to make them.

An additional pair of variables, artifactually established as a mutually exclusive dichotomy by most health care funders, affects surgical decision making: *reconstructive* versus *cosmetic* operations. Operations performed exclusively or primarily to improve physical function are labeled *reconstructive;* operations performed exclusively to improve the psychological well-being of the patient are labeled *cosmetic.* This simplistic formulation fails to appreciate the difference between the kinds of psychosocial benefits achieved by reconstructing an abnormal body part and the kinds of psychosocial benefits achieved by altering a body part that is perceived as normal by the rest of society. In the first case, the positive effect is on both the affected individual and other members of society; in the second case, the effect is usually restricted to the individual who has sought the surgery. This failure can adversely impact funding for health care for affected individuals because of the pervasive assumption that whereas reconstructive operations are *necessary,* cosmetic operations are not. This does not merely impact funding for surgery but also for services such as psychological counseling, speech/language therapy, physical therapy, occupational therapy, and restorative dentistry. That assumption at least sometimes rests on the further, problematic assumption that physical function is more important than psychosocial function. Health care professionals, unlike health care funders, define *reconstructive* surgery as that surgery intended to restore or make whole, with respect to both physical and mental functions, body parts that are abnormal due to birth defect, trauma, or medical/surgical treatment. In contrast, *cosmetic* surgery is that surgery that alters a normal body part purely to please the patient or her parents.

The nonholistic artificiality of the physical benefit=reconstructive=necessary versus psychosocial benefit=cosmetic=unnecessary is easily appreciated when considering cleft lip and palate, where the aim is simultaneously to improve both types of function. We repair cleft lips, for example, both to improve the physical functioning of the mouth and also, by improving the appearance of the mouth, to improve psychosocial functioning. We repair cleft palates both to improve the physical functions of eating and speaking and also, by removing nasal regurgitation during eating and improving speech intelligibility, to improve psychosocial functioning. It is important to note that there are currently no outcome assessment tools to gauge the relative value of improved physical function versus improved psychosocial function for a specific operation or an individual.

Having obtained sufficient information to make an informed decision about surgical management of their child's condition, the parents then either give their permission to have the operation performed or not. And, if the child is old enough, assent is also obtained. Ideally, the surgeon's role in this process should be that of unbiased educator. Reality usually has the surgeon assuming the dominant role, both as the advocate of surgery and as the source of authority deferred to by the parents and, at times, the child.

Following what I perceive as a balanced discussion of the treatment I propose, alternative treatments, and comparative benefits and risks, parents frequently ask me: "What would you do if it were your child?" This desire for me, the surgeon, to assume a paternalistic role is unrelated to parental educational or socioeconomic level. As a young surgeon, I assumed such a question meant that I had failed to explain adequately in comprehendible language the choices I was offering. As a mature surgeon, I now assume that the question reflects the inability of most individuals to process meaningfully inadequate and at times contradictory information, especially when it involves surgery on their child. They assume I know what to do and are confused and distraught by an honest discussion of the uncertainties of the real world of medicine. Such individuals want a black-and-white binary choice, not alternatives and multiple shades of gray.

Why Do Surgeons Advocate Surgery?

Some surgeons prefer the uncomplicated binary choice of "the operation I am offering" versus "go elsewhere," which leads me to some thoughts on the personalities of surgeons. It is a commonplace belief among medical trainees that individuals choose that field of medicine for their avocation whose practitioners either match the established or the desired behavior and lifestyle of the trainee. Surgery attracts the fixers: those who have already known the personal pleasure of manual labor associated with problem solving or creation. These individuals are interventionists: they need to be the active agents in resolution of situations to obtain personal satisfaction. The process of transforming a new medical school graduate into a surgeon remains rather militaristic compared to other postgraduate medical training programs. Surgical residents are expected to take orders without question, to spend long hours doing non-stimulating tasks ("scut"), and slowly to ascend an almost medieval hierarchical ladder, the rungs of which are based on time served rather than knowledge acquired and skills mastered. Furthermore, in the operating room, the surgeon is "captain of the ship" and her decisions and wishes are rarely questioned. These factors combine to make most surgeons proactive, positive, enthusiastic individuals who strongly advocate the treatment they perceive to be the best. Not surprisingly, that treatment usually is surgery.

I believe that when most surgeons advocate surgery it is because they are convinced that surgery is the best treatment option. However, one cannot discount the ego-inflating aspect of surgery for the surgeon, or the potential for economic reward. The surgeon who considers himself a "miracle worker" clearly has an ego problem. The surgeon who solicits business through slick media advertisements clearly is in search of augmented income.

An additional concern is that surgeons sometimes say that they will "correct" or "reconstruct" differences, without the use of the modifier *partially.* Yet it is rarely the case that the operation is so perfect that there is no residue of the original difference. This terminology may cause cognitive dissonance for the patient and family when the discrepancy between result and expectation becomes apparent. During four years of medical school, including two three-month rotations on Surgery, during seven years of residency (five of General Surgery, two of Plastic Surgery), and during twenty-five years as a full-time academic surgeon, I have not heard a formal presentation on these issues. Surgeons are trained to think and perform as "surgeons," but not to contemplate the psychosocial implications of surgery for the patient and her immediate family.

What's in a Name? Difference, Deformity, Defect

During my initial presentation to the Surgically Shaping Children working group, I first showed a slide of a birth photograph of a female infant with an unrepaired unilateral cleft lip and palate, and then displayed her high school graduation picture, portraying a smiling, confident-appearing, attractive 18-year-old without visible facial difference. At the bottom of that slide I wrote that "[the goal of surgery] for the baby with a craniofacial deformity is for that individual to function in society as if the deformity had not happened." I was surprised that a few members of the working group were offended by the idea that health care professionals, parents, affected individuals, and society would want the deformity not to have happened. Furthermore, as I returned home and reflected on my experience at The Hastings Center, I was even more surprised by my reaction to their reaction: How could they question what seemed self-evident to me? As I noted in my introductory comments in this chapter, English does not have a neutral descriptive phrase for the conditions for which I am consulted. They are craniofacial deformities, craniofacial anomalies, or birth defects of the head and neck. These terms necessarily imply "something is not right" or "something went wrong" and those denotations suggest the need to "fix" or "correct" or, in plastic surgical jargon, "to make whole."

I question whether the more politically correct use of the noun *difference,* as in "an individual with a facial difference," is truly less stigmatizing or less strongly suggests the need to fix or correct. Egalitarians may wish all language to be neutral, but is that the nature of humans and language? How dull the spoken and written word, literature in its broadest sense, would be, were we to try to rid it of all color.

In my second presentation to the working group, I spent some time sharing my reflections as noted above and discussing the concept of normalization. I believe that normalization is noxious if "normal" really is code for "ideal"; the pursuit of normalization in that sense raises the specter of homogenization. In cosmetic facial surgery and to some degree reconstructive craniofacial surgery, normalization can label the belief in and pursuit of some ideal mathematical set of traits that defines beauty. Art historians, anthropologists, orthodontists, and facial surgeons have published on this subject. Surgeons who accept such a Platonic ideal surgically alter faces to coincide with the ideal as closely as possible. The hypothesis, that ideally proportioned faces produce psychosocial benefit for those who have or acquire them, is not validated.

But "normal" isn't always code for "ideal." An alternative sense of *normalization,* and the one I employ, concerns the bell-shaped curve. "Normal" in this sense refers to a range of human variation with respect to both physical and functional characteristics. Individuals with differences outside the +/−2 standard deviation limits are easily recognized as *other,* even by small children, while those within the limits are less likely to be so stigmatized. Surgical normalization in this sense means moving the individual with a visible difference into the expected range of physical form.

The hypothesis that a psychosocial benefit accrues to persons whose faces are made less different by surgery has been partially validated for only one of the craniofacial deformities, that is, cleft lip/palate. In my own surgical practice, I make a distinction between those facial differences that, if unoperated on, I expect will induce negative psychosocial reactions in others versus those that are more likely only to impact the affected individual, if at all. In the former case, I recommend surgery to the parents when I can offer what I consider to be significant improvement, that is, destigmatization. In the latter case, I defer consideration of surgery until the affected individual is old enough to participate actively in the decision-making process, which I believe is about 8 years of age for most children, and empower them accordingly. Extending this formulation to individuals with short limbs, I would encourage discussion of surgery for limb-lengthening as one treatment option with parents of an affected child once the condition is diagnosed. However, I would defer such intervention until the affected individual is old enough for assent, since current surgical technology cannot destigmatize the condition. With respect to ambiguous genitalia, I would defer surgical alteration until the affected individual is old enough to understand personal anatomic status, personal gender identity, and the actualities and limitations of state-of-the-art genital surgery. I make this recommendation since there is no visible difference that stigmatizes the affected individual in society, and since current operations fail to normalize genitalia either structurally or functionally.

As a practicing plastic surgeon, who for the past twenty-five years has focused on the evaluation and management of children with birth defects of the skull and face, I have addressed several aspects of surgically shaping children in this chapter, including the initial consultation with the child and parents or legal guardians; the process of surgical decision making; and the reasons why surgeons advocate surgery. I also have offered personal reflections on the reactions some members of the Surgically Shaping Children working group had to my initial presentation.

The primary hypothesis motivating surgery to alter children with differences—that such surgery will improve their psychosocial function in later life—remains unvalidated for all but a few conditions. Even when provided with a complete inventory of all possible treatments with benefit-risk analysis for each as well as for the proposed intervention and an honest appraisal of the state of uncertainty regarding that information, many parents want the surgeon to tell them what to do. While consultation with similarly affected adults who have and have not undergone the proposed treatment may provide an important counterbalance to the opinions and advice of health care professionals, methodology to validate the assessments and advice of laity are lacking as well.

As a surgeon who regularly alters children with differences, I found the opportunity of discussing the ethics of such alterations illuminating. While I do not have answers, I now do have questions that I look forward to continuing to explore.

CHAPTER NINE

What's Special about the
Surgical Context?

Wendy E. Mouradian, M.D., M.S.

This essay aims to contribute to the understanding—and ultimately improvement—of decision making for surgeries that involve children. I explore the nature of the patient-surgeon relationship in general and, more specifically, the difficulties that arise when the patient is a child. I also describe salient features of the childhood-surgery context, including the often elective, quality-of-life goals of such surgeries and the considerable uncertainty that often surrounds their outcomes.

The Surgeon-Patient Relationship

Trust between physicians, patients, and families is a crucial element in all medical decision making and care (Katz 1984; Pellegrino 1986). Trust can be defined as an "assured reliance on the character, ability, strength, or truth of someone or something . . . a charge or duty imposed in faith or confidence or as a condition of some relationship."[1] In the surgical setting, it is crucial to believe that the surgeon will act in your (or your child's) best interests. Trust enhances good communication and hence patient exercise of autonomy, thus increasing the chances for a "healing" relationship (Spiro 1998). The need for trust grows out of, and is a reminder of, the vulnerability of all patients and of the fiduciary relationship between physicians and patients.

So what makes the *surgeon*-patient relationship special? How can we avoid unnecessary harms and take advantage of the positive aspects of this relationship? To answer those questions, I discuss the surgeon-patient relationship in the craniofacial setting, but the concerns that arise in that field do so in other clinical settings as well.

Models of Care and Severity of Clinical Circumstances

Trust in the physician-patient relationship can develop over time, or very quickly when urgent circumstances require it. Although factors such as the personality of the surgeon and family and sociocultural factors influence the development of trust, I consider those factors that can be identified across individual cases and are especially relevant to the discussion of surgeries to shape children.

The primary care model. Continuity and regularity of care promote the development of trust in the physician-patient relationship. Continuity and regularity are characteristic of primary care, especially during childhood. In the early years, children and families typically have regular and frequent contact with their health provider, creating opportunities for the development of this trust. Well-child care and the normal illnesses of childhood can be anticipated, so most families seek primary care providers to be available for such needs. If and when serious problems and emergencies come up, families then have someone to turn to they know and trust to help them through the crisis. At least that is the ideal of primary care, even if current health care delivery mechanisms keep it from being the reality.

Surgical encounters. By contrast, families usually don't anticipate the need for surgeries, and may meet surgeons for the first time during a crisis. When the need for surgery is urgent, or is presented that way, parents are called on to make high-stakes decisions rapidly. They must move forward, whether or not they have a preexisting relationship with the surgeon. Parents are very vulnerable to the recommendations of the surgeon at such a time. Part of that parental vulnerability relates to their emotional needs in such a crisis, and part of it relates to the special relationship that is needed with the surgeon (discussed further below).

When surgery can be anticipated. Something of an intermediate situation occurs when a child with a cleft lip and palate—the most common craniofacial condition (CFC)—is born. Although the problem is noted at birth, or increasingly by prenatal ultrasound, surgery is generally not scheduled for several months to give the child a chance to grow larger. However, the child and family are typically referred to a surgeon early to discuss future plans and establish a relationship.

Surgery in the context of interdisciplinary team care. If the child is brought to a craniofacial team—as opposed to a surgeon operating outside of a team context—the family also will be scheduled to visit with other team members, such as the pediatrician, social worker/psychologist, nurse, feeding therapist, and dentist, to address the child's particular medical needs, including feeding problems. (Babies with a cleft palate typically cannot feed from a normal bottle or be breast fed since they cannot generate suction.) Parents receive information and support from the other team members and this can increase their comfort with and trust in the whole team, including their surgeon. These visits can help to reassure parents that their child's needs—and their own—will be attended to in a comprehensive way. This also helps to keep the surgical care in the context of the other medical and psychosocial needs.

Coordinated interdisciplinary team care is the preferred way of handling the complex needs of the family who has a child with a CFC and has been the standard of care in the craniofacial community for sixty years (American Cleft Palate-Craniofacial Association 1993). Team care aspires to provide continuity and regularity of care related to the craniofacial condition; this helps to promote trust and ongoing sharing of information, and provides support for families.

Importance of psychosocial support. The importance of psychosocial support cannot be overemphasized, even when no surgical decisions need to be made immediately. The birth of a new child is typically an overwhelming and exhausting experience for families, but when the infant is diagnosed with an impairment it can be traumatic. Parents are often very raw early on, with guilt, anger, sadness, and fear for the child and themselves. These feelings can be part of healthy adjustment to a new situation, but also can lead to withdrawal, depression, or an inability to cope with new roles. To be able to care for their infant (and themselves) and to be able to make decisions about surgery and other treatments, families need support and time to process their feelings and the new information they have received. Families often consult others outside of the surgical team to help them make decisions; other providers, friends, and clergy have all been cited as providing help to parents when they decide on surgeries (Lashley et al. 2000). Parents may also need psychosocial support at later times, such as when children enter school, when additional surgeries are contemplated, or during times of special family stress.

Providing psychosocial support and information for parents is one of the most important functions of the craniofacial team and should be an important role of any health care team. Such care still can receive somewhat short shrift in a field historically driven by surgery, but interdisciplinary team care, including psychosocial support, remains the standard of care recommended by professionals and parent advocates in the craniofacial field (Strauss 1998). In fact, interdisciplinary, family-centered approaches to care are recommended for all children with special health care needs,[2] as outlined in the landmark U.S. Surgeon General's report, *Children with Special Health Care Needs* (U.S. Department of Health and Human Services 1987).

Problems with surgical decision making related to team care. While team care is clearly the best option for children with complex medical conditions, it is not a panacea. For one thing, when many providers are involved, responsibility can be diffused and families may receive incomplete or inaccurate information. Surgeons may assume that other providers have emotionally and cognitively prepared the family for surgery. Thus the surgeon may take less time with explanations. Patients may assume they have received all the information, or not know what else to ask. This diffusion of responsibility and care may interfere with the development of an effective relationship between the surgeon and family.

Other problems can arise in the interdisciplinary care environment when health professionals disagree about care for the child. How team decision making and surgical recommendations are handled within the team and with the family is important. Presenting a "united front" to families may be preferable to health care professionals, but it can also be very intimidating to patients and families who may be afraid to challenge team authority. In addition, it may oversimplify the real complexities, differences of opinions, and uncertainties that more nuanced team discussions can reveal.

Another potential problem in the interdisciplinary team context has to do with unequal power relationships among surgeons, other physicians, and nonphysician team members. In a well-functioning interdisciplinary team, the full circumstances of the child and family are discussed with all the relevant providers and a consensus is reached and shared with the family. Despite these pitfalls, the interdisciplinary approach is still the best one to ensure a balance between the surgical and nonsurgical aspects of care.

Ideally, then, new parents are provided with information and have a chance to process their feelings and acquire the skills and knowledge they need to help their newborn baby thrive. By the time the first surgery takes place for the infant with cleft lip and palate, parents usually have achieved a certain level of adaptation, are committed to the surgery, and are ready to meet their baby's special needs through the recovery period. Introducing families to surgeons early on and providing a team for support can assist families enormously in their adjustment. It also helps to widen the net of trust that families need.

Severity of the medical condition and the need to trust. Under serious and urgent circumstances, the vulnerability of patients and parents is very high and their need to trust the physician is correspondingly great. The amount of trust the family needs seems to be directly related to the severity of the problem and thus to the family's vulnerability. If a physician is able to support a family through a difficult time, and respond to them with empathy and concern, the relationship is cemented. The physician, in turn, often develops a sense of attachment to the patient and family and an appreciation for the gift of sharing this intensely human experience. I illustrate this point about vulnerability and trust with two personal experiences, one nonsurgical and the other surgical.

I was first exposed to the powerful relationship between vulnerability and trust as a new pediatrician in my first year in a rural practice. I had answered a call to see a 9-year-old girl, Sara, in the emergency room. I had no real relationship with the family, and had only met them briefly once before.

Sara had a persistent sore throat and fatigue, and I ordered some blood tests. Within the hour I received a call from the pathologist that the blood count suggested leukemia. Probably the hardest thing I have ever had to do was break the news to this family and make arrangements for her care. That interaction—the extremity of the circumstances—evoked something in me and something in the family, and the relationship was cemented immediately.

Sara died in less than a year. I did not provide most of her care, which was managed through the distant children's hospital. But with time I became friends with the family, something that happens easily in small towns, and I took care of their other children. Sara's mother started to write about her experience, and I encouraged her. Eventually she wrote a book that was published and later chosen for the *Reader's Digest* condensed series (Kruckenberg 1984). In the book all the physicians caring for Sara were described—with more grace, I admit, than we really deserved. I was amazed to find myself on the first page. The experience will never be erased from my mind, and no doubt it will never be erased from this family's memory. My point is that a patient or family's vulnerability can evoke an intense intimacy between them and their providers as well as an intense need to trust their providers.

My second experience, several years ago, was as a patient, the recipient of a liver transplant. I refrain from discussing the several years of misdiagnosis and mistreatment that preceded the correct diagnosis of my progressive and fatal liver disease in 1997, although I still have anger about those experiences. And I refrain from describing the myriad diss-appointments (dissatisfying medical appointments), except to say, because it is relevant to the discussion, that I am not an easy patient to please. I know too much, ask too many questions, challenge fuzzy thinking. I force my physicians to conjecture, to explain contradictory opinions from different sources, and am generally a nuisance. I become positively incensed when I am not being heard, and will seek out second and third opinions and order my own lab tests and X-rays if necessary when my physicians disagree with me. Unfortunately, this habit has been strongly reinforced, since I have discovered how replete with errors, misunderstanding, and plain ignorance some of the best health care systems are. Too many times, my interpretations and suspicions have proved correct. In fact, I am sure I would not be alive today had I not taken this approach to my care. So I will continue to behave this way in my own care, and on behalf of family members, because it seems necessary. I don't think it is because I know more than my physicians, although sometimes I do. Nor is it just because I hate losing control, although that's true, too. Sadly, it just seems to be necessary. Good doctors though they are, I trust none of them fully.

Except my transplant surgeon. *Maybe*, I think to myself, it is just because he is truly astounding and wonderful and the kindest and best there is—except, that long before I knew I would have a liver transplant, I heard patients in the craniofacial clinic say similar things about their surgeons. In fact, most of the discussion in this chapter was framed years before my transplant experience. I watched myself reach out to this man like the drowning person I was. I remember talking with him before surgery, watching him the morning of surgery, how reassuring his voice and touch were to me in the operating room, mask and all. I had a sense of extreme letting go and turning myself over to this person who would open me up, cut me stem to stern, and leave me on the table waiting while the liver was harvested. The imagery it evoked before the surgery was powerful. I felt like the epitome of a fallen world on Good Friday, waiting for the Resurrection when I would receive my life-saving organ. And so I did.

Afterward many members of the surgical and medical team attended to my care, but he was the only one I ever really listened to. After I woke up in the recovery room I sobbed—partly out of relief, but partly because the denial necessary to get me to that place finally dropped and I knew that my life would always be different, that I would live in the vulnerability of a transplant patient, babysitting a liver precariously set in a new home that could reject it at any time. For weeks and months after the surgery I had nightmares; the bodily invasion, the trauma, was enormous. But through all this I never had any negative feelings for my surgeon. There is something so powerful about willingly giving your body so fully over to someone else—completely acknowledging your helplessness while unconscious. I still have the highest regard for this man, despite some postoperative difficulties, despite mistakes made in my care. In fact, I feel positively attached to this man for life. I had to trust in him, and still do. And I have a profound sense of gratitude for his skills as a surgeon and a human being.

Vulnerability of Patients in the Surgical Setting

Vulnerability is the source of the patient's need to trust and thus of the inequality in the patient-doctor relationship. Nowhere is that inequality greater than in the surgical context. My case is extreme because of the life-threatening nature of my health condition and the technical complexity of a liver transplant. But something like this is always going on in a surgical setting. There are always high risks in a surgical setting—the anesthesia, the technical complications that can happen in "ordinary" cases, in elective cases. The patient—and usually the family—cannot participate in decision making while the surgery is happening. The aura of the operating room can be strange and frightening: the mysterious and concealed nature of things, people wearing masks, gowns, funny smells, instruments clicking. The patient and family's lack of control could hardly be greater. And though the setting was not frightening to me personally, and I had lots of understanding about what was going on, I still experienced the vulnerability and the desperate need to trust. I had never experienced to this depth what I had written about so many times. I had never fully understood certain words from Dr. Pellegrino, even though I had referred to them many times. He reminds us that a doctor's commitment to patients

> flows from the nature of illness and the promise of service made by individual physicians and the profession as a whole. That commitment has a basis in the empirical nature of the healing relationship in which a sick person—dependent, vulnerable, exploitable— must seek out the help of another who has the knowledge, skill and facilities needed to effect cure. It is inevitably a relationship of inequality in freedom and power in which the stronger is obliged to protect the interest of the weaker. (Pellegrino 1986, 34)

This vulnerability and inequality are nowhere greater than in the surgical setting, and result in the tremendous need to trust the person in whose hands you place your life or your child's. That trust seems to happen, not because we providers are so good at engendering it (although no doubt some of us are better at this than others), but because our human psyche requires it.

In the more ordinary medical encounters we try and test our physicians, and find them human. But in the surgical setting, the need for trust is compelling. We need our surgeons to be godlike, infallible. We must believe they will be successful. (Is it any surprise that surgeons sometimes act like gods?) Comparing my surgical experience with my experience with other physicians over the years, I am led to believe that there is really something very different going on here, perhaps not unlike the transference relationship described by psychiatrists (Katz 1984).

Ironically, though patients need to trust and become attached to their surgeons, surgeons need to detach from the emotions of the moment if they are to cut open their patients. Too much empathy might jeopardize this task and make it dangerously difficult. Thus what we ask of surgeons is in a way fundamentally paradoxical. We wish surgeons to be empathetic and compassionate with patients and families, yet we need them to put these emotions aside to work effectively in the operating room. I am amazed at the surgeons I know who are able to accomplish this with sincerity and grace, and who retain their humanity and humility through the process. I could never be a surgeon—I could not muster the detachment nor would I want the responsibility.

Yet so much good can come out of this situation where power is so unequal. Very little attention has been paid to the possibility of good beyond the process of the surgery and the surgical outcomes. The encouragement, respect, and attention of someone held in such high esteem can be truly healing—especially for patients who are particularly vulnerable. Undergoing a surgery to shape a body part that is importantly related to one's identity and thus human interactions (as is the face) can create such vulnerability (Mouradian 2000). Where such vulnerability is present, it is also important to acknowledge the possibility of physicians manipulating patients and families. This is particularly a threat when outcomes are very uncertain, such as when surgeries aim to "improve quality of life," as they often do in the craniofacial context.

Uncertainties in Craniofacial Outcomes: The Case of Quality of Life

I have sat in a lot of rooms over the years and listened to a lot of surgeons talk with families about surgeries. The main thing I find lacking is honesty about what we do and don't know regarding the long-term impact of many surgical procedures. We do have a fair amount of information about the most common procedures, like repairing cleft lips and palates (although even here the debates rage and we don't have as much evidence as we should; see Mouradian et al., this volume). But we have far less information about the effectiveness of many other craniofacial interventions, like secondary cleft surgeries, which aim to improve appearance and thus psychosocial functioning or quality of life. As incomplete as our knowledge is in this area, we do know that physical appearance is only one parameter—and possibly not the most important one—in determining psychological or quality-of-life outcomes (Robinson 1997; Rumsey 2002) . The phrase *quality of life* is used continuously in the craniofacial setting, but few providers have a clear definition in mind when they use this term. I have heard providers say, "that's for the family to determine." Of course it is for the family to determine. But it is we who offer up the surgery as an intervention to improve the quality of life. It is we who collect the data or fail to collect data on patient outcomes. And it is we who sometimes imply the child is not okay the way she looks now, that she will be "better off" after surgery. And we just do not know that.

Sometimes we walk away in disbelief when a family or adolescent refuses additional surgeries. We may think they are in denial about the severity of their condition and ignorant about the help and hope we can offer. Sometimes we fail to suggest other kinds of interventions, such as psychological counseling, social skills training, and vocational and educational counseling. Offering these sorts of interventions, which emphasize the strengths of the individual, sends a very different message to patients and families.

In some cases, both medical and quality-of life-outcomes are uncertain. Take, for example, the release of a single prematurely fused cranial bone. We have very unclear knowledge about risks to the child from leaving the bone fused. The data surgeons cite include reports of increased pressure on the brain from the fused bone, but none of these studies would pass muster in the evidence-based environment of today. (In fact, given current ethical standards, it is unlikely such research will be done unless or until technology creates accurate, noninvasive measures of pressure on the brain, and prospective multicenter longitudinal studies are carried out on children including controls.) Nor do we know the quality-of-life outcomes. What, for example, is the toll on a child of an unusually shaped head?

We do know, however, that in addition to the possibility of brain damage, there are very substantial risks with such surgeries, including those associated with a general anesthetic, with blood loss, and with transfusion. I have seen things go wrong in these cases. The level of uncertainty in the craniofacial setting seems particularly high— given the difficulty of acquiring certain kinds of data and the subjective nature of "quality-of-life" data.

Medical Uncertainty

These specific uncertainties regarding craniofacial outcomes are embedded in the more general issue of medical uncertainty. It has been said that the problem with medicine is not that it is lacking in science, but that it has been confused with science (Beresford 1991). Even with the best of science, there is the uncertainty of extrapolating from population studies to the case of an individual child. There is always uncertainty related to the skills and judgment of the individual surgeon, the anesthesiologist, the rest of the operating room team, and the quality of postoperative care. Whenever we intervene with any surgical procedure we are increasing uncertainty and adding certain irreducible risks. At every step of the way, clinical judgments are made by fallible human beings. Yet our faith in science and technology is so strong that we often overlook this.

The language we use to present information and the manner in which we present it can profoundly influence people's perceptions of risk and the decisions they make (see Lustig and Scardion's 1998 work on so-called framing effects). For example, in the current context, we may believe we can improve on the results of earlier surgeries and make things "better." But the patient may hear "*all* better," and have unrealistic expectations for surgical outcomes and ignore potential complications (Partridge 1997). Such subtleties are more problematic when fewer outcome data are available. In that situation, the discussion of uncertainty depends heavily on the personal experience and opinion of the surgeon, who may not wish to discuss the enormous uncertainty in outcomes in many craniofacial surgeries.

Why do surgeons fail to disclose uncertainty? I will not reiterate Katz's classic work (1984) on this question. I will say, however, that over the years I have noted that when surgeons share information with families, they often skirt issues of uncertainty. I have come to the conclusion that either (1) the surgeons in question are not familiar with a critical appraisal of the literature on a certain subject; or (2) they possess the knowledge about the uncertainty of the data but do not to share it because either they believe that the patient doesn't really need it or perhaps because they don't want to think about it themselves; or (3) they share the uncertain data with the family but don't take the time to determine whether the patient/family has absorbed the information. Moreover, there is a tendency for some surgeons to influence the discussions and decision making with their style, by the tone and certainty with which they present their viewpoints. Some surgical providers so concisely outline the facts and so emphasize the hoped-for positive outcomes that it is hard to understand there are any uncertainties at all.

This problem is only partly addressed by having patients/families discuss possible interventions with the other craniofacial team members. Subjecting complex cases to team review does provide a sort of internal audit on the reasonableness of the recommendations. But questions of lines of authority may arise: What happens when the team recommends against a surgery and the surgeon still offers it to families? Should teams operate solely on a consensus basis? Should these recommendations be considered binding? Who bears the responsibility—and liability—for team decisions?

Of course, a surgeon's confidence in her recommendations is also a good thing. Who would want a surgeon who appeared to lack confidence, or did not seem ready to take charge in an emergency in the operating room? What does it take to believe you can accomplish complex surgical goals? Does the desire to avoid self-doubt unconsciously drive the denial of uncertainties with patients? What about the "thrill" of surgery, of challenging yourself in a high-risk setting? There is a fine line between handling to the best of one's ability the high-stakes setting of the operating room and pressing the challenge for the thrill of it. On one side of the line, one uses her "nerves of steel" to steer through all sorts of surgical "weather"—anticipated or not; on the other, she seeks out the surgical "weather" for the sake of the challenge. Other professionals, like aviators, must know the same fine line. However, in the operating room suite, there is not the safeguard of air travel, where poor handling of the aircraft brings equal risk to the pilot and passengers.

Why patients fail to acknowledge uncertainties. Surgeons are not the only ones who dislike uncertainties. When uncertainties and risks are candidly acknowledged, patients and families may be less likely to agree to surgery. Given their vulnerability and need to trust the surgeon, patients and families may not be able to hear clearly those uncertainties that are acknowledged. Or if they do hear them clearly, they may feel more vulnerable and thus worse. At least for some patients and families, it may be easier to go through surgeries with a sort of tunnel vision.

In fact, before my transplant, I simply grew unable to hear about how complex my surgery would be, how my liver was wrapped around the aorta, how they might have to dissect the whole thing out and put me on a bypass pump. My brain heard the words, processed terms like *stroke risk,* and saw the images as in a dream. But I could not get emotionally near them—and this is what is necessary if we are to really understand risks. If the ideal of truly informed consent entails getting emotionally near to those risks, then it should be clear how difficult it will be to achieve that ideal.

There are circumstances in which patients or parents would like to give up the right to know and *authorize* a surgeon to make the best judgment, such as when the decision for medically necessary care has essentially been made ("just do the right thing, doctor"). But in the sorts of circumstances I'm discussing here, where what is at issue are highly subjective, quality-of-life goals, such authorization is not possible. The decision must be made by the parent and/or patient, and one or both must accept responsibility for it (Beauchamp and Childress 1994).

So the reasons that medical uncertainties are not always discussed are many, and stem from both physician and patient needs. But the uncertainties surrounding many interventions to surgically shape children must be acknowledged. In fact, it is not at all clear that surgery always confers benefits that are commensurate with the risks these children take. Furthermore, we may serve children badly by believing that surgery is the key to successful adjustment, and by foregoing the kinds of psychosocial interventions and support that may in fact be more valuable in the long run.

When Patients Are Children

Much of what I have said up until now could apply equally to an adult patient or parent making the decision for the child. But the elective, quality-of-life nature of many craniofacial surgeries really requires us to look at decision making for children in more detail (Buchanan and Brock 1990; American Academy of Pediatrics 1993, 1995;

Mouradian 1999; see also the chapters by Nelson, Alderson, and Dreger in this volume). Quality-of-life judgments are difficult to make for others, although parents must make them all the time. When quality-of-life issues related to appearance are pivotal in deciding on surgical interventions, these are often deferred until the child is old enough to participate in decision making.

When are children thought to be old enough to participate? The strict developmental model proposed by Piaget (1952)—and adopted to discussions of minor decision making—suggests the child can understand and reason about risks and benefits only after acquiring abstract-thinking skills, presumably after about age 12. However, as Alderson (1993 and in this volume) and Scott (1992) and others have pointed out, a strict Piagetian model is not borne out by experience on either side of that magic moment: younger children who have experienced chronic illnesses are often very articulate about their experiences and clear about their desires. And you don't have to know too many teenagers to see their difficulty in making decisions.

However, there can also be problems with deferring interventions until the child is older. For one, the child may experience considerable teasing and social derision in the formative years, with the potential for negative impact on self-esteem. By the time the procedure is offered, the damage may have already been done. In addition, some procedures are much easier when performed earlier. Unfortunately, it is not possible to preserve an entirely open future for children; certain paths are chosen and others are not. Medical uncertainty begets moral ambiguity, making it very difficult to determine what is in the child's best interests.

The Parent-Child-Surgeon Triangle

Another special aspect of surgical interventions with children relates to psychological influences at work when parents make decisions for children and interpret their best interests. The younger the child, the more the physician-patient relationship is mediated through the parent(s). The parent is vulnerable, but in a way that's very different from the way a competent adult is vulnerable in seeking care for herself. My own experience as a parent suggests that, if anything, the vulnerability is much greater: the sheer terror one experiences in the face of threats to the health and well-being of one's children is far worse than what one experiences for oneself. I remember thinking as I went through my transplant that it would have been far worse for me to watch a child of mine face this illness and surgery than to face it myself. And indeed the greatest pain to me through the process was the possibility that I might be separated from my children, and they from me, if I did not make it.

There are powerful relationship issues that emerge when parents consider putting their children through surgical procedures. Such an event calls up all one's inner parental protectiveness—and it brings up our deepest relationship issues and fears. The maximal investment in outcomes, coupled with parents' minimal control in the surgical arena, can be a recipe for agony. I have watched many parents go through this in my years as a pediatrician.

The younger the child is, and particularly if this is a first baby, the more one's own experiences, expectations, and insecurities play into the decision-making process, the more that child represents the infant inside the parent. The desire to rescue one's child from future pain (and perhaps from the parents' past pain), and the desire of most parents to see their children's lives be better than their own, are also factors that can heighten the parents' vulnerability to the surgeon's influence. The less support parents receive, the more vulnerable they are to the surgeon's recommendations. Conversely, the more supported parents feel, the more opportunity they have to prepare themselves internally, the better they will be able to cope, to analyze the surgeon's recommendations, to make decisions, and to support their child.

With older children, the parent's sense of vulnerability—though not caring—is generally lessened. The parent now experiences and respects the growing child's emerging sense of self and notion of the "good," and the parent desires to support what are increasingly the child's own goals. When the child reaches adolescence, the parent-child-surgeon triangle includes a host of different dynamics that can affect the decision-making process. Adolescence is a time of heightened concerns about appearance and the opinions of peers. Teens typically experience insecurity in relationships, emerging identity issues, conflicts with authority, and emotional ups and downs. Although cognitively adults, adolescents may make decisions more impulsively, with different attitudes toward risk taking and future orientation (Scott 1992).

These issues, superimposed on the adolescent's experience of the medical condition, underline the need for great caution. When teens present with depression or significant emotional distress, psychological assessment should take place before more procedures are scheduled. While surgeons motivated by compassion may try to rescue such patients, reconstructive surgery may not be the only or even most effective means of helping them, and may obfuscate the underlying issues. Thus the exceedingly complex psychological dynamics among the patient, family, and surgeon can make the surgical decision-making process exceedingly complex. At each stage of that process it is necessary to consider what the developmental and psychological needs of children and parents are, and how they are affecting the surgical decision-making process.

The surgical context presents special risks and challenges to children and parents who have to make decisions about appearance-normalizing surgeries, which aim at improving psychosocial functioning or quality of life. Among the salient features of that context are the vulnerability of patients and families in their relationship with surgeons; the uncertain and subjective nature of the quality-of-life outcomes these surgeries aim to achieve; and the fact that the patients are children. The special psychological dynamics that parents bring to surgical decisions for their children may further heighten their vulnerability and complicate decision making.

One of the most basic steps to improve the quality of the decisions made in this special context will be to ensure the provision of interdisciplinary team care, which, among other things, can facilitate the discussion of these complex issues as well as provide psychosocial support for children and families. Only if such discussions and support are in place will decision making be truly informed. The risks and challenges of the surgical setting call for special caution on the part of all medical practitioners involved in providing care to children and families.

ACKNOWLEDGMENTS

This work was made possible by a grant from the National Institute for Dental and Craniofacial Research to the University of Washington Comprehensive Center for Oral Heath Research #P60DE13061 and by a grant from the National Endowment for the Humanities to The Hastings Center (RZ-20715).

NOTES

1. Merriam-Webster dictionary on line: www.m-w.com/cgi-bin/dictionary.
2. Children with special health care needs are defined by the federal Maternal and Child Health Bureau as "those who have or are at increased risk for a chronic physical, developmental, behavioral, or emotional condition and who also require health and related services of a type or amount beyond that required by children generally" (McPherson et al. 1998, 137–40). Children with achondroplasia, intersex, and craniofacial conditions all fit this definition children with special health care needs.

REFERENCES

Alderson, P. 1993. *Children's Consent to Surgery.* Philadelphia: Open University Press.
American Academy of Pediatrics. 1993. Committee on Bioethics: Treatment of critically ill newborns. *Pediatrics* 72:565–66

————. 1995. Committee on Bioethics: Informed consent, parental permission and assent in pediatric practice. *Pediatrics* 95 (2):314–17.

American Cleft Palate-Craniofacial Association. 1993. Parameters for the evaluation and treatment of patients with cleft lip/palate or other craniofacial anomalies. *Cleft Palate Journal* (suppl.):1–34.

Bartholome, W. G. 1989. A new understanding of consent in pediatric practice: Consent, parental permission and child assent. *Pediatric Annals* 18 (4):262–65.

Beauchamp, T., and J. F. Childress. 1994. *Principles of Biomedical Ethics.* New York. Oxford University Press.

Beresford, E. B. 1991. Uncertainty and the shaping of medical decisions. *The Hastings Center Report* 21 (4):6–11.

Buchanan, A., and D. Brock. 1990. *Deciding for Others: The Ethics of Surrogate Decision Making.* New York: Cambridge University Press.

Katz, J. 1984. Why doctors don't disclose uncertainty. *The Hastings Center Report* (February):35– 44.

————. 2002. *The Silent World of Doctor and Patient.* New ed with foreword by Alexander Capron. Baltimore: Johns Hopkins University Press.

Kruckenberg, C. 1984. *What Was Good about Today.* Seattle: Madrona.

Lashley, M., W. Talley, L. C. Lands, et al. 2000. Informed proxy consent: communication between pediatric surgeons and surrogates about surgery. *Pediatrics* 105 (3):591–97.

Lustig, A., and P. Scardino. 1998. Elective patients. In *Surgical Ethics,* edited by L. McCullough, J. W. Jones, and B. Brody, 133–51. New York: Oxford University Press.

Marsh, J. L. 1990. When is enough enough? Secondary surgery for cleft lip and palate patients. *Clinical Plastic Surgery* 17:37–47.

McCullough, L. B., J. W. Jones, and B. A. Brody, eds. 1998. *Informed Consent: Autonomous Decision-making of the Surgical Patient.* New York: Oxford University Press.

McPherson, M., P. Arango, H. Fox, et al. 1998. A new definition of children with special health care needs. *Pediatrics* 102:137–40.

Mouradian, W. 1999. Making decisions for children. *Angle Orthodontist* 60 (4): 300–306.

————. 2000. Deficits vs strengths: Ethics and implications for clinical practice. *Cleft Palate-Craniofacial Journal* 38 (3): 255–59.

Partridge, J. 1997. The experience of being visibly different. *Visibly Different: Coping with Disfigurement,* edited by R. Lansdown, N. Rumsey, E. Bradbury et al, 3–9. Oxford: Butterworth Heinemann.

Pellegrino, E. D. 1986. Rationing health care: The ethics of medical gatekeeping. *Journal of Contemporary Health Law & Policy* 2: 23–45.

Piaget, J. 1952. *The Origins of Intelligence in Children.* New York: International University Press.

Robinson, E. 1997. Psychological research on visible differences in adults. In *Visibly Different: Coping with Disfigurement,* edited by R. Lansdown, N. Rumsey, A. Bradbury, A. Carr, and J. Patridge, 102–11. Butterworth Heineman.

Rumsey, N. 2002. Body image and congenital conditions. In *Body Image: A Handbook of Theory, Research and Clinical Practice,* edited by T. Cash and T. Pruzinsky, 226–33. New York: Guilford.

Scott, E. 1992. Judgment and reasoning in adolescent decision-making. *Villanova Law Review* 37: 1607–69.

Spiro, H. 1998. *The Power of Hope.* New Haven: Yale University Press.

Strauss, R. 1998. Cleft palate and craniofacial teams in the United States and Canada: A national survey of team organization and standards of care. *Cleft Palate-Craniofacial Journal* 35 (6): 473–80.

U.S. Department of Health and Human Services, Public Health Service. June, 1987. Surgeon General's report. *Children with Special Health Care Needs.* Campaign 87. Washington, DC: Public Health Service, U.S. Department of Health and Human Services.

Ward, C. 1999. The technological imperative in craniofacial surgery. (Editorial). *Cleft Palate-Craniofacial Journal* 36 (1):1–2.

CHAPTER TEN

Are We Helping Children?

Outcome Assessments in Craniofacial Care

Wendy E. Mouradian, M.D., M.S., Todd C. Edwards, Ph.D.,
Tari D. Topolski, Ph.D., Nichola Rumsey, M.S.C., Ph.D.,
and Donald L. Patrick, Ph.D., M.S.P.H.

How we answer the question, Are we helping children with craniofacial interventions? depends on how we approach health outcomes. We can measure the size of the scar, but is the child better off? We need a much broader view of health to answer that question. The World Health Organization defines health as "a state of complete *physical, mental,* and *social* well-being, and not merely the absence of disease or infirmity" (World Health Organization 1948). Such a robust understanding of health directs researchers to consider not only the biological state of an individual's body, but also psychosocial adjustment and a myriad of other variables that affect the individual's well-being, including family context, geographic location, educational opportunities, economic standing, the values that predominate in her culture, and the medical care she receives (Patrick 1997).

We hope and believe that by surgically improving a child's appearance, we improve her "psychosocial functioning" or "mental and social well-being." Unfortunately, there is little systematic data on psychosocial outcomes after appearance-normalizing surgeries. This is partly because we have not sought to collect such data, which in turn may be because doing so is very difficult.

This chapter places craniofacial outcome assessments in the context of current guidelines for assessing evidence, comments on barriers to generating an adequate evidence base in the craniofacial field, and briefly summarizes approaches to assessing psychological and psychosocial outcomes for individuals with craniofacial conditions (CFCs).

Assessing Evidence

How much evidence is necessary before an intervention is recommended or withheld? What counts as evidence? And who determines that? Current approaches to rating evidence draw on systematic reviews of the literature (Cochrane Collaboration 2004; Agency for Health Research and Quality 2004). Evidence is rated from level 1, the highest level of evidence for effectiveness of an intervention (supported by multiple randomized control trials), to level 3 (supported only by clinical opinions of experts, case reports, etc.). In the case of preventive interventions, such as those rated by the U.S. Preventive Services Task Force (USPSTF), data are subjected to high degrees of scrutiny because of the policy and cost implications of recommending an intervention for everyone. Recommendations for preventive care are then generated based on the levels of evidence available, and only those with proven effectiveness are recommended; those with no evidence of benefit or of harm are proscribed. When subject to this level of scrutiny, few clinical interventions pass muster; nor are there ever likely to be the resources to study *all* clinical areas with the high level of rigor demanded by such criteria. Most craniofacial clinical guidelines are supported by level 3 evidence, and are quite general (American Cleft Palate-Craniofacial Association 1993; Cleft Lip and Palate 2003). (The few more rigorous outcome studies are summarized below.)

If rigorous evidence is not easily obtainable, in which clinical circumstances should we accept less than ideal evidence? One might argue that as the seriousness of the patient's medical condition increases, the rigor of the evidence we require can decrease. Under these circumstances we might accept higher risks and lower evidence of benefit. (Yet we must be cautious about the vulnerability of patients in desperate circumstances—and thus the potential for manipulating them—as well as the cost of providing futile treatments.) By contrast, to the extent that craniofacial surgeries are more elective and less urgent, they would seem to require the opposite: high evidence of benefit and low risks. But even if the risks are truly low, can we accept a lower promise of benefit as well?

There are at least three reasons why, even if the risks are low, we should require a high level of evidence of benefit from elective surgeries (such as those that occur in the craniofacial setting). First, investing hope in a surgical intervention that has only a small promise of benefit to a child's mental and social well-being may actually create harms. It can raise false expectations and may keep the family focused on an endless stream of surgical maneuvers that will never eliminate the craniofacial condition. Fixing the child's face will not "fix" the adolescent's or family's life, if there are other dysfunctions. Furthermore it may give the child or adolescent or family the message that the child is really not okay the way she currently looks. Focusing on surgical interventions may well inhibit healthy adaptation and the pursuit of other kinds of treatments, resources, and opportunities (for example, education, counseling, social skills training, artistic/recreational activities, etc.) that promote resilience and personal growth (Mouradian 2001). Second, such elective surgeries may not always be a reasonable allocation of resources: surgical interventions are costly and burdensome, and use up the resources of children, families, and health systems. (This includes financial resources as well as time and energy and hence the ability to pursue alternative opportunities.) Finally, surgical procedures are never risk-free; we cannot eliminate the risks of bleeding, infection, and adverse reactions to anesthesia. In the surgical setting there is always "something to lose."

One could also ask how many negative outcomes must be reported before recommending against an intervention. It would seem that fewer reports of adverse outcomes (especially if they are serious) should be necessary before an intervention is proscribed, or at least scrutinized carefully. We believe case reports and patient or family narratives are very important, especially in the absence of other systematic outcome data, and should carry heavy weight when adverse experiences are reported. But how is an adverse outcome defined? Is it an unexpected problem? In the surgical setting it is common practice to provide an exhaustive list of possible consequences for patients and families, including death. With this framing, no outcome would be truly unexpected, perhaps making it difficult for families or others to identify an adverse event.

While recognizing that clinical interventions may not always be supported by the highest levels of evidence, we have argued that craniofacial surgeries that are elective and intended to improve appearance should be supported by reasonable evidence of benefit and of low risk. Yet there are many barriers to obtaining such evidence.

Difficulties Developing an Evidence Base in Craniofacial Care

One major obstacle to developing evidence in craniofacial care is the relatively small numbers of patients with any single CFC, leading to the need for large multicenter studies. Only two major outcome studies have been completed to date: the European multicenter study on cleft lip and palate outcomes (the Eurocleft study) and an audit by the United Kingdom's Clinical Standards Advisory Group (CSAG). The Eurocleft study assessed physical outcomes in patients with complete unilateral cleft lip and palate (CLP) ages 8–10 at six different centers. They reported on craniofacial form, soft tissue profile, dental arch relationships, and appearance of the nose and lip (Shaw et al. 1992a, 1992b). They did not use patient-centered outcome measures.

The CSAG study looked at patients ages 5 and 12 with unilateral CLP across the United Kingdom and assessed dental arch and skeletal relationships, success of alveolar (gum) bone grafting, esthetic appearance, and speech intelligibility (Clinical Standards Advisory Group 1998). Auditors were very disappointed with physical outcomes and additionally noted that many clinical centers had inadequate records and too few patients to even permit a genuine review of outcomes. CSAG also assessed parent and patient satisfaction with a semistructured questionnaire. Of note, parents (N=432) and 12-year-old children (N=214) were almost all satisfied with or moderately satisfied with the treatment provided. These results contrasted with the much lower rating of *"success of treatment"* by the auditors (Williams et al. 2001).

Both CSAG and Eurocleft found that high-volume operators had better outcomes; high volume also allowed for review of outcomes. It is estimated that, to maintain clinical skill and provide for meaningful audit, centers need from thirty to sixty new cleft cases per year (American Cleft Palate-Craniofacial Association 1993; Shaw et al. 1996). Auditors recommended carefully planned collaborative studies among those centers where a significant numbers of patients are treated; the creation of a common database for all cleft patients in the United Kingdom; centralization of services and training; and more complete multidisciplinary teams and the inclusion of psychologists as team members.

Of note, the publicity surrounding the generally poor results of the audit disturbed a number of families who had been relatively satisfied until they discovered their care or outcomes may have been "suboptimal." This raises the issue of the impact of outcome studies on patients and families themselves. Also, the report's emphasis on physical outcomes may have undermined patients' satisfaction with *overall* outcomes. Finally, in assessing patient/family satisfaction, it may be difficult to distinguish between *gratitude* to the team and *satisfaction* with surgical results and psychosocial outcomes.

Obstacles to outcomes assessments in craniofacial care include but are not limited to:

- the relative rarity and heterogeneity of conditions
- the fact that single treatments can have effects in multiple health areas, making it difficult to decide which outcomes should be prioritized in determining overall benefit
- lack of well-defined, reproducible, agreed-on outcome measures
- lack of consensus within the field as to preferred treatment regimens (and thus which should be studied)
- the lack of multidisciplinary research teams to assess outcomes[1]

Many of these obstacles to generating evidence in the craniofacial area arise in the other two areas the Surgically Shaping Children project has considered: achondroplasia and intersex conditions. In fact, these issues plague research on chronic and complex health conditions of childhood, many of which are rare and must be studied with multicenter protocols. Since children are constantly changing, costly and arduous longitudinal studies are often needed. Ethical concerns in research with children present additional barriers. Finally, competition for limited resources often drives the choice of variables to study. Some outcomes are easier to measure than others: mental and social well-being is more difficult to assess than physical outcomes, and as a result it may be more difficult to fund such studies. Yet these are the very studies that are needed to assess outcomes of surgeries to improve appearance.

Variables to Address in Outcome Studies

The kinds of outcomes we measure should be driven by the goals of the craniofacial surgery. Although it can be difficult to distinguish neatly among craniofacial surgeries, which often have multiple goals, we can roughly divide surgeries by those intended to preserve or improve physical functioning, and those intended to improve psychosocial function (such as improving the appearance of a child's face to make her look more normal and thereby less subject to stigmatization). In the case of cleft lip and palate, the most common CFC, surgeries aimed at improving basic physical functioning include:

- closing the palate to improve speech and reduce ear infections
- bone grafting to allow normal eruption of teeth
- orthodontics and jaw surgery to improve chewing

Appearance-normalizing surgeries, which can be used to improve psychosocial functioning, include:

- initial repair of cleft lip and nasal cartilage
- later revisions of lip and nose surgeries
- jaw surgeries primarily intended to improve appearances

Assessing Psychological and Psychosocial Outcomes

Psychological measures have been used the most to assess mental well-being—or, more commonly, psychopathology. Many of these instruments have been well validated and provide normative data for comparison. Psychological studies can be a valuable adjunct to an individual's psychological evaluation and treatment, and they may provide clues to outcomes for groups of patients. By necessity such measures are usually deficit-oriented, and may not fully capture sources of strength and resilience. In addition, psychological measures have not been commonly used to measure *changes in response to specific treatments* (except those assessing developmental gains, such as linguistic and cognitive outcomes) (Speltz et al. 1997; Kapp-Simon 1998).

Current Literature on Psychological Outcomes

With these considerations in mind, we briefly review psychological outcome studies in patients with CFC. As a group, individuals with congenital CFCs seem to experience a modestly elevated risk of psychological, educational, and social problems across the lifespan, although the lack of comparison with controls renders even this conclusion tentative, as reviewed in several studies (Speltz et al. 1995; Tobiasen and Speltz 1996; Rumsey 2002). Adolescents with CFCs have been reported to show, for example, an elevated risk of both externalizing (disruptive, impulsive) and internalizing (shy, withdrawn, despondent) behavior problems (Harper et al. 1980; Richman 1976; Tobiasen et al. 1992). In one study focusing on the subjective perspectives of adolescents with CFCs, Strauss and colleagues found that a significant number of adolescent patients with CLP and their parents have concerns about the appearance of their repaired lip, speech results, and overall appearance (Strauss et al. 1988). Psychological studies that have examined self-esteem have yielded inconsistent results, suggesting these constructs may not be the most useful ones for this population, or that the constructs are useful but the technology of the instruments is poor.

Of note, many studies in the craniofacial literatures report the lack of correlation between the severity of facial defect and the psychological adjustment of patients (Rumsey 2002; Tarnowski and Rasnake; 1994; Lansdown et al. 1997; Robinson 1997). More recent evidence suggests that levels of appearance-related concern are at least as high, if not higher, in the noncleft adolescent population. In a fifteen-year longitudinal cohort of children with CFC and control group there are many fewer differences than anticipated between the two groups (Emerson et al. 2004).

Limitations of some of this research include the use of convenience samples, the use of retrospective methodologies and small sample size, and the lack of comparison groups. There are very few well-controlled, prospective longitudinal studies of individuals with craniofacial conditions and most research has been done on patients with cleft lip and palate or isolated craniosynostosis.

Newer studies contrast with older ones, which presented very negative impacts on dating, marital/family status, SES, and increased rates of suicide (Peter and Chinsky

1974; Peter et al. 1975; McWilliams and Paradise 1973; Heller et al. 1981; Van Demark and Van Demark 1970; Herskind et al. 1993; Nash 1995). The older studies reflect the earlier state of the art of treatment of craniofacial conditions, which has improved with advances in craniofacial surgical technique and other modalities. It is not known whether these technical improvements have led to improved overall well-being for individuals with CFCs, or whether societal changes, differences in study design, or other factors are responsible for the observed differences.

Given the methodological shortcomings of many of the studies and the inconsistency of results, it is still not clear to what extent children and adolescents with CFC experience increased psychological distress as a result of their underlying medical condition. Certainly these children are at risk for social and psychological problems—if for no other reason than the numbers of medical interventions and absences from school. But there appears to be no simple relationship between craniofacial appearance and psychosocial functioning (or "mental and social well-being"). Clinicians have seen many well-adjusted children with CFCs, even quite severe ones, and others who are mildly affected but seem devastated.

A Developmental Model for Risk: Longitudinal Study of Individuals with CLP

In a longitudinal study of children with CLP, Speltz and colleagues are addressing the relationship between craniofacial appearance and psychosocial functioning (mental and social well-being) (Speltz et al. 1994). They hypothesize that craniofacial conditions can impact children's experiences at key developmental periods as the child progresses through a series of *age-specific socioemotional tasks* (for example, formation of effective attachment relationship with the parent during infancy; development of same-sex friendships and academic competence during middle school years, etc.) (Cicchetti and Schneider-Rosen 1984; Sroufe and Rutter 1984). In this developmental model, the child's probability of success or failure at each new task is dependent on his or her previous adaptations to earlier tasks (Cicchetti and Toth 1992). The child's ability to negotiate these developmental tasks is influenced by key variables, including infant/child characteristics (temperament, cognitive abilities); medical factors (diagnosis, treatments/surgeries, functional limitations); quality of parent-child relationship including attachment; parenting skills; and family environment (SES, marital stability, social supports, etc.) (Speltz et al. 1994).

It is easy to see how cleft-related factors can have potential negative effects on the child's ability to negotiate important socioemotional tasks. For example, difficulties feeding a child with a cleft palate can challenge parental confidence and potentially interfere with parent-child attachment. Parents' emotional responses, such as over-protectiveness, might interfere with the acquisition of age-appropriate tasks and the development of self-confidence in later years. On the other hand, Speltz postulates that positive factors like a secure attachment to the primary caretaker and good psychosocial supports would have a *protective* effect on psychosocial development.

Despite the plausibility of this model, so far this approach has not demonstrated a disruption of maternal attachment in infants with the group of children with clefts compared with controls (Maris et al. 2000; Coy et al. 2002). Facial appearance of infants with cleft lip was much less of a risk factor than hypothesized. Paradoxically, in these studies children with visible clefts appeared to be more securely attached to their mother, leading to the speculation that parents may compensate and develop especially close bonds when they perceive special vulnerabilities in their children. Limitations of these studies include the relatively small size of the cohort and the fact that infant temperament was not considered, which may affect attachment behaviors in young children.

This type of work could help identify children at risk for problems so that appropriate therapeutic psychosocial support and interventions could be offered early. On the other hand, this approach does not easily lend itself to understanding the role of surgeries per se in psychosocial outcomes.

Quality-of-Life Outcome Measures

Another approach to assessing psychosocial outcomes is to utilize a much broader construct—quality of life. The World Health Organization defines quality of life (QOL) for individuals as the "perceptions of their position in life in the context of the culture and value systems in which they live, and in relation to their goals, expectations, standards, and concerns" (WHOQOL Group, 1994, 1995, 1997). Ideally, a QOL instrument should include: (1) the individual's perspective, (2) a universal definition of QOL, (3) a multidimensional definition of the QOL construct (not just health), and (4) a consideration of the positive as well as negative aspects of QOL. The use of QOL measures in children and adolescents has lagged behind usage in adults, in part because of obvious difficulty in obtaining subjective perceptions in young children and the dynamic nature of child and adolescent development (Bullinger and Ravens-Sieberer 1995; Pal 1996; Spieth and Harris 1996; Starr 1983; Schor 1998). Some efforts have been made to apply the QOL paradigm to craniofacial outcomes. Rumsey has adapted the Short Form of the SEIQoL (Hickey et al. 1996) for the clinical setting, using a semistructured interview format, which allows respondents to generate those dimensions that are important to them (Rumsey 1998). This tool allows for following individual patients over time, but may be less useful in population comparisons.

YQOL Collaborative Studies: QOL in youth with CFC

Recently Patrick and colleagues developed an adolescent QOL instrument (Youth Quality of Life Instrument Research tool, the "YQOL-R") (Edwards et al. 2002; Patrick et al. 2002) and additional modules specific to youth with CFC (the YQOL-Facial Difference module [YQOL-FD] and the YQOL-Facial Surgery module [YQOL-FS)]) (Edwards et al. 2005; Topolski et al. in press). The questions used in these craniofacial modules were generated from extensive interviews and focus groups with adolescents with CFCs, to uncover the themes and words individuals themselves use in talking about their lives (consistent with "grounded theory" methodology) (Glaser and Strauss 1967; Strauss and Corbin 1990). These were augmented with focus groups with young adults with CFCs, parents of adolescents with CFCs, and an advisory group of clinical and academic experts in the field. These interviews and focus groups led to the identification of seven important themes or clusters of concern: (1) coping; (2) intimacy, trust; (3) negative emotions; (4) positive consequences; (5) self-image; (6) stigma, isolation; and (7) surgery. The generic instrument (YQOL-R) domains include (1) sense of self; (2) social relationships; (3) culture and community; and (4) general quality of life. Currently, the YQOL-R and the newly developed CFC modules (YQOL-FD/FS) are being field-tested in a multicenter cross-cultural international study of youth with CFCs (Patrick, Principal Investigator). If this approach is validated, then the next phase will be to determine if the measure can detect changes in relationship to surgeries. A significant issue will be how to apply this to work with younger children.

To have a sense of what the QOL approach captures, we consider the responses of adolescents when discussing their experiences with surgery. Some adolescents were angry about having had to spend a significant portion of their vacation time in the hospital or recuperating. Others were angry at their parents for making them go through surgeries, which made it difficult to go out and be seen in public. One youth said, "I mostly have a grudge toward my mom because she made me go to school looking like a monster, and everyone staring at me . . . I hated her because she brought me into the world and I looked different." Other expressed an appreciation for what surgery had done for them, and their ability to participate in decision making.

Many youths expressed the positive aspects of their life experience as a "different" kind of individual. Several reported that they felt that their facial difference made them "stronger," and better able to accept other people for who they are. As one adolescent put it, "I'm more sensitive of other people's needs, and . . . it's more easy to, like, accept people for who they are because of how I've been." Preliminary findings from the YQOL craniofacial conditions study have been recently reported (Edwards et al. 2005; Topolski et al. 2005).

Practical Interventions

The lack of rigorous outcome studies notwithstanding, there is still much that can be offered to individuals and families with CFCs to cope with the difficulties they experience. In addition to or instead of surgeries, there is individual counseling, social skills interventions, peer-group support, education, and vocational interventions. The University of Illinois's social skills training program, developed by Kapp-Simon and others (Simon and Kapp-Simon 1992) includes workbooks, support groups, and class activities. The program helps youngsters by teaching them to be proactive in handling social situations. A similar emphasis has been given by the U.K. charitable group Changing Faces, which was started by James Partridge, who suffered severe and life-threatening burns in a car accident as an adolescent (Changing Faces 2004; Partridge 1990). This U.K. group has also developed a program that goes into the schools and provides training to classes and teachers about individuals with facial differences (Robinson et al. 1996).

Craniofacial surgeries are often undertaken with the goal of altering facial appearance to improve the individual's well-being or psychosocial functioning. However, little systematically collected outcome data are available to demonstrate that these interventions actually improve well-being. Reviews of the literature to date suggest that individuals with CFCs may be at increased risk for psychosocial difficulties, but limitations of available research make such conclusions tentative. Moreover, there is no simple correlation between craniofacial appearance and psychosocial outcomes. Providing surgical interventions (even "low-risk" surgeries) without evidence of benefit interventions can do harm. Such interventions may focus patients and families on surgical interventions to the exclusion of other health-promoting resources and opportunities; such surgeries may also reinforce assumptions about the importance of physical appearance and the child's need for improved appearance.

Research in this area is urgently needed, although there are substantial practical and conceptual obstacles to carrying out such research, including the complexity and rarity of such conditions and the length of time and cost of longitudinal, multicenter studies. Information can also be gleaned from narratives and case reports that may capture important elements not included in more typical studies. In addition to traditional psychological measures, there is a need for more patient- and family-centered outcome measures that assess areas of strength and resilience, and prioritize the individual's subjective experience (such as QOL measures). Finally, conceptual frameworks are needed for generating testable hypotheses on the causation of psychosocial difficulties, and for predicting which children are at high risk for problems so interventions can be offered early.

In the meantime, craniofacial care continues. Safeguards must be in place to ensure that patients and families understand the lack of evidence to support the view that normalizing surgeries improve psychosocial functioning. It is also critical that families be provided with information about nonsurgical means of achieving the end of positive psychosocial adjustment. Our systems of care could benefit from an ethos that strengthens the psychosocial component of care and focuses more on patient- and family-centered outcome assessments.

ACKNOWLEDGEMENTS

In addition to support from the National Endowment for the Humanities, this work was made possible by grants from the National Institute for Dental and Craniofacial Research to the University of Washington (1) Comprehensive Center for Oral Heath Research (Mouradian) (#P60 DE13061); and (2) Quality of Life in Youth with Craniofacial Conditions project (Patrick, Edwards, Topolski, Mouradian), R01 DE13546-01 (Phase I) and R01 DE13546-03 (Phase II).

NOTE

1. For example, the craniofacial quality-of-life research project discussed above includes expertise in psychology/psychometrics, public health, health policy, sociology, developmental pediatrics, dentistry, orthodontics, child psychology, social work, behavioral genetics, ethics, craniofacial molecular biology, as well as a parent/patient with a craniofacial condition.

REFERENCES

Agency for Health Research and Quality. 2004. U.S. Preventive Services Task Force, Clinical Pocket Guides to Clinical Preventive Services. Available at www.ahrq.gov/clinic/uspstfix .htm, accessed August 22, 2005.
American Cleft Palate-Craniofacial Association. 1993. Parameters for the evaluation and treatment of patients with cleft lip/palate and other craniofacial anomalies. *Cleft Palate-Craniofacial Journal* 30 (suppl. 1):S1–16.
Bullinger, M., and U. Ravens-Sieberer. 1995. General principles, methods and areas of applica-

tion of quality of life research in children. *Praxis der Kinderpsychologie und Kinderpsychiatrie* 44:391–99.

Changing Faces. 2004. www.changingfaces.co.uk/default.html, accessed August 22, 2005.

Cicchetti, D., and K. Schneider-Rosen. 1984. Theoretical and empirical considerations in the investigation of the relationship between affect and cognition in atypical populations of infants: Contributions to the formulation of an integrative theory of development. In *Emotions, Cognition and Behavior,* edited by D. Izard, J. Lagan, R. Zajonc, et al., 366–406. New York: Cambridge University Press.

Cicchetti, D. and K. Toth. 1992. The role of developmental theory in prevention and intervention. *Developmental Psychopathology* 1002 (4):489–93.

Cleft Lip and Palate: Critical Elements of Care, The Center for Children with Special Health Needs Children's Hospital and Regional Medical Center, Revised May 2003. Available at www.cshcn.org/forms/CLP5–03.pdf, accessed August 22, 2005.

Clinical Standards Advisory Group. 1998. Martin Harris, Chair. London: The Stationery Office, Crown Copyright.

The Cochrane Collaboration. 2004. www.cochrane.org/index0.htm, accessed August 22, 2005.

Coy, K., M. L. Speltz, and K. Jones. 2002. Facial appearance and attachment in infants with orofacial clefts: A replication. *Cleft Palate-Craniofacial Journal* 39 (1):66–72.

Edwards, T. C., C. E. Huebner, F .A. Connell, and D. L. Patrick. 2002. Adolescent quality of life, Part I: Conceptual and measurement model. *Journal of Adolescence* 25(3):275–86.

Edwards, T. C., D. L. Patrick, T. K. Topolski, C. Aspinall, W. E. Mouradian, et al. (2005). Approaches to craniofacial-specific quality of life assessment in adolescence. *Cleft Palate-Craniofacial Journal* 42 (1):19–24.

Emerson, M., T. Owen, and N. Rumsey. 2004. Auditing the psychosocial adjustment of children affected by a cleft. Presented at the annual meeting of the Craniofacial Society of Great Britain and Ireland, April, 2004, Bath, UK.

Glaser, B. G., and A. L. Strauss. 1967. *The Discovery of Grounded Theory: Strategies for Qualitative Research.* New York: Aldine De Gruyter.

Harper, D. C., L. C. Richman, and B. C. Snyder. 1980. School adjustment and degree of physical impairment. *Journal of Pediatric Psychology* 5:377–82.

Heller, A., W. Tidmarsh, and I. B. Pless. 1981. The psychosocial functioning of young adults born with cleft lip or palate. A follow-up study. *Clinical Pediatrics* 20 (7):459–65.

Herskind, A., K. Christensen, K. Juel, and P. Fogh-Anderson. 1993. Cleft lip: A risk factor for suicide. [Abstract]. 7th International Congress on cleft palate and related craniofacial anomalies. Australia, 156.

Hickey, A., G. Bury, C. O'Boyle, F. Bradley, et al. 1996. A new short form individual quality of life measure (SEIQoL-DW): Application in a cohort of individuals with HIV/AIDS. *British Medical Journal* 313 (7048):29–33.

Kapp-Simon, K. A. 1998. Mental development and learning disorders in children with single suture craniosynostosis. *Cleft Palate-Craniofacial Journal* 35 (3):197–203.

Lansdown, R., N. Rumsey, E. Bradbury, et al. 1997. *Visibly Different: Coping with Disfigurement.* Oxford: Butterworth-Heinemann.

Maris, M. A., M. C. Endriga, M. L. Speltz, et al. 2000. Are infants with orofacial clefts at risk for insecure mother-child attachment? *Cleft Palate-Craniofacial Journal* 37 (3):257–65.

McWilliams, B. J., and L. P. Paradise. 1973. Educational, occupational, and marital status of cleft palate adults. *Cleft Palate Journal* 10:223–29.

Mouradian, W. E. 2001. Deficits versus strengths: Ethics and implications for clinical practice and research. *Cleft Palate-Craniofacial Journal* 38:255–59.

Nash, P. 1995. *Living with Disfigurement: The Psychosocial Implications of Being Born with a Cleft Lip and Palate.* Avebury: Aldershot.

Pal, D. K. 1996. Quality of life assessment in children: A review of conceptual and methodological issues in multidimensional health status measures. *Journal of Epidemiology and Community Health* 50:391–96.

Partridge, J. 1990. *Changing Faces.* London: Penguin Group.

Patrick, D. L. 1997. Rethinking prevention for people with disabilities, part I: A conceptual model for promoting health. *American Journal of Health Promotion* 11:257–63.

Patrick, D. L., T. C. Edwards, and T. D. Topolski. 2002. Adolescent quality of life, part II: Initial validation of a new instrument. *Journal of Adolescence* 25 (3):287–300.

Peter, J. P., and R. R. Chinsky. 1974. Sociological aspects of cleft palate adults: I. Marriage. *Cleft Palate Journal* 11:295–309.

Peter, J. P., R. R. Chinsky, and M. J. Fisher. 1975. Sociological aspects of cleft palate adults. III. Vocational and economic aspects. *Cleft Palate-Craniofacial Journal* 12:193–99.

Richman, L. C. 1976. Behavior and achievement of the cleft palate child. *Cleft Palate- Craniofacial Journal* 13:4–10.

Robinson, E. 1997. Psychological research on visible differences in adults. In *Visibly Different: Coping with Disfigurement,* edited by R. Lansdown, N. Rumsey, E. Bradbury, A. Carr, and J. Partridge, 102–11. Oxford: Butterworth Heineman.

Robinson, E., N. Rumsey, and J. Partridge. 1996. An evaluation of the impact of social interaction skills training for facially disfigured people. *British Journal of Plastic Surgery* 1 (49):281–89.

Rumsey, N. 1998. Quality of life issues in complex craniofacial care. Presented at the 55th annual meeting of the American Cleft Palate and Craniofacial Association, April, Baltimore.

———. 2002. Body image and congenital conditions. In *Body Image: A Handbook of Theory, Research and Clinical Practice,* edited by T. Cash and T. Pruzinsky, 226–33. New York: Guilford.

Schor, E. L. 1998. Children's health and the assessment of health-related quality of life. In *Measuring Health-related Quality of Life in Children and Adolescents,* edited by D. Drotar, 25–37. Mahwah, NJ: Erlbaum.

Shaw, W. C., et al. 1992a. A six-center international study of treatment outcomes in patients with clefts of the lip and palate: Part 1. Principles and study design. *Cleft Palate-Craniofacial Journal* 29 (5):393–97.

———. 1992b. A six-center international study of treatment outcomes in patients with clefts of the lip and palate: Part 5. General discussion and conclusions. *Cleft Palate-Craniofacial Journal* 29 (5):413–18.

Shaw W., A. Williams, J. Sandy, and B. Devlin. 1996. Minimum standards for the management of cleft lip and palate: Efforts to close the audit loop. *Annals of the Royal College of Surgeons of England* 78:110–14.

Simon, D. J., and K. Kapp-Simon. 1992. *Meeting the Challenge: A Social Skills Training Program for Adolescents with Special Needs.* Available from Kapp-Simon, University of Illinois.

Speltz, M. L., M. T. Greenberg, and M. C. Endriga, et al. 1994. Developmental approach to the psychology of craniofacial anomalies. *Cleft Palate-Craniofacial Journal* 31 (1):61–67.

Speltz, M. L., H. Galbreath, and M. T. Greenberg. 1995. A developmental framework for psychosocial research on young children with craniofacial anomalies. In *Developmental Perspectives on Craniofacial Problems,* edited by R. Elder, 258–86. New York: Springer-Verlag.

Speltz, M. L., M. C. Endriga, and W. E. Mouradian. 1997. Presurgical and postsurgical mental and psychomotor development of infants with sagittal synostosis. *Cleft Palate-Craniofacial Journal* 34 (5):374–79.

Spieth, L. E., and C. V. Harris. 1996. Assessment of health-related quality of life in children and adolescents: An integrative review. *Journal of Pediatric Psychology* 21:175–93.

Sroufe, L., and M. Rutter. 1984. The domain of psychopathology. *Child Development* 55:17–29.

Starr, P. 1983. *Cleft Lip and or Palate: Behavioral Effects from Infancy to Adulthood.* Springfield, IL: Charles C. Thomas.

Strauss, A., and J. Corbin. 1990. *Basics of Qualitative Research.* Newbury Park, CA: Sage.

Strauss, R. P., H. Broder, and R. W. Helms. 1988. Perceptions of appearance and speech by adolescent patients with cleft lip and palate and by their parents. *Cleft Palate Journal* 25 (4):335–42.

Tarnowski, K .J., and L. K. Rasnake. 1994. Long-term psychosocial sequelae. In *Behavioral Aspects of Pediatric Burns,* edited by K. J. Tarnowski, 81–114. New York: Plenum.

Tobiasen, J. M., A. Perkins, J. Weaver, et al. 1992. Incidence of psychological adjustment problems in children and adolescents with cleft lip and palate. Paper presented at the 49th annual meeting of the American Cleft Palate-Craniofacial Association, Portland, OR.

Tobiasen, J., and M. L. Speltz. 1996. Cleft palate: A psychosocial developmental perspective. In *Cleft Lip & Palate: Perspectives in Management,* edited by S. Berkowitz, 2:15–23. Singular Publishing Group: San Diego.

Topolski, T., T. C. Edwards, and D. L. Patrick (2005). Quality of life: How do adolescents with facial differences compare with other adolescents? *Cleft Palate-Craniofacial Journal* 42 (1):25–32.

Van Demark, D. R., and A. A. Van Demark. 1970. Speech and socio-vocational aspects of individuals with cleft palate. *Cleft Palate Journal* 7:284–99.

Williams A., D. Bearn, S. Mildinhall, et al. 2001. Cleft lip and palate care in the UK—The CSAG Study Part 2: Dentofacial outcomes and patient satisfaction. *Cleft Palate-Craniofacial Journal* 38 (1):24–29.

WHOQOL Group. 1994. The development of the World Health Organization Quality of Life Assessment Instrument (the WHOQOL). In *Quality of Life Assessment: International Perspectives,* edited by J. Orley and W. Kuyken, 41–57. Berlin: Springer-Verlag.

———. 1995. The World Health Organization Quality of Life Assessment (WHOQOL): Position paper from the World Health Organization. *Social Science and Medicine* 41 (10):1403–9.

———. 1997. *Measuring Quality of Life: The World Health Organization Quality of Life Instruments* (The WHOQOL-100 and the WHOQOL-BREF). Geneva, Switzerland: World Health Organization.

World Health Organization. 1948. *Constitution of the World Health Organization.* Geneva: World Health Organization.

PART IV

CHILDREN AND PARENTS DECIDING ABOUT APPEARANCE-NORMALIZING SURGERY

CHAPTER ELEVEN

Who Should Decide and How?

Priscilla Alderson, Ph.D.

"With leg lengthening, only the person who is going to have it can decide whether to have it. I decided when I was eight."

(Amy, age 10, whose mother agreed) (Alderson 1993, 30)

"I would like to see the age limits completely scrapped, and maturity brought in. As you grow up, your age has a stereotype. I'm trying to escape from that stereotype."

(Robin, age 13) (ibid., 43)

"He is an exceptional and unique person. He likes to maintain his integrity as a human being, and he felt violated by the way they treated him, dirty. I found that he had put the clothes that he had worn at the clinic and even his teddy in the rubbish bin. I felt his refusal [of proposed treatment] was right. He may have a small body, but he has a great personality."

(Mother of a 10-year-old boy) (ibid., 39)

The questions, Who should decide about children's surgery? and How? involve further questions: Who is informed enough to decide? Who is competent to decide? Who ought to decide? And may competent people choose to refer that responsibility to others? How are decisions about surgery made, and possibly shared? And could we promote more just, benign, and efficacious ways of making decisions about surgically shaping children? The replies to these questions rest on different kinds of knowledge and authority in research evidence, law, and ethics. (The term *children* refers to minors ages 0 to 17, from babyhood to young adulthood, and in this chapter usually involves children and young people ages 4, 5, or 6 onward.)

Evidence, Law, and Ethics

Discussion about consent and competence is informed by research evidence of how people understand and make decisions, and here I draw mainly on my sociological research with children having surgery or talking about their impairments, and with their parents and professionals who care for them (Alderson 1990, 1993; Alderson and Goodey 1998).

Competence is partly a legal issue. American states tend to set 18 or 19 as the age of consent to medical treatment, except for "mature minors," such as those needing treatment for drug or alcohol abuse. Paradoxically, they can consent at a younger age than their seemingly more responsible peers. In some parts of Canada the age of consent is 13. In the United Kingdom, although young people have the right to consent from 18 and often from 16, there is no specified lower age. Children can give valid consent if they understand fully what is involved, and have the discretion to make a wise decision in their best interests, and if the doctor treating them considers that they are competent (*Gillick* All ER [1985]; Age of Legal Capacity Act 1991). Although an earlier court ruling, that parents' rights "terminate" when the child is competent (*Gillick* [1985]) was later challenged, English law recognizes that the competent child's consent to treatment can override parents' refusal, although a parent's consent can override a ("Gillick") competent child's refusal (*In re* R [1991] 4 All ER 177; *In re* W [1992] 4 All ER 627). Children have more rights to confidentiality and to make treatment decisions if they use free state services, as in the United Kingdom, than when their parents pay for them directly or indirectly. However, whereas adults' self-destructive and seemingly irrational decisions are respected in English law, legally valid decisions for and by children must respect the child's welfare and best interests. As with patients of any age, choices are limited to what treatments the doctor decides to offer. The consent of competent children is controlled by adults' discretion and determinations about whether the child is "competent or mature"; the choice is in the child's "best interests"; the treatment is available; and the treatment is paid for.

Ethical questions—Who ought to decide? How? and Why?—invoke principles and values, which I approach in three main ways: by reviewing a range of ethical positions and authorities; by analyzing some of the moral assumptions about children and parents that reflect and reinforce current values; and by aiming to justify respect for children's views and decisions as a logical conclusion.

The next section discusses theories and research methods. These inevitably and inextricably shape all research evidence and conclusions, as well as debates about the contentious topic of consent to children's treatment.

Research on Decision Making about Children's Surgery

Very little research on this topic has systematically observed and listened to groups of children having surgery, their parents, and other adults caring for them, or has critically analyzed the related theories and data. A comprehensive overview of empirical research on informed consent, for example, includes only patients over 18 years old (Sugarman et al. 1999). In their analyses, ethicists and psychologists tend to accept outdated child development theories, and either ignore children's consent (Ramsey 1970; McCormick 1974; Murray 1996; Faden and Beauchamp 1986) or almost wholly dismiss the consent of younger children (Buchanan and Brock 1989; Melton et al. 1983; Gaylin and Macklin 1982; Kopelman and Moskop 1989).

It is widely assumed that research interviews should not be conducted with child surgery patients. The reasons given include the following, listed here with brief replies.

"There are no valid methods for researching children's decisions about surgery." This is a problem with adults' decisions too. In research about any complex, potentially distressing, fairly rare, and partly unique experiences, traditional methods tend to provide misleading results. The methods include questionnaire surveys, discussion of hypothetical questions and vignettes, and standardized tests of knowledge and competence. Representative groups of children are tested for their general health knowledge (Wilkinson 1988). "Representative" (healthy, normal) children (and adults) tend to give ignorant and cautious replies because they lack direct experience of surgery. Psychological assessments tend to screen, and give higher scores, for failures, deficits, and problems, rather than identifying achievements and competencies—for which the highest score may be zero. When standardized surveys, unsurprisingly, elicit limited knowledge from inexperienced children, researchers may then infer that children cannot and should not have to understand complex and distressing matters. Most survey research about young people is still guided by, and reinforces, dominant Piagetian theories of children as deficient, not yet fully developed human being (James and Prout 1997).

Statistical research uses standardized, quantifiable data, whereas children's decisions about surgery are individual. Each child is unique; indeed, this book is concerned with children who look unusual. Their social and family background, age and ability, conditions and courses of treatment, personality and values, perceptions and experiences, all vary too much for their reactions to be standardized usefully. When quantitative research analyzes all the variables separately, instead of also as interactive aspects of whole experiences, it risks producing unhelpful generalizations. I could not, in my research, set the same test of informed competence for all the 120 people ages 8 to 15 having surgery for a wide range of conditions and needs, because I could not determine which pieces of knowledge or attributes of competence were most relevant and essential in each case. Instead, I asked the children and adults involved when and why they thought the child concerned became, or would become, as competent to decide about the proposed surgery as the parents were. The children's replies were slightly more cautious than the adults'.

Another limitation of much research on informed consent is that it is not about consent, but about how patients recall and recount medical information. And these research reports often omit to say what patients were actually told, or to explain why any omissions and inaccuracies are attributed solely to the patients' recall, whereas some might have originated in doctors' explanations. Much of the research that claims to be about decision making instead concerns tests of competence, and does not examine the actual process of deciding (Sugarman et al. 1999).

Decision making and consent are partly invisible, elusive processes of reflection, which entail evaluating information in the light of personal values and weighing alternatives. People may also make an emotional journey from shocked rejection of proposed surgery toward hope and trust in the clinical team, and faith that treatment will be less awful than the untreated disease (Alderson 1990; see Mouridian, this volume). Alison, age 14, for example, fainted on first hearing about surgery to straighten her spine. "To faint, I must have wanted not to know. I was laughing, having hysterics . . . I had a little cry but I still wasn't absorbing it." Alison had the surgery weeks later, and she recalled that at the time "[the information] hit me then, but by then it was all right." She met a girl who had been paralyzed by spinal surgery and was slowly learning to walk with crutches. "I'm glad I knew. It was very worrying, but I'd have been really upset if I hadn't known and it had happened" (Alderson 1993, 126).

Traditional research methods tend to collect impersonal, standardized, observable, static data—snapshots rather than film. In contrast, methods of research about decision making are needed that capture the personal, individual, invisible, and dynamic process. These methods include semistructured interviews, which encourage detailed narratives, contextualized within each person's life. Respectful, trusting rapport between interviewer and interviewee, including young children, encourages rich accounts.

The power of this research is not statistical but analytical, aiming to enable readers to see the depths of meaning in each case, in the accurate descriptions, and in the common themes they illustrate. Only a few research examples are needed to refute false generalizations; such as that all young children cannot understand or share in making surgery decisions. Yet many people still demand the certainty that generalizations seem to offer. Doctors ask, "If it is not 18 or 16 years, then what is the age of consent?" An alternative is to attend to each child and context, instead of to numbers. This involves assessing competence not by status (such as age of minority/majority) or outcome (the assessor agrees with the child's decision), but by function (how well the child can take part in the decision making) (Brazier 1987).

"Children would be distressed by research." Yes, I have found that occasionally children, and also adults, become distressed during my research interviews about surgery. I offer to stop or to pause. However, most people say they want to continue; they move on to more positive or tranquil moods later, and tend to say that they valued the opportunity to talk. The danger of attempting to protect children from the challenges of taking part in research is that they are silenced and excluded, and it is then often assumed that they cannot and should not be involved in useful research that could influence policy and practice.

"The parents' authority could be undermined." The data-collection stage involves interviewing children and parents, with their consent, and listening respectfully to both viewpoints. It involves asking questions and not making comments or intervening deliberately in individual cases. Later on during data analysis and report writing, parents' authority in general might be critically reviewed. Surely such an important issue is a legitimate topic for research? A great challenge in writing up any research is to respect all the individuals who generously contributed, while also analyzing their data rigorously.

"Children are unreliable witnesses and research participants." Research on children as legal witnesses has found them to be as reliable as adults (Dent and Flin 1992). The past fifteen years or so have seen a rapid increase in childhood research that observes and interviews children directly as active participants, rather than as research subjects (Christensen and James 2000; Mayall 1994). There is new respect for children's reliable and articulate accounts and their own explanations about their motives, values, and behavior. I have found that the parents' and clinicians' accounts rarely disagreed with the children's, and even if they did, the child's view could look reasonable. A foster mother thought that her daughter ought to have a toe amputated, because a surgeon advised that this would improve the girl's balance and weight-bearing, and thus reduce the pressure when she had to lean on her caregivers. The girl was not convinced, and felt that her views about her bodily integrity, besides many other aspects of her daily life, were dismissed and overridden because her body was already so impaired (Alderson 1993, 151).

"Evidence of children's competence is irrelevant when it has no legal validity." Competence involves the person's intrinsic knowledge and ability as well as extrinsic rules or laws that respect certain groups as competent. History provides many examples of groups now believed to be competent who used to be denied legal capacity—women,

ethnic minorities, disabled people, and Russian refusniks, to name just a few. It is fair and logical to check for evidence to support assumed legal incapacity, rather than to regard the law as a realistic guide to human ability.

"Children's lack of competence is too obvious to be worth researching." The newer childhood research critiques beliefs that childhood is essentially a precompetent state and a series of Piagetian stages (James and Prout 1997; Christensen and James 2000; Morss 1990; R. and W. Stainton Rogers 1992; Burman 1994). The growing evidence of young children's sophisticated social and moral competence shows that people become competent far more through experience than because of their age, "stage," or ability (Alderson 1993; Gardner 1993; Hutchby and Moran-Ellis 1998; Dunn 1988; Damon 1998; Alderson 2000; Kagan and Lamb 1987). Children who live safe, secure, fortunate lives may not need to realize or demonstrate latent strengths and capacities, which children may reveal when they are exposed to serious risk, such as major surgery or severe adversity (Butler 1998).

Since the 1970s, many people ages 12 to 14 have been acknowledged to have "adult" cognitive abilities (National Commission for the Protection of Human Subjects of Biomedical and Behavioural Research 1997). Yet over the twentieth century, the status of young people in Western societies generally regressed from young working adults to hormonally challenged dependents, while middle-class women were gradually emancipated from this role. Women became emancipated partly by reconceptualizing their supposed biological weaknesses as social constructions, and their ascribed personal inadequacies as political oppressions, through the slogan "the personal is political." They also gained independence when their domestic and childcare duties were increasingly recognized and paid as work. Women's economic power grew as they joined the new armies of professional child-work experts and agents, which multiplied as new "needs" and deficiencies were identified in young people (Qvortrup et al. 1994; Zelizer 1995).

Among the complex reasons for the modern infantilizing of young people is control of the labor market, keeping them in low-paid or unpaid positions; their domestic and school work is not recognized as "work." Another reason is the view since the 1900s that, with the high immigration rates, young American citizens need time to develop through two decades of education and assimilation (Hall 1904; Musgrove 1984). This political expedience became repackaged as essential support for inevitably deficient youth, a paradoxical mirror opposite, yet also reinforcement, of feminism. Childhood research identifies generation, like gender, as a key explanatory theory to analyze and clarify the underlying working of these policies and relationships (Mayall 2002). It examines differences between the long-shared histories of women's and children's presumed incompetence, the economic and political interests these theories have served, how authentic the theories are for understanding the reality of people's daily life, and the power the theories still exert when children's incompetence is presumed (Alderson 1993, 2000; James and Prout 1997; Christensen and James 2000; Gardner 1993; Hutchby and Moran-Ellis 1998; Dunn 1998; Damon 1998; Butler 1998; Qvortrup et al., 1994; Zelizer 1995). Locke and Kant assumed that women as well as children were incapable of being autonomous rational agents (Kennedy and Mendus 1987). If they were so wrong about women—the topic for twentieth-century research—the question for twenty-first-century research is: Were they so right about children?

Hilde Lindemann reviews (in this volume) three dangerous master narratives: the self-absorbed consumer, the ugly outcast, and the scientific "fix" that can sway parents' surgical decisions for their children. James Edwards reviews (also in this volume) powerful assumptions about the technological imperative that also dominate our thinking. The "vulnerable child" is another master narrative of our time, as if all children are as helpless and ignorant as infants. Yet by around 9 years, many children are bigger and stronger than many adults. In war-torn, AIDS-torn Africa and Asia, children as young as 8 years run small businesses and households. Severe misfortune and adversity reveal strengths and competencies in them, which are hardly imaginable in the protected 8-year-olds who live in the minority wealthy societies. Another master narrative, the theory that children require years of learning to be socialized, denies their early sophisticated social competencies that are acquired mainly through children's active imitation, and their interpretation of the countless subtle hidden rules that structure daily life (Hutchby and Moran-Ellis 1998; Waskler 1991). Children quickly begin to absorb their families' values, and in societies where different ethnic groups live together, or where there is conflict, they show early awareness of social differences and tensions (Connolly et al. 2002). Even young children live in interdependent relationships with their parents. Lisa Hedley in this volume beautifully describes her young daughter LilyClaire's gracious competence in dealing with unwanted inquiries, and Nelson comments on LilyClaire's lucidity, integrity, and grace.

Who Is Informed Enough?

If children are to be able to share in making informed decisions, they need to be told as much as they can understand about the medical details, the purpose and nature of the surgery, the risks, benefits, alternatives, and likely outcomes, as in Arthur Frank's analysis of consumer-protection bioethics (in this volume). Whereas surgeons tend to concentrate on describing surgical procedures, children especially want to know how the whole course of treatment might affect them, possibly for weeks, months, or years, what they will have to endure, what they can hope for, and how their life and identity might be affected. This relates to Frank's Socratic bioethics. To acknowledge and include these issues in the dialogue between the adults and child also involves recognizing the complexities in practitioner-patient relationships considered by Wendy Mouradian in this volume.

Nurses, psychologists and child-life workers begin to inform young children from their second year, such as when telling them the story of their treatment and showing them photographs, surgery dolls, and puppets. When children about 3 years old are drastically reshaped, for example, by limb amputation because of injury or cancer, it is possible to help them to understand, prepare, and adapt (Alderson 1993).

It is crucial to convey the adults' benign intention to help the child. Far from having no understanding, young children interpret and search for meaning. Babies at 6 months show surprise during experiments when cause appears to follow effect (Siegal 1997). Without constant reassurance, children will logically believe that unpleasant, painful, or mutilating treatments are worse than the original condition, of which they may be unaware. They are then liable to perceive treatment as deliberate cruelty, with adults abandoning them to punishment, to torture (Melzak 1992). Even premature babies react with less crying and stress (shown, for example, by desaturation levels) during painful procedures if an adult gently talks and holds them throughout, as if the baby can find very helpful reassurance in the human tones and touch and can distinguish these from the simultaneous painful intervention (Als 1999).

Contrary to theories of infant egoism (Bradley 1989) babies communicate with other people and respond to their smiling or depression long before they try to handle inanimate objects. Babies learn other people's names and discuss other people's mental states before beginning to talk about their own (Eibl-Eibersfeldt 1971). Relationships are their framework of meaning. This consciousness distinguishes children from property, however much it is valued and cherished. Property cannot interpret, interact, suffer, or hope. These capacities raise questions about whether children are persons in their own right, or whether their parents may or ought to exercise, in effect, property rights over their children, as considered later.

Some children, for example, 8-year-old Linda, were highly informed (Alderson 1993, 30, 127–28). She felt the decision about surgery was jointly made. "My doctor and my mummy decided about my operation. They knew what I wanted. After all she is my mum and I do trust her." She kissed her mother. She added that the doctors should inform her mother, "And auntie should hear too, so she doesn't get worried [she kissed her aunt]. But particularly me, so I can face up to it if I'm frightened." Serious and painful complications had occurred during Linda's previous operation, her fourth, and she had been very upset that she had not been warned. Her mother said, "I usually tell her everything, she wants to know exactly what is entailed."

Yet Linda's mother felt that she could not explain everything, and Linda was not told that her fifth and partly cosmetic operation had a 10 percent mortality rate. Although cosmetic surgery is rarely so risky, Linda's example is relevant in showing some young children's maturity and courage in coping with complex, distressing information. Like children who have cancer (Bluebond-Langner 1978), Linda may have known or sensed this risk, and protected her mother from her own fears. She had asked why the neighbors cried when they said goodbye to her before she came into hospital. She spoke cheerfully to me in front of her mother and aunt, "I say, thank goodness I'm getting it over and done with." But later when they had gone she said, "They'll be in tears for me." Linda's surgeon described how he believed that he could ensure that patients from age 6 or 7 understood some of the major risks of surgery, through comparing these to crossing the road, and "being very careful" (Alderson 1993, 108–9).

The children I interviewed often had to endure frightening, painful ordeals. Even if they were not warned in advance, they became deeply informed during the course of treatment. Children are able to have informed views about surgery that alters their appearance because they can see the condition and the highly visible difference that surgery might make. Only the child can fully experience, perceive, and understand life within the particular body shape, and continuously receive and have to deal with the stream of reactions from other people during the daily presentation of self (Goffman 1959). From an early age, the person with unique and essential insight into any need, risk, and benefit incurred in reshaping a body is the person who lives in and also is that mindful body. This daily experience helps children to realize what they want to gain from surgery, and what costs of pain and potential failure they are prepared to endure. The patient is far more directly affected than anyone else. There may be preverbal signs, such as when children with ambiguous genitalia begin to indicate whether they feel themselves to be a boy or a girl.

Socratic bioethics (to use Arthur Frank's phrase) involves much more than the one-way process of doctors informing families. It is a two-way exchange of clinical and personal knowledge. If doctors and parents are to be able to make informed decisions, they have to listen to the child's unique insights into what "the good life" means, as far as these can be ascertained, to consult, and sometimes be led by, the child.

Who Is Competent?

There are four levels of involvement in decision making: (1) being informed; (2) expressing a view; (3) contributing to and influencing a decision; and (4) being the main or sole decision maker (Alderson and Montgomery 1996). The third and fourth levels require greater competence to reflect on information in the light of lasting values, and discretion to decide in the child's best interests. Level 4 involves having the resolve to form and stick to a decision, and to bear responsibility for risks without blaming others if these harms occur.

Lasting values may link to broader political awareness. Is the impaired person being unnecessarily pressured by other people to conform to social norms? Is a genuine and fairly independent choice being made, such as from a disability rights perspective? This awareness is not age related. Many adults are unaware of the political dimensions of surgical reshaping; some children are aware of them, such as when they learn from a parent who also has their condition and is a disability activist. Some children appear to work out the principles for themselves, such as Tina, who refused treatment for short stature (Alderson 1993, 38). By age 12, she had new confidence after her house was adapted, enabling her to reach doorknobs and light switches. "I was afraid they'd go out and leave me. I feel much safer now it's adapted."

Tina came to feel that people and society should also adapt, and accept her for herself, instead of expecting her to change her shape to accommodate their prejudices. In this volume, James Edwards, paraphrasing Martin Heidegger, writes that truth is "disclosure, that seeking the truth is not about matching up our ideas with the reality they purport to represent, but about letting our ideas call attention to aspects of what appears, aspects that we are likely otherwise to overlook." Then, he adds, perhaps we can see "theories" not as solving problems but as "indicators of salience." I suggest that Tina's hard experiences had led her to see new salience, new authenticity in her body and her self. One example is her sense of moral responsibility about medical decision making: "If I make the wrong decision, it's my fault, not my mum's," whereas if the treatment is enforced against her will and goes wrong, "If anything happens to me it's going to be your fault," she said to her mother.

Tina's interest in the reshaping of society rather than of herself resonates with Ellen Feder's example in this volume of the mother who was concerned that poor surgical outcomes "robbed" children with ambiguous genitalia of the "normal kid stuff" such as "running around naked in sprinklers in hot summers." Through supportive friendships, she found that her son could run with friends in sprinklers. "Kids knew he was different, but that was okay, and he learned that everyone, really, looks different from everyone else no matter what mold they come from."

To alter attitudes and relationships instead of bodies is to move on from the "fix-it response" and returns us to Frank's Socratic questions about "the kind of person that I want to be . . . and the kind of community of which I seek to be a responsible member." However, in Tina's case, the child rather than the parent is taking the initiative in asking these questions about the good life based on the social justice model of disability (instead of the medical model). Tina's mother argued with Tina, as if she thought she should play devil's advocate and force Tina to think through her dilemma rigorously, but she accepted Tina's decision. "To a large extent I agree with [Tina]. Society should change to be more open-minded and accept people in all shapes and sizes."

Amy was equally thoughtful, articulate, and determined; she began leg-lengthening treatment at 8 years to resist being dismissed for her short stature and being "treated as if I'm 4 years old." Amy's mother also supported her daughter, by giving up her work as a physiotherapist to care for Amy through years of treatment. In their complicated reflections and balancing of present and potential future needs and values with medical, personal, and social information, and for their courage and resolve, both girls were treated as competent by their parents and doctors. Amy's mother explicitly said that no one else could make such a decision except the child concerned. Four years later, the girls spoke at a conference, and each held firmly to her own original view. Their acceptance of the different significant costs and problems that each decision brought suggests that some children are competent to decide about reshaping surgery.

Among the hundreds of children with long-term disability or illness whom I have interviewed, I have met many remarkably stoic, mature children. They may have capacities that are perhaps latent in all children but, as mentioned earlier, are especially called on and revealed during adversity. While no one would wish for children to have such conditions, James Edwards's questioning about why we should see "life as a problem and a challenge [rather than] as a gift" is relevant.

Edwards adds, citing Thoreau, "it's what the fact does to you that's important; not what you do to the fact." During interviews, many children spoke with realism, humor, and determination about living with disability and "the moral language of personal authenticity" (Alderson 1993; Frank, this volume). They tended to see disability, in their narratives, as a problem and also a daily reality that to some extent they just had to accept, describing how disability affected them, was affected by them, and was part of their identity and life. Their agency challenges any light assumption that either the impairment, or indeed the child, can be regarded as *Bestand,* a standing reserve or resource waiting to be shaped to suit the parents' values, without regard for the child's own views once these begin to be formed. Questions about surgical shaping are set within questions and assumptions about all other forms of shaping and socializing children, which need to be addressed if the surgery questions are to be understood.

Frank (2003) also discusses "ambiguous voices" citing Myerson (2000):

"You'd better start trusting the ambiguous ones, the voice which cannot be defined. If you want to understand these new facts, then try imagining them from the perspective of the [Frank adds here adults who have had limb surgery]. Seek out the most ambiguous viewpoint, and re-view the facts from there . . . Facts are not what they used to be."

A central voice in discussions about surgically shaping children is the voice of the child whose voice is ambiguous in several ways. Younger children are not even expected to have voices; "infant" means without speech. They are expected to be not yet rational, wise, or worth hearing. Child development theory has trained us all to think in quite rigid age-stage stereotypes, to tend to hear what we expect the age group to say and be deaf to the children who do not match these prejudices. Most ambiguous of all, if children are to be heard, is to have to suspend the age-stage theories we rely on for rapid, efficient interactions, and instead enter a "nonagist" arena, without secure beliefs in a moral order of adults protecting and controlling helpless, ignorant children, without the rules and laws such as age of consent that protect adult authority and regulate the adult-child dichotomy. This involves the risk of listening to the child instead of the ascribed age level, hearing some children speak in "adult" voices, and exploring with them how far they can and wish to share in making decisions about surgery.

Who Ought to Decide?

Being able to decide does not mean that children must decide. Like women having breast cancer treatment (Alderson et al. 1994), most of the well-prepared children in our elective surgery study (Alderson 1993) wanted to share the decision making with their doctors and family, a few wanted others to decide for them, and a few wanted to be "the main decider," almost always supported by their parents. This was not age or ability related.

Adults deciding about surgery for themselves may say, "I don't want to hear all the gory details, I'll accept your advice, doctor, and sign the form." However, parents or guardians deciding for or with another person, their child, have an extra obligation to take the information sharing, risk taking, and decision making extremely seriously.

Some authors agree that children may be competent, but believe that parents should retain their right to decide for their minor child. This has important justifications: to protect and support children, to promote their future flourishing and open choices (Feinberg 1980; Davis 2001), and to sustain family harmony through respecting parents' rights to decide what is best for the whole family (Ross 1998).

However, to enforce parents' rights and control over children who are able and willing to make competent (and for minors this must include wise) decisions implies anxiety that children are liable to be foolish and must be protected from their self-destructive decisions. Contrary to media and psychological (Erikson 1971) stereotypes of rebellious or inadequate young people, parents and their children appear usually to agree more or less on major issues. With education, for example, only a minority of young people refuses to go to school, despite the many problems they often encounter there. It is not reported that families usually fight over serious health care decisions, especially once they have had time to reach a shared decision. Many parents report, with surprise, harmony rather than conflict with their growing children (Apter 1990). An important unresearched question is whether children and parents should have greater freedom to question and possibly resist treatment and surgery that are likely to be ineffective or harmful, as other chapters in this volume discuss.

This book is mainly concerned with children who have long-term problems and treatments and exceptional experiences, as with the children I interviewed. They took their health and medical care very seriously. Through having one or more chronic conditions, and an average of four to five previous operations, many of them had intense knowledge of disability, of looking different, and of treatment that could fail. They tended to be realistic and courageous, knowing that their parents and doctors could not ensure successful surgery or protect them from suffering.

One reason given for excluding children from decision making is that they cannot, and should not have to, bear risk and blame—even though if things go wrong, the child is the main bearer of any practical, bodily consequences. This argument unnecessarily implies that children who are competent decision makers will be on their own, and even in opposition to the adults. However, where there are serious risks, instead of a single, obvious, correct choice, there are usually complicated, uncertain risk-benefit equations, which people balance in different ways, and some of the adults concerned may share the child's view. Even if they disagree with their child's view, parents may eventually decide to support it. One mother spoke of having "cried buckets" over some of her children's lifestyle choices, but if they persisted after much discussion, she would support them (Alderson 1993, 157). A hospital chaplain and former head teacher thought this support called for great maturity and courage in adults and asked:

> But are you going to lay on children the weight of their future? . . . These are impossible questions, but hospital staff have to find the answers. Am I big enough to say, "Whatever you choose will be valued, even if you decide against the tide, o.k., you've made that decision, I'll do all I can to support you, and we'll go forward together"? It's such a big step for the adult to surrender power to the child. (Ibid., 143)

In cases of uncertainty and disagreement, are parents always the best choice makers? Surgically shaping children throws into extra sharp relief questions about coercion, rights, moral choice, and the "intimate family" (Ross 1998). All families may be "intimate" in contrast to the impersonal public domain of justice, rights, contracts, and formal accountability. But if parents override children's reasonable views about their own body, the family is hardly intimate in terms of loving equality. True intimacy involves moving beyond dichotomies of justice versus care and recognizing how the ethic of justice complements the equally important ethic of care (Gilligan 1982). This complementary enmeshing of care and justice offers useful ways of conceptualizing ethical principles within family relationships. The discourse of the intimate family that tries to exclude a public ethic of justice, by denying children's rights, paradoxically invokes public concepts of parents' rights, and thereby invites justice to reenter by the back door in its most dangerous form of defending a status quo, in which unaccountable power falls to the powerful.

The questions "Who ought to decide about surgery?" and "How can decisions be shared?" are finally answered by deep assumptions about justice and care, and these will be considered further in the final section.

More Just, Benign, and Efficacious Ways of Making Decisions

Ethical progress often depends on changes of attitude. The first step is to move on from theories that perceive children as not-yet-persons but as possessions over which their owners/parents have rights; that regard children as developing projects who ought to be shaped and reshaped; and that assume children do not suffer as real persons do. Those old theories are liable to feed and lead into assumptions that surgery is a desirable benefit, instead of encouraging such cautious questions as, "How can the surgery be justified, especially if the child is unwilling or not yet able to understand?" An orthopedist (orthopedics means correcting children) summed up these views when he said, "We can do limb lengthening up to about 30 years of age, but we prefer to do it much earlier because adults seem to have more psychological problems than young children do" (Alderson 1993, 28). The repeated casual assumption that genetic and other experimental enhancements should primarily "benefit" children, instead of volunteer adults, dangerously aligns moral parenting with avid reshaping of the child (Alderson 2002).

Child development theories collapse the moral and social into the biological, in mistakenly assuming that children's minds grow as slowly as their bodies, and that young children cannot have social and moral views worth respecting. As reviewed earlier, feminist scholarship has shown the dangers for women and their rights when they were similarly consigned to a natural (biological, given, nonpolitical) domain.

The supposedly large difference between child and adult appears to justify unequal rights. Too often rights are seen as adult prerogatives that license selfish individualism, lonely Kantian autonomy, and zero-sum conflict. Rights are thus incompatible with childhood dependence and family harmony. A far more positive conception of rights, enshrined in a UN treaty that has been ratified by every government except the United States (United Nations 1989), sees rights as collective, inalienable to all members of the human family, and expressions of equality and solidarity that lay the foundation of freedom, justice, and peace. These rights respect the worth and dignity of every child. "Your rights" are not just "my rights" but "our rights." The key article 12 assures to children who are capable of forming and expressing their own views "the right to express those views in all matters affecting the child" and for "due weight" to be given to those views (ibid.).

This respect does not prevent conflict—between children and adults, or between adults—but it offers means of resolving conflicts of interests, and conflicts between justice and care. Seyla Benhabib (1986) gives a fine example of detailed new ways of thinking beyond the old conflicting dichotomies in moral philosophy. She contrasts the traditional impersonal generalized and *disembodied* other, an empty mask that is everyone and no one, with the individual concrete other: the embodied, feeling person, with memories, history, and relationships, living and telling his or her own identity and history. Benhabib argues that before we can integrate justice with care, we have to enlarge the moral framework. Recognizing the dignity and worth of the generalized other is necessary but not sufficient without also recognizing the individual concrete other. Benhabib writes about including "all," though she does not mention children. Yet she offers a far richer and fairer way of relating to children whose bodies and identities may be reshaped by surgery, and who therefore stand between the private intimate family and the political economy of the health services and public values. Benhabib argues that moral understanding is informed through being contextualized within people's needs, desires, and rights, their feelings and thoughts, and their own life story.

The Socratic perspective proposed by Benhabib enables vital questions about reshaping surgery to be raised that, for example, Mary Winkler has raised about enhancement. Does it "enhance the whole person or offer only a palliative substitute for wholeness? Does it serve our desires for completeness and connection, or pander to our anxieties and our short-sighted demands for control? Finally, does the technology and its application help us to love and honor the body in all its fragility, imperfection and finitude?" (Winkler 1998, 249). The questions take on new gravity when adults ask them of decisions about another person's body, the child's.

A further way to enlarge moral theory that enfranchises children is to attend far more to voluntariness in consent. Voluntariness is very rarely mentioned. Faden and Beauchamp dismiss it as too confusing and better retermed as "noncontrol" (Faden and Beauchamp 1986, 257). Yet voluntariness *is* control, the person as agent and pilot in her own life, without the constraints of force, fraud, deceit, duress, or other coercion (Nuremberg Code 1947). Voluntariness fuses reason, emotion, and will, as children such as Amy and Tina demonstrate that they can do. Respect for the voluntary consent of the concrete other protects children who are meaning makers from being coerced through ignorance or fear, and from the risks of having to endure rage and terror (Melzak 1992) about the processes and effects of unwanted and enforced treatments.

This chapter has mainly discussed theories about children, rights, and decision making, since deeply held theories or assumptions block change in policies and practices until the theories themselves change. New attitudes toward women transformed their status during the past century. However, in conclusion, to move from theory to practice, here are a few practical examples of respectful approaches used by many clinicians and parents. They listen carefully to children, an integral part of therapeutic care and of avoiding harm. They start by assuming that the (school-age) child might be competent to understand and decide, because it is easier to check for and identify incompetence than competence (Royal College of Paediatrics and Child Health 2000; British Medical Association 2001). If children seem not to understand, they ascertain whether this is due to the child's inability to understand or to the adults' lack of skill in explaining. They regard tests of competence as a test of how far the adults are able to increase the child's understanding and willing involvement in decision making. They look for the sense and reasoning in the child's views that may help to resolve children's and adults' misunderstandings. And they recognize the expertise of the child who is living in the body and who is the body that might be reshaped.

ACKNOWLEDGMENTS

I am grateful to all the children and adults who contributed to my research on consent to surgery, and to the members of the Surgically Shaping Children project at The Hastings Center for their inspiring ideas and discussions.

REFERENCES

Age of Legal Capacity (Scotland) Act 1991, 423.

Alderson, P. 1990. *Choosing for Children: Parents' Consent to Surgery.* Oxford: Oxford University Press.

———. 1993. *Children's Consent to Surgery.* Buckingham: Open University Press.

———. 2000. *Young Children's Rights.* London: Jessica Kingsley/Save the Children.

———. 2002. The new genetics: Promise or threat to children? *Bulletin of Medical Ethics* 176:13–18.

Alderson, P., and C. Goodey. 1998. *Enabling Education.* London: Tufnell.

Alderson, P., M. Madden, A. Oakley, et al. 1994. *Women's Views of Breast Cancer Treatment and Research.* London: Institute of Education.

Alderson, P., and J. Montgomery. 1996. *Health Care Choices: Making Decisions with Children.* London: Institute for Public Policy Research.

Als, H. 1999. Reading the premature infant. In *Nurturing the Premature Infant,* edited by E. Goldson, 18–85. New York: Oxford University Press.

Apter, T. 1990. *Altered Lives: Mothers and Daughters During Adolescence.* Hemmel Hempstead: Wheatsheaf Harvester.

Benhabib, S. 1986. The generalized and concrete other. In *Feminism as Critique,* edited by S. Behabib and D. Cornell, 77–95. Oxford: Polity.

Bluebond-Langner, M. 1978. *The Private Worlds of Dying Children.* Princeton: Princeton University Press.

Bradley, B. 1989. *Visions of Infancy.* Cambridge: Polity.

Brazier, M. 1987. *Medicine, Patients and the Law.* Harmondsworth: Penguin.

British Medical Association. 2001. *Consent, Rights and Choices in Health Care for Children and Young People.* London: British Medical Association.

Buchanan, A., and D. Brock. 1989. *Deciding for Others.* New York: Cambridge University Press.

Burman, E. 1994. *Deconstructing Developmental Psychology.* London: Routledge.

Butler, M. 1998. Negotiating place: The importance of children's realities. In *Students as Researchers: Creating Classrooms that Matter,* edited by S. Steinberg and J. Kincheloe, 94–112. London: Falmer.

Christensen, P., and A. James, eds. 2000. *Research with Children: Perspectives and Practices.* London: Routledge Falmer.

Connolly, P., A. Smith, and B. Kelly. 2002. *Too Young to Notice? The Cultural and Political Awareness of 3–6 Year Olds in Northern Ireland.* NI Community Relations Council with TV Channel 4.

Damon, W. 1998. *The Moral Child.* New York: The Free Press.

Davis, D. 2001. *Genetic Dilemmas, Reproductive Technologies, Parental Choices, and Children's Futures.* New York: Routledge.

Dent, H., and R. Flin. 1992. *Children as Witnesses.* Chichester: Wiley.

Dunn, J. 1988. *The Beginnings of Social Understanding.* Oxford: Blackwell.

Eibl-Eibersfeldt, I. 1971. *Love and Hate.* London: Methuen.

Erikson, E. 1971. *Identity, Youth and Crisis.* London: Faber.

Faden, R., and T. Beauchamp. 1986. *A History and Theory of Informed Consent.* New York: Oxford University Press.

Feinberg, J. 1980. The child's right to an open future. In *Whose Child? Children's Rights, Parental Authority, and State Power,* edited by W. Aikin and H. La Fallette, 124–53. Totowa, NJ: Littlefield.

Frank, A. 2003. Surgical body modification and altruistic individualism. *Qualitative Health Research* 13 (10):1407–18.

Gardner, H. 1993. *The Unschooled Mind.* London: Fontana.

Gaylin, W., and R. Macklin. 1982. *Who Speaks for the Child?* New York: Plenum.

Gillick v Wisbech & W Norfolk AHA [1985] 3 All ER 402.

Gilligan, C. 1982. *In a Different Voice.* Cambridge, MA: Harvard University Press.

Goffman, E. 1959. *The Presentation of Self in Everyday Life.* Harmondsworth: Penguin.

Hall, G. S. 1904. *Adolescence: Its Psychology and its Relations to Physiology, Anthropology, Sociology, Sex, Crime, Religion and Education.* New York: Appleton.

Hutchby, I., and J. Moran-Ellis, eds. 1998. *Children and Social Competence: Arenas of Action.* London: Falmer.

In re R [1991] 4 All ER 177.

In re W [1992] 4 All ER 627.

James, A., and A. Prout, eds. 1997. *Constructing and Reconstructing Childhood.* London: Routledge Falmer.

Kagan, J., and S. Lamb, eds. 1987. *The Emergence of Morality in Young Children.* Chicago: University of Chicago Press.

Kennedy, E., and S. Mendus, eds. 1987. *Women in Western Political Philosophy.* Wheatsheaf: Brighton.

Kopelman, L., and J. Moskop, eds. 1989. *Children and Health Care: Moral and Social Issues.* Dordrecht: Kluwer.

Mayall, B. 2002. *Towards a Sociology for Childhood.* London: Routledge Falmer.

Mayall, B., ed. 1994. *Children's Childhoods: Observed and Experienced.* London: Falmer.

McCormick, R. 1974. Proxy consent in the experimental situation. *Perspectives in Biology and Medicine* 18 (1):2–20.

Melton, G., G. Koocher, and M. Saks, eds. 1983. *Children's Competence to Consent.* New York: Plenum.

Melzak, S. 1992. Secrecy, privacy, survival, repressive regimes and growing up. *Bulletin of Anna Freud Centre* 15:205–24.

Morss, J. 1990. *Biologising of Childhood.* Hillsdale, NJ: Erlbaum.

Murray, T. 1996. *The Worth of a Child.* Berkley: University of California Press.

Musgrove, F. 1984. *Youth and Social Order.* London: Routledge.

Myerson, G. 2000. *Donna Haraway and GM Foods.* London: Totem.

National Commission for the Protection of Human Subjects of Biomedical and Behavioural Research. 1977. *Research Involving Children* (DHEW, 77–0004). Washington, DC: President's Commission.

Nuremberg Code, 1947.

Qvortrup, J., M. Bardy, G. Sigritta, et al., eds. 1994. *Childhood Matters.* Aldershot: Avebury.

Ramsey, P. 1970. *The Patient as Person.* New Haven: Yale University Press.

Ross, L. F. 1998. *Children, Families and Health Care Decision Making.* New York: Oxford University Press.

Royal College of Paediatrics and Child Health, Ethics Advisory Committee. 2000. Guidelines on the ethical conduct of medical research involving children. *Archives of Disease in Childhood* 82:177–82.

Siegal, M. 1997. *Knowing Children: Experiments in Conversation and Cognition.* New York: Erlbaum.

Stainton Rogers, R. and W. 1992. *Stories of Childhood: Shifting Agendas in Child Concern.* Hemmel Hempstead: Harvester.

Sugarman, J., D. McCoy, D. Powell, et al., 1999. *Empirical Research on Informed Consent.* The Hastings Center Report Special Supplement.

United Nations. 1989. *Convention on the Rights of the Child.* New York: United Nations.

Waskler, F. 1991. *Studying the Social Worlds of Children.* London: Falmer.

Wilkinson, S. 1988. *The Child's World of Illness.* Cambridge: Cambridge University Press.

Winkler, M. 1998. Devices and desires of our own hearts. In *Enhancing Human Traits: Ethical and Social Implications,* edited by E. Parens, 238–50. Washington, DC: Georgetown University Press.

Zelizer, V. 1995. *Pricing the Priceless Child.* New York: Basic.

CHAPTER TWELVE

The Power of Parents and the Agency of Children

Hilde Lindemann, Ph.D.

The power relationship between parents and children is necessarily asymmetrical. It is a relationship in which physically, emotionally, and socially vulnerable persons must depend on others to keep them safe, nurture them, and teach them how to live within their society. In this chapter I argue that parents are morally remiss if they do not use the power they have over their children, but then I map out some of the moral dangers that beset parents who contemplate wielding that power by authorizing body-shaping surgery for children with physical anomalies. My hope is that by attending to these dangers, parents who face such decisions will be better able to exercise their power responsibly.

The Practice of Childcare

Let me begin by considering, in the most general terms, what parents are doing when they care for their children. In *Maternal Thinking*, Sara Ruddick points out that caring for children is a *practice*—that is, a socially recognized set of behaviors that is governed by rules and has a point (Ruddick 1989). She argues that the point of the practice—to preserve the child's life and health, to nurture the child's growth, and to teach the child how to live well among others—determines the kind of thinking in which its practitioners must engage. Keeping the child safe from harm, Ruddick believes, is "the central constitutive, invariant aim" of parental practice. Parents who are committed to achieving that aim do what they can to keep their children from drowning, wandering out into the traffic, eating poisonous substances, falling out the window, running afoul of a child molester, and so on. Children's need for protection does not automatically guarantee a response on the parents' part, but parents who engage in the practice of child care must see "the fact of biological vulnerability as socially significant and as demanding care" (ibid., 18, 19).

Children grow naturally, given favorable conditions for growing, but producing and maintaining those conditions, Ruddick believes, is an integral part of caring for one's child. Intellectual and emotional growth can be stunted as readily as physical growth if parents do not attend to it. Parents foster intellectual growth not only by sending their children to school, but by providing a climate in which the children are encouraged to ask questions and to develop their imaginations. Parents foster emotional growth by maintaining an atmosphere in which their children are allowed to express themselves and to know that they are loved.

If the point of the practice of caring for one's children includes preservation and nurturance, then we are already in a position to explain why parents are morally obliged to use their power: failure to do so could leave their children warped, stunted, or dead. The aims of preservation and nurturance do not, however, tell us very much about the moral risks attached to the exercise of parental power. For that, I suggest, we must look at the third part of the point of childcare—socialization.

Socialization involves such matters as teaching children to use the toilet, to eat with the proper fork, and to say please and thank you, but more broadly, it involves interacting with one's children on the basis of some rich and comprehensive notion of what life is about. In socializing their children, parents show them how, according to their own understanding of these matters, the children should live within and make sense of the society in which they are reared. They teach them what usually happens, how they can expect others to behave, what is expected of them, how things are supposed to be—all of which is governed by powerful social norms. They also teach them the consequences of violating these norms.

In the process, parents inevitably encumber their children with their own "thick" normative framework. It is thick in the sense that it comprises a complicated and extensive set of beliefs about how to live, covering everything from the behavioral standards of a particular social class or religious community to (for some of us) the principle that one should always replace the cap on the tube of toothpaste. And while grown children may repudiate some of the beliefs in the web that constitutes their parents' approach to life, they not infrequently find that remnants of their parents' precepts for living linger on in their own outlook. Many of us with adult children have experienced something like what happened to me a year or two ago, when my daughter rang me up one Saturday in October to accuse me of having forced her to wash her windows that morning. She says this happens to her every autumn, and probably will keep on happening long after I am gone.

Parents cannot help but encumber their children with their own understanding of how to live because, in a society where parents are assigned the responsibility for their children's upbringing, that is the only one available, at least until the child is old enough to realize that not everyone lives the way his father or mother does. This encumbrance is not, however, something that ought to be regarded as a regrettable necessity—not even if a part of the conception is that daughters are supposed to do women's work while sons are entitled to special treatment, that prayer is always more effective than medicine, that creationism is true, that the white race is superior, that people with AIDS deserve what they get, that war is glorious. Whatever it is, and no matter what we may think of certain components of it, the parental conception is the child's birthright, giving shape and color to his location in the world and furnishing crucial elements of his identity. In encumbering their children with their own normative framework, parents provide them with the conceptual resources that allow them to understand who they are, what their place within—or outside—the social order is, what they may expect from that, and how they are supposed to behave there.

The only altogether reliable way to foreclose the possibility that parents might saddle their children with a morally repugnant notion of how to live is to prevent them from socializing their children at all, and that is no real alternative. Children need to be socialized because human lives are inherently and necessarily social. People need their relationships with others not only so that they may flourish, but so that they may survive. Infants die without someone to tend them; adulthood involves interaction with others for even such supposedly solitary pursuits as reasoning and intending (Baier 1997). No human life can be lived at all, let alone well, outside some sort of social arrangement, and as navigating these arrangements requires training, socialization too is a central aim of parental practice.

Conceptions of How to Live

Authorizing surgery for children with congenital anomalies is a significant exercise of parental power. The decision is relatively unproblematic, from an ethical point of view, in those cases where the aim of the surgery is to *preserve* the child from physical harm or to *foster* the child's growth. Craniofacial surgeries, for example, that permit the child to eat or breathe normally, or rectal surgeries that allow the child to evacuate her bowels seem fairly straightforward responses to the child's needs. It is when parents request surgery for the purpose of *socializing* their children that they are at special risk of using their power irresponsibly. Because parents' conception of how to live is so central to how their children are socialized, it is bound to play a major role in their thinking about surgery whose purpose is to make their children's bodies conform more closely to the norms for acceptable appearance, so it matters a great deal what the parental conception is like.

Master Narratives

The social norms that inevitably form some part of a parental conception of what life is about are not the product of rational individual reflection and personal choice: it would be a staggering coincidence if millions of Americans all decided, independently, that women look good in high-heeled shoes but men look ridiculous. Instead, the standards for how things are supposed to be circulate widely throughout particular cultures by means of images and stories that are familiar to everyone in those cultures. The stories—Richard Delgado has dubbed them *master narratives* (Delgado 1995)—consist of the plot templates and character types that people use to make sense of their social worlds. Richard Nisbett and Lee Ross offer the example of one such plot template—the "restaurant script," which contains "entering," "ordering," "eating," "paying," and "exiting" scenes (Nisbett and Ross 1994). Because all of these scenes are very familiar, a person needs to observe just one of them to infer with a high degree of accuracy what happened earlier or will happen next. The restaurant script can be thought of as a stock plot in miniature, a story cliché that is an old cultural standby. The character types who populate these plot templates are equally familiar, and as Nisbett and Ross point out, a reference to the character is often sufficient to convey much of the action of the story—think of the whore with a heart of gold, for example, or the rebel without a cause.

Information about what to expect from certain types of people, as well as a society's standard operating procedures, is conveyed in the form of images and narratives that capture our imagination without our ever having to think about them. Master narratives are seductive, often absorbed unconsciously as they both guide and justify our sense of how things are supposed to be. It is the unconscious absorption of these images and stories that gives them so much of their hold over us. We take them for granted, which means we do not think about them, which means we need not explicitly criticize, accept, or reject them. And what often escapes us altogether is that these representations are *prescriptive*. Under the guise of description, they tell the members of a particular group how they are expected to act, and they tell everyone else how the group is supposed to be treated. "A lady never raises her voice" looks like a statement of fact, but there is a suppressed "should" in the statement that gives it the force of a command. In just that same way, a movie that appears simply to depict

African American men as drug dealers subtly reinforces the sense that most African American men can be *expected* to be drug dealers. (For Bourdieu's version of the master narrative idea, see Ellen Feder's chapter in this volume.)

A second reason why master narratives are so powerful is that they are evidence resistant. It makes no difference if you have never met anyone who behaves the way the master narratives show members of that group behaving, because what the master narratives say about the group is only common sense, what everybody knows, what one does not have to think about, what is necessarily and naturally true. Evidence to the contrary—even a great deal of evidence—has little power to alter what everybody knows. Worse yet, even when we *realize* that a master narrative is false, it can still exert power over us. Most people in contemporary American society do not really believe, for example, that African American men in general are drug dealers or that ladies never raise their voices, and if asked whether we believe these things we would vigorously deny it. All the same, these things that we do not believe have a propensity to influence us, subtly infecting our attitudes toward and expectations of the groups in question—even when we ourselves are members of those groups. We are apt to find ourselves reacting to the people these master narratives depict as if the stories had the ultimate say over who those people are.

Because master narratives cannot help but enter into everyone's conception of how to live, the question arises as to which of these narratives might put the parents at particular risk of misusing their power over their children as they contemplate body-normalizing surgery. There are many possibilities here, but I content myself with describing three: the master narrative of the Self-Absorbed Consumer, the master narrative of the Ugly Outcast, and the master narrative of the Scientific Fix. I do not claim that parents whose normative frameworks include one or more of these narratives will necessarily abuse their power if they consent to surgery aimed at making their children more socially acceptable, but I think that they have a special reason to reflect long and hard before permitting the surgery to go forward.

The Master Narrative of the Self-Absorbed Consumer

The philosopher Carl Elliott describes what he calls the consumption ethic in his book *Better than Well.* "Today," he writes, "buying has come to be seen as a legitimate, even obvious way to achieve well-being . . . Advertising is no longer just a means of selling goods; it is also an instrument for the transmission of values. Like television and the movies, advertising teaches us how to dress, how to furnish our homes, how to eat well, and how to be cool. It also tells us what kind of people deserve respect and which deserve ridicule, what romantic love looks like and how to find it, how to lead a successful life and how to be a failure. Many Americans today learn who they want to be not by listening to a Methodist minister or a civics teacher but by watching advertisements for The Gap" (Elliott 2003, 127).

The consumption ethic is installed and maintained by a system of interlocking stories that corporations use to promote their products and that, taken together, form the master narrative of the Self-Absorbed Consumer. Many of the stories are only a few seconds long, and some are tacit: advertising images that seem to stand on their own actually carry with them, like comets' tails, subtle but familiar stories embodying the norms to which consumers are encouraged to conform.

Consumption, Elliott observes, is part of a larger moral system that involves a number of capitalist values. It is a system that promotes *self-fulfillment:* the narrative of the Self-Absorbed Consumer represents people as aiming at a certain lifestyle open to only a few, buying things so that they can become the kind of person who attains that lifestyle, and being self-fulfilled when they have attained it. The system promotes *self-expression:* the Consumer narrative represents people buying luxury items as a way of expressing who they are, as if owning a Porsche were akin to celebrating Passover or composing a symphony. And the system prizes *authenticity:* the narrative connects consumption not only to self-expression, but to the expression of one's "real" self; the woman exclaims that this house, sofa, shade of lipstick "is really me," and we see that the Prozac she purchases makes her feel more like herself.

In sum, the master narrative of the Self-Absorbed Consumer depicts an ethos whose "locus of meaning is the self, not any higher commitments outside the self" (Elliott 2003, 141). It portrays the world as valuable only for what it can do for me, bidding me to achieve my interests in the most economically efficient way. This kind of reasoning, which focuses solely on means rather than ends, is what the philosopher Charles Taylor calls "instrumental rationality" (Taylor 1989). Elliott's example of instrumental thinking is the rationale behind suburban housing. These houses, he says, rather than being places of "engagement with the world," are designed to satisfy the need for sleeping, eating, safety, entertainment, and to satisfy this need efficiently, they make use of all sorts of technologies—central heating, electric garage-door openers, dishwashers, garbage disposals, riding mowers, and answering machines—that "transform the house, in Corbusier's famous phrase, into a 'machine for living'" (Elliott 2003, 148).

The philosopher Albert Borgmann calls this the transformation of a "thing" into a "device." Things, he argues, are inseparable from their contexts, so our engagement with the thing is also an engagement with its context. By contrast, devices, which are the product of instrumental rationality, are merely efficient means of achieving an end result. Devices are designed to accomplish their purpose with minimal skill and effort, so their appeal quickly wears out and they are then replaced by other devices. They are not meant to be cherished or valued—they are just supposed to be used. (For the Heideggerian roots of this analysis, see James Edwards's chapter in this volume.)

Notice that it is the employment of garage-door openers and other gadgets that, on Elliott's account, turns a house—or a wilderness area, or an eating establishment—from a thing into a device. I am not sure he is right about this, but I do think that when the master narrative of the Self-Absorbed Consumer circulates widely in one's culture, it is amazingly easy to transform things—and people—into devices, to see them in an important sense as instruments meant to serve one's own purposes. (Again, see James Edwards's chapter for more on this idea.) And this raises a serious moral worry about socially normalizing surgeries. If the master narrative of the Self-Absorbed Consumer is a part of the parents' thick vision of how to live, then might their motivation for using these surgeries stem partly from regarding their own children as "devices" for self-promotion? Might they, for example, be ashamed of a son or daughter whose appearance is abnormal, feeling that the child sends the wrong message about who they themselves are? And there is a further worry: Might the widespread use of these surgeries actually *reinforce* the power of this master narrative? (Little 1998).

My concern here is not that such parents have failed to mark a clear boundary between themselves and their children. In a properly loving relationship that boundary ought to be blurred in at least as many places as it remains distinct. The personal pride the parent feels in the deeds of the child, like the personal distress occasioned by the child's pain, are evidence of the intermingling of selves that is love at work. What poses a danger when the master narrative of the Self-Absorbed Consumer is a part of parents' view of the good is not love but *arrogance:* the parents are at risk of consuming their children by arrogating to themselves the children's looks and social success.

The Master Narrative of the Ugly Outcast

Parents are not likely to acknowledge to themselves, let alone to their children or their children's physicians, that their concern about their children's appearance is grounded in parental self-absorption. A far more common justification for surgery is the child's own well-being. Children who are visibly disfigured face rejection by their peers; they are teased, laughed at, taunted, and made to feel ashamed. Loving parents quite rightly worry that a serious scar, blemish, or deformity will severely affect their child's ability to lead a normal social life.

The master narrative of the Ugly Outcast enters into almost everyone's conception of a good life. It consists of the stories—from "The Ugly Duckling" to *Pretty Woman*—

that link social acceptance to looking good. The narrative shows us the friendless 90-pound weakling who muscles up and finds himself surrounded by a bevy of beautiful women. It shows us the lonely spinster who casts off her spectacles, lets down her hair, and lives happily ever after with the leading man. It shows us that the most popular high school girls are thin and wear designer clothing and that rising corporate executives look like Tom Cruise. It shows us that blondes have more fun.

Primarily, however, the narrative of the Ugly Outcast portrays the social rejection of the physically deformed. Frankenstein's monster, the Hunchback of Notre Dame, and *To Kill a Mockingbird*'s Boo Radley are only a few of the characters in the popular imagination who are exiled from their community and feared by their neighbors on account of their looks. Often, too, the narrative depicts physically ugly people as morally ugly. The humpbacked Richard III falls at the Battle of Bosworth, reaping the fruits of his villainy and shouting for his horse. The hag-ugly Cruella DeVille nearly succeeds in her plot to murder 101 defenseless puppies for their fur. Stories like these connect with other stories on similar themes, to produce an extensive network of intertwining ideas about the role of good looks in winning social acceptance.

Empirical data suggest that the master narrative of the Ugly Outcast reflects a sorry social reality. The economists Daniel Hamermesh and Jeff Biddle reported in 1993, for example, that beautiful people earn more than ugly ones. Their study indicated that while good looks increase one's hourly income by about 5 percent, ugliness decreases it by 7 percent (Haiken 1997). Another study suggests that something similar happens in the classroom, where teachers' expectations regarding their pupils' academic achievements are influenced by how the pupil looks. Teachers do not merely expect their good-looking students to be academically successful—they grade the work of disfigured students less favorably, punish them more harshly, and give them less in-class attention (Walters 1997, 27).

Master narratives are often deeply enmeshed with other master narratives, and this one is no exception. There is a master narrative of Women's Place in Society, which assigns social recognition to men's deeds, but to women's looks. According to this master narrative, the work associated with women, such as housekeeping, childcare, teaching, and care of the sick, is less important than the work associated with men, such as national defense, running corporations, and scientific research. Women, then, are not valued for the work they do (though they are expected to do it)—they are valued, or scorned, for the way they look. The narrative of Women's Place in Society strongly features the view that girls and women must monitor themselves carefully so that they will appear as attractive as possible, dieting, exercising, caring for their skin and hair, and dressing in ways that feature their strong points and camouflage unsightly defects. All girls and women feel the force of this master narrative, even though many resist it. A girl whose body presents an abnormal appearance may therefore find herself subjected to two sets of master narratives at once: because she is deformed, she can expect to be an outcast, and because she is female, she is required to police her appearance anyway.

Parents whose vision of the good life is informed by the master narrative of the Ugly Outcast may be able to disentangle it to some degree from the narrative of Women's Place. They may reject the story that conditions women's worth on looking good, and resist the temptation to pressure a daughter who is disfigured to "make up for it" by keeping her weight down or steering her toward particularly feminine clothing. But they may still want to do everything humanly possible to gain social acceptance for their child. The danger posed by this desire, however, is that *even if* body-shaping surgery produces that acceptance (and more about that in a moment), it is apt to misfire.

Recall that the parents we are now talking about do not (at least consciously) view their children as extensions of themselves, but are instead concerned with their children's well-being. They therefore do not seek social acceptance for their children as an end in itself, but rather as a means to an end: they value it because their children cannot live well without it. Their children, however, may find it difficult to grasp this distinction between inherent and instrumental value—it is, after all, a distinction that eludes many adults. When children see their parents spending (or having spent) serious amounts of time, money, and effort to ensure that they will be more like everyone else, they might interpret that expenditure as a sign of parental love and commitment. But they are at least as likely to see the need for social acceptance as evidence that they are unacceptable. Or they may see it as evidence that what others think of them is far more important than what they themselves think (Asch, this volume). Either of the negative interpretations will make it much harder for the children to acquire self-respect. And that is how the parental desire misfires, for self-respect is even more necessary to a good life than social acceptance is. To sacrifice self-respect in the hopes of gaining social acceptance is to pay far too high a price for that acceptance.

The Master Narrative of the Scientific Fix

The stories portraying science as holding the whip hand over nature go back at least to the seventeenth century. One of the founders of modern science, Francis Bacon, wrote that his "only earthly wish" was "to stretch the deplorably narrow limits of man's dominion over the universe to their promised bounds." He spoke of science's ability to help mankind unite "against the Nature of things, to storm and occupy her castles and strongholds," and declared, "I am come in very truth leading you to Nature with all her children to bind her to your service and make her your slave . . . The mechanical inventions of recent years do not merely exert a gentle guidance over Nature's courses, they have the power to conquer and subdue her, to shake her to her foundations" (Farrington 1970, 92, 93, 129–30).

In one variation of the story representing science as nature's conqueror, it is engineering science that defeats nature, allowing people to defy the force of gravity, communicate instantly with one another over great distances, store and retrieve vast amounts of information, and travel at enormous speed. The most common version of the narrative, however, features medical science as the protagonist. In the person of the white-coated or green-gowned doctor, medical science conquers disease, repairs broken bodies, unlocks the secrets of the human genome, and increases the human lifespan. In all its variants, the master narrative of the Scientific Fix shows science not merely overpowering nature, but using that power to correct nature's flaws. The handicap of winglessness is overcome by aeronautical engineering; the malfunctioning kidney is replaced by biomedical technology.

The master narrative of the Scientific Fix is embodied in many stories of sickness. The characters and diagnosis may vary widely, but the plot remains the same: the person is congenitally abnormal, badly injured, or seriously ill; nature, under the guidance of science, is bound to the doctor's service and made his slave; and the person is either restored to health or made whole for the first time. This plot, which Arthur Frank has dubbed the *restitution narrative,* is by no means the only one a story of sickness can have (Frank 1995). But it is certainly the most popular one, and it is the plot required by this particular master narrative.

My concern about the narrative of the Scientific Fix is not that it is false. Indeed, it is *not* entirely false, though health care practitioners and bioethicists alike have tended to greet it with skepticism. What worries me, rather, is that it is *dangerous,* not so much for what it represents as for what it conceals. Parents whose normative framework includes this narrative and who are faced with the decision to subject their children to normalizing surgery may abuse their power over their children if they do not attend to the morally relevant details that the story hides from view.

In the first place, the master narrative does not reveal the many instances in which the surgery fails to make the child look normal, or how this failure keeps the goal of social acceptance from being fully achieved. Craniofacial surgeries will usually leave visible scars, and while parents and children alike may prefer them to gross deformities, the child who has undergone surgery may nevertheless find herself the object of taunts, rude questions, and teasing. Limb-lengthening surgery likewise can do no more than lengthen limbs; it cannot remove all visible manifestations of achondroplasia.

In the second place, the master narrative does not describe what children may have to go through to achieve even the more modest results of diminished teasing and greater social acceptance. Often, they undergo repeated surgeries, suffer many bouts of pain, endure long periods of mind-numbing immobility, require continuous medical monitoring, and miss a considerable amount of school. After one kind of normalizing genital surgery, they are subjected to painful dilation several times a week to keep their surgically constructed vaginas open. And, as I mentioned previously, there is always the possibility that the child will not be able to attain self-respect, either because she believes she is not acceptable as she is or because she has learned that what others think of her matters far more than what she herself thinks. The master narrative of the Scientific Fix is silent about all of these matters.

In the third place, the master narrative conceals the damage that the surgery itself can do. Even the most technically sophisticated sex-assignment surgeries performed in infancy can later produce sexual dysfunction, loss of sensation, and pain during intercourse. Limb-lengthened bones can break easily. Craniofacial surgical scalpels can accidentally nick a nerve and cause a muscle to sag. Parents are of course warned of most of these risks, but the narrative of the Scientific Fix can exert so much power over their imaginations that the danger of iatrogenic damage might seem negligible or remote.

Fourth and perhaps most crucially, the master narrative of the Scientific Fix keeps the parents' attention focused firmly on *fixing,* as though that response to a child's disfigurement were the best and only one. Behind the impulse to fix, however, lies the presumption of control—the faith not only that human beings have the power to correct nature's mistakes, but that they have a responsibility to exercise that power. The converse assumption is also taken on faith: human beings have no responsibility for the things they cannot control. Because loving parents want to take responsibility for bringing it about that their children have good lives, they cling to the hope that they can control the disfigurements or disabilities that threaten to stand in the way of the child's living well.

Parents do, of course, have a responsibility to try to bring it about that their children's lives are good, but a part of what this involves is teaching their children how to respond to circumstances that are *beyond* their control. The philosopher Margaret Urban Walker identifies three virtues that figure prominently in that response. *Lucidity* is the virtue of grasping the fact that the world does not always bend to our will. It is the clear understanding that despite our best efforts, our responsibilities sometimes outrun our control, and that much of what befalls us, for good or for ill, is a matter of luck. *Integrity* is the virtue of preserving one's moral self, keeping that self from shattering, corruption, or decay. From the perspective of others, Walker observes, integrity amounts to dependability in one's moral conduct, "not just in the long run or in the sphere of the everyday, but more especially in trying times where unwanted circumstance proposes more severe tests"(Walker 2003, 27). *Grace* is the virtue of living with what cannot be fixed, resisting fantasies of repair or restitution and accepting the limits of one's own effectiveness. Parents whose vision of the right way to live is heavily infused by the master narrative of the Scientific Fix may find it difficult to teach their children these crucially important virtues.

No society could function without master narratives that are known to all and that serve as summaries of socially shared understandings. Without such narratives, the members of the society would not be able to make sense of themselves, their neighbors, or their world. The narratives of the Self-Absorbed Consumer, the Ugly Outcast, and the Scientific Fix are morally suspect, then, not because they are master narratives, but because they bid us to understand ourselves, our neighbors, and our world in morally defective ways. Parents of children with serious physical abnormalities would do well, when considering the power they have over their children, to reflect on the power these narratives have over them.

Coda

Elsewhere in this volume, Lisa Abelow Hedley recounts her struggle with the seductive master narrative I have called the Scientific Fix, as she and her husband contemplate limb-straightening surgery for their daughter LilyClaire. LilyClaire at age 7 is bowlegged due to achondroplasia, and her doctor recommends the operation to avoid damaging misalignment and wear and tear on cartilage. Like all good parents, Hedley takes seriously her responsibility to protect her child from damage, though questions remain about whether to proceed now or to wait until there is clearer evidence that the damage will in fact occur. But then comes the temptation: given that LilyClaire will undergo the surgery and endure the attendant pain and months of immobility, why not lengthen the limbs as well as straightening them, and add between 2 and 4 inches of extra height? Here the goal is not just protection and nurturance, but socialization: LilyClaire will look more like other children, and this will enhance her chances of blending in better.

Hedley realizes that her vision of the good life is informed by the master narrative of the Scientific (or, as she puts it, "Surgical") Fix, and she admirably fends off its seduction. Perhaps at 3:00 in the morning she might also feel the pull of the master narrative of the Self-Absorbed Consumer, though she would certainly repudiate that one as well. It is the narrative of the Ugly Outcast that I suspect haunts her daily, as it presumably haunts all good parents whose children present an unusual appearance. But if Hedley and her husband act on that narrative, LilyClaire would, as Hedley herself acknowledges, "bloody well get the very message I know we must never send: We love you, you're perfect the way you are . . . now change."

Hedley needs a counterstory that can first uproot and then replace the bedeviling Outcast narrative. She is fortunate, however, because very close by her is the resource for such a story. I refer to LilyClaire herself, who has already fashioned a counterstory to offer when inquisitive strangers ask her about why she is so small, why her head is big, why she looks the way she does. The story has two parts. First, as she tells her mother, nobody has the right to explain her to people. And second, if *she* feels like explaining, "I will say that I fell out of a tree and broke my legs and shrank." The story is a delightful bit of nonsense that says in the politest way possible that inquisitive people should mind their own business. As Hedley's essay reveals, she is blessed with a fair amount of lucidity, integrity, and grace. But should these virtues fail her momentarily, she can rely on those of LilyClaire.

REFERENCES

Baier, A. 1997. *The Commons of the Mind,* Paul Carus Lecture. Chicago: Open Court.

Delgado, R., ed. 1995. *Critical Race Theory: The Cutting Edge.* Philadelphia: Temple University Press.

Elliott, C. 2003. *Better than Well: American Medicine Meets the American Dream.* New York: W. W. Norton.

Farrington, B. 1970. *The Philosophy of Francis Bacon.* New York: Haskell.

Frank, A. 1995. *The Wounded Storyteller: Body, Illness, and Ethics.* Chicago: University of Chicago Press.

Haiken, E. 1997. *Venus Envy: A History of Cosmetic Surgery.* Baltimore: Johns Hopkins University Press.

Little, M. O. 1998. Cosmetic surgery, suspect norms, and the ethics of complicity. In *Enhancing Human Traits,* edited by E. Parens, 162–76. Washington, DC: Georgetown University Press.

Nisbett, R., and L. Ross. 1994. Judgmental heuristics and knowledge structures. In *Naturalizing Epistemology,* edited by H. Kornblith, 261–90. 2d ed. Cambridge: MIT Press.

Ruddick, S. 1989. *Maternal Thinking: Toward a Politics of Peace.* Boston: Basic.

Taylor, C. 1989. *Sources of the Self.* Cambridge, MA: Harvard University Press.

Walker. M. U. 2003. Moral luck and the virtues of impure agency. In *Moral Contexts,* 21–34. Lanham, MD: Rowman & Littlefield.

Walters, E. 1997. Problems faced by children and families living with visible differences. In *Visibly Different: Coping with Disfigurement,* edited by R. Lansdown et al., 112–20. London: Oxford University Press.

CHAPTER THIRTEEN

"In Their Best Interests"

Parents' Experience of Atypical Genitalia

Ellen K. Feder, Ph.D.

In a study conducted by psychologist Suzanne Kessler, college students were asked to imagine that they had been born with clitoromegaly, a condition defined as having a clitoris larger than one centimeter at birth. In response to the question as to whether they would have wanted their parents to sanction clitoral surgery if the condition were not life-threatening, an overwhelming 93 percent of the students reported that they would not have wanted their parents to agree to surgery. Kessler reports that "women predicted that having a large clitoris would not have had much of an impact on their peer relations and almost no impact on their relations with their parents . . . They were more likely to want surgery to reduce a large nose, large ears, or large breasts than surgery to reduce a large clitoris" (Kessler 1998, 101).[1]

These findings, Kessler reflects, are not surprising given that the respondents characterized genital sensation and the capacity for orgasm as "very important to the average woman, and the size of the clitoris as being not even 'somewhat important'" (ibid. 101–2). Men in the study were faced with a different dilemma, the one facing parents of boys with "micropenis," a penis smaller than the putative standard of 2.5 centimeters at birth. Their question was whether to stay as male with a small penis or to be reassigned as female. More than half rejected the prospect of gender reassignment. But, according to Kessler, that percentage increases to almost all men if the surgery was described as reducing pleasurable sensitivity or orgasmic capability. Contrary to beliefs about male sexuality, the college men in this study did not think that having a micropenis would have had a major impact on their sexual relations, peer or parental relations, or self-esteem (ibid.).

In a separate study, Kessler and her team asked students to imagine that their child was born with ambiguous genitalia. Students in this study indicated they would make what Kessler describes as "more traditional choices" to consent to "corrective" or cosmetic surgery. Their rationales mirrored those of parents that can now be found on Internet bulletin boards devoted to parenting intersexed children: students reported that they did not want their child to feel "different," and believed that early surgery would be less traumatizing than later surgery (ibid.). Like parents over the last forty years who have been faced with these difficult decisions, students did not reflect on the somatic experience of the child, and with it, the possibility of lost sensation that so concerned the students in the first study.

Kessler's paired studies confirm a kind of common sense that individuals, as individuals, are disinclined to compromise their erotic response for the sake of cosmetic enhancement. At the same time, parents, as parents, want "what is best for their child," and the promise of a "normal life" figures prominently in that conception. The juxtaposition of the two studies raises the obvious, if nonetheless vexing, question: Why would parents consent to procedures on behalf of their children that they would refuse for themselves?

The work of social theorist Pierre Bourdieu, I suggest in the first part of this chapter, provides a powerful descriptive framework that can account for what might be characterized as the ambivalence that marks parents' experience, and the heavy responsibility they must bear to conceal that ambivalence from others, and from themselves. I then turn in the second part to parents' own stories. What is most salient in the stories, as they tell them, is the acute vulnerability that attends their efforts to do what is best for their children. All parents are, as parents, vulnerable; they must rely on others to do their work as parents. And yet, this vulnerability can be masked by parents' roles as protectors of their children (Kittay 1999; Nelson, this volume). Though the parents I interviewed live thousands of miles away from one another, and a thirty-year difference separates the birth of their children, their experiences are remarkably similar. All speak of intense isolation: they carry the burden of the secrets doctors encouraged them to keep from their child, their neighbors, and their extended families. Those with grown children recount the anger and despair of their sons and daughters who cannot have normal sex lives and who hold them responsible for the silence to which they were also subject. Parents' situation, as I propose in the third section, presents a conflict in the intention to ensure the best interests of the child. The guilt and shame that typically characterize parents' experience is owing, I conclude, to a situation in which parents' caring identification with their children is forsaken in the well-intentioned effort to tend to these best interests.

The Imperative of Normality

While obvious on its face, the question of why parents would consent to cosmetic genital surgeries is really one of the most difficult raised by the conventional management of intersexed infants. Its difficulty lies, I think, in the fact that seeking answers demands that we investigate areas of understanding resistant to critical examination—areas we call "common sense," or "what goes without saying." This is the realm that Pierre Bourdieu has called the *habitus*. It is not so easy to objectify a structure that, on Bourdieu's analysis, natively resists such objectification, but understanding something of the mechanics of *habitus* promises genuine insight into parents' experience. Bourdieu provides a number of ways of getting at how *habitus* works. It functions, he says, as "durable . . . dispositions," or "principles which generate and organize practices and representations that can be objectively adapted to their outcomes without presupposing a conscious aiming at ends or an express mastery of the operations necessary in order to attain them." It is at once a stable framework, a "structured structure," and a dynamic "structuring structure" (Bourdieu 1990, 53) ordering action and understanding in the seamless ways that we take for granted in ordinary life. As Bourdieu describes it, the understanding that is sustained by *habitus* is not then, for the most part, a reflected understanding. Playing by the rules of *habitus*, in other words, does not entail an *intention* to follow the rules, and moreover does not require understanding or conscious recognition of the rules.[2]

For example, we take for granted the fact of sexual difference. That the world is comprised of men and women, boys and girls, orders our world and regulates practices in countless unreflected ways. That is not to say that there isn't disagreement where questions of sex and gender are concerned. Indeed, controversy concerning what it means to be a man or a woman, what social roles and political rights these entail, is a thriving concern. But sexual difference *as* sexual difference is not for the most part in dispute. In fact, sexual difference could be said to be the primary structure that itself structures the social order in which we move and make sense of the world. As such, it is also a structure that can be understood, at the same time, to make sense of us, that is, to place us in the world in ways that render the positions we occupy, the roles we play—as girls and boys, daughters and sons, mothers and fathers—intelligible; sexual difference provides order for the world and for our place in it.

Parents' wishes to have normal children and their fears about the consequences— for themselves and for their children—of living outside the norm, are also products of this structuring structure. *Of course*, we might say, one wishes to have normal children; one could not wish for one's children anything but the easy path that normality promises. The concept of *habitus* marks this realm of the taken-for-granted, what is not questioned, what might be understood, in philosophical terms, as a kind of implicit normative order—a normative order that nowhere spells out the rules, that nowhere commands obedience to rules, but works, at the same time, to regulate practices in conformity with a prevailing social order. If the management of intersexed children suggests that there are in fact rules of normality that must be followed, these rules are not the rules of mere social convention, but something more along the lines of what might be described as a "cultural unconscious," conventions that are not considered and weighed, thoughtfully enacted *by* individuals but conventions that could more precisely be understood to work *through* individuals.[3]

What Kessler's paired studies suggest is that even as these conventions powerfully enforce a discernible regularity in individuals' responses to given situations, these regularities, forceful as they are, can also be in conflict—an instance of competing *habituses*. Following Bourdieu, the conflict presented by the very appearance of ambiguous genitalia must be concealed lest it disrupt the taken-for-granted conceptions of "normality" that ground social practices. Parents of children with ambiguous genitalia, then, must not only bear the burden of the secret of their children's difference, but are also responsible for masking the tension produced by the necessity of concealing this difference. They must do so not only for themselves and their children, but for the sake of the preservation of the prevailing *habitus* itself.

Parents' Stories

In the literature on surgical correction of ambiguous genitalia in children, parents make the briefest of appearances.[4] The leading roles go to doctors, who recommend and execute surgical decisions, and the children themselves, who appear not so much as children as discrete body parts (see Dreger 1999, 18–19; Dreger 2000): a hypospadiac penis in a "before" picture displayed urinating from a new meatus in an "after" picture; a phallic clitoris that is then shown after recession or trimming; or even a whole child with eyes concealed by a black patch to preserve anonymity. Neither sons nor daughters, but pure organs or subjects, such representations resist association with living children, complete with parents and communities. Despite the distorted images represented in the pictures, despite the difficulty one might face in imagining lives in place of body parts, parents' absence nevertheless becomes conspicuous when we consider the emphasis placed on parental response as a determining factor in the success of corrective surgery measured by the adjustment of children to their assigned gender (Money and Erhardt 1982). The silence surrounding parents' experience, then, mirrors the silence parents are asked to, and willingly maintain, regarding their children's condition.

When I tried to make contact with parents in the spring of 2000, I encountered significant resistance and suspicion. Many parents thought that my interest couldn't really be in their stories or in their experience, but a ploy to gain access to their children of whose welfare they were so rightly protective. It was difficult for many parents, and particularly parents of younger children, to understand why there would be any interest in their own stories. One reason may be owing to the unusual degree of isolation they experience, isolation consistent with the treatment protocol first advocated by the psychologist John Money and accepted for more than three decades. While parents of children with other congenital problems are urged to seek help, to join or form support groups, and to bring their children in contact with others like themselves, parents of children with ambiguous genitalia have not been given the opportunity to meet with other parents; the possibility of consultation with mental health professionals with expertise in intersex or even gender development is not presented to them. At the same time that they are urged to keep the truth about their children to themselves, they are led to believe that the intersex condition has been corrected, and that their children will grow up to be normal girls or boys. In this context, it is easy to see why parents find it difficult to understand themselves as subjects of interest in their own right.

I was introduced to many of the parents of older and adult children I interviewed between May 2000 and August 2001 by personal contacts; others, and particularly those with younger children, were contacted through new Internet bulletin boards devoted to parents of children with medical conditions associated with ambiguous genitalia. Starting in 1995, adults with intersex have been speaking publicly about the debilitating physical and emotional effects of cosmetic genital surgeries; the disturbing questions raised by these stories had begun to be taken up by parents who faced, or who had recently consented to, surgeries for their children. Parents posting to these boards demonstrate considerable diversity of experience—some speak with confidence and certainty that their children have been "fixed," while others express anguish and confusion associated with their decisions. The parents who agreed to speak with me demonstrated a similar diversity, with a majority of those with older children critical of decisions they may have once embraced.

The mother I call "Ruby" was the first who agreed to speak with me, breaking a silence maintained for more than two decades. Both of Ruby's daughters were born with congenital adrenal hyperplasia (CAH).[5] While most intersex conditions are not associated with medical conditions as severe as those suffered by Ruby's children, I begin with this story because it also highlights the distinctive nature and consequences of the treatment of medical issues associated with intersex on the one hand, and the cosmetic issues on the other. It is telling also for the reason that, despite significant refinements in cosmetic surgical techniques, Ruby's story presages the experience of parents ten, twenty, and even thirty years later.[6]

Ruby's Story

The first was born in 1961. Doctors thought she was a boy. Her clitoris was enlarged, her labia fused. She was given a male name. But she became sick almost immediately. She couldn't breastfeed, she lost weight, and on New Year's Eve we took her to the ER. The doctors thought she was going to die, but one doctor knew about pediatric endocrinology, and transferred her to the children's hospital in the city. They diagnosed her with CAH and explained that she was female. She had no testicles, but a uterus and ovaries.

At 3 months, she hemorrhaged; her urethra was connected to her vagina. She had surgery, and they performed a clitorectomy at the same time. She had another surgery when she was 2.

The same thing happened with my second daughter. Everyone thought, "This one's the boy," but I knew. I just knew it was a girl, but we gave her a boy's name. When we brought her home she became very sick. So I insisted that we be sent to the children's hospital again. She was kept in the hospital for a long time, because the doctors thought that any talk about a son would upset my older daughter. At 3 months she had the clitorectomy. This was a female, and she needed to look like a female. They did leave tissue, but she had a series of infections and she had more surgeries—five by the time she was 5 years old. She has almost no clitoris left, and massive scarring.

My daughters received medical care throughout their childhood. Once a month, sometimes more, we drove a whole day to get to the hospital. Fifteen hours there and fifteen hours back, with two active children in the back seat. And at the hospital I would have to fight the doctors. They would conduct a study on the salt levels, and make my children sick, and I had to yell at them to stop. The doctors almost gave up on my younger daughter, and I took over a lot of her care. I had to dilate her urethra, and it was so hard. I did cultures for the doctors, too. I grew the bacteria, and the doctors would tell me what antibiotics to give her. I was the one who had to coordinate her care, and I was determined that my daughter not die because her mom didn't fight for her. We were lucky to be part of these studies, though. As my daughters got older, they started to complain about the examinations. But somebody before my first child was born allowed these doctors—many doctors—to examine their child, to figure out what all this was about. My younger daughter is angry with me as an adult. She felt that she was raped, medically raped. And she's right. And I know how she feels. When you have a baby, you lose your right to modesty, and everyone is looking everywhere. But it was necessary, in my mind, just like when I gave birth. I told my daughters I wish we didn't have to do this. How would you feel having seventeen doctors look at you all at once? But it wasn't just that I felt a responsibility. This was a teaching hospital, and their treatment was being subsidized.

No one wanted to talk about the gender issues, how my daughters wouldn't play with their dolls. Both girls are gay. No one wanted to talk about that. Their father didn't want to deal with the gender issues at all, and his family thought that we had turned two little boys into girls. We divorced in 1976.

I had pastors who told me that they didn't know how to pray for me. And I told them I know how you can pray for me. You imagine a God who is bigger than all of these problems and you ask Him to help me.

As infants and young children, humans are vulnerable. Others, most often parents, must provide what dependent beings cannot provide for themselves. Children who are ill or medically fragile are not exceptions in this respect; their needs magnify the needs—for preservative love, fostering growth, and training for social acceptance (Ruddick 1989)—that are common to all children. As the needs of these children are magnified, so too are the corresponding demands on parents with ill or medically fragile children. Those engaged in the practices of mothering will recognize the love that motivates Ruby's determination that her "daughter not die because her mom didn't fight for her." Ruby's explanation to her daughters of the need to consent to invasive examinations reveals both an attempt to foster moral growth and to teach a difficult lesson in training for social acceptance: other parents sacrificed their children's comfort so that doctors could help you, she tells them, and now we are obliged to do the same. And in life there are times that you must "go along to get along." Sometimes there's no choice.

Such lessons are ones with which Ruby herself must grapple in the day-to-day care of her children. Having experienced the withdrawal of the support of her family—first by her in-laws, who believed she had robbed them of a grandson two times over, and then by her husband, who failed in so many ways to stand by his wife—Ruby finds herself not only alone, but completely dependent on the individual physicians managing the medical studies that subsidized her children's care. Refusal to consent to experimental treatments or yet another examination of her children's genitals would have put Ruby and her family at considerable financial, and thereby medical, risk. Caught in a bind of financial and medical exigency, Ruby could not really be understood to have a choice in the matter. To refuse a medical intervention would have effectively constituted a risk to her children's lives. This was a risk she would assume only at those times when she clearly perceived that an intervention itself posed a worse threat. That a mother would be faced with such a dilemma starkly underscores the special vulnerability to which Ruby is subject.

The "gender issues." What Ruby calls the "gender issues" form a part of any parent's raising of a child. Training for social acceptance may require a mother to direct her daughter to behave at times more like a girl or teach her son to behave more like a boy. In some cases, a parent may come to believe that a social script dictating a particular gender behavior is not appropriate for her child. Parents with convictions concerning the problematic nature of gender scripts may resist the imperative that encourages them to direct their children to behave according to norms linked with a particular gender. For the most part, however, mothers generally harbor no doubts or anxieties about the "true sex" of their children. Absent such doubts or questions, a mother might shrug off a daughter's aversion to dolls. She needn't question whether her lack of interest is a sign that her daughter isn't really a girl or wonder whether she did the right thing in treating her as a girl. Anxiety that parents may feel if a daughter prefers trucks or a son prefers dolls may be concerned not so much with their child's sex but with the possibility that their child might experience homosexual desire. The difference between the kind of gender panic manifested by parents afraid that their otherwise normal girl or boy might be gay, and that experienced by parents of children with ambiguous genitalia is the apparent tangibility of the diagnosis of intersex.[7]

As Ruby tells it, the "gender issues" first emerged in the criticism directed at her by her husband's family following the discovery that the children first announced as boys were, in fact, girls. They came up again when the children were just about school age; Ruby remembers the support group that doctors had finally permitted parents involved in the long-term study to form. While parents spoke about the challenges involved in staving off adrenal crises and coping with communicating their children's needs to teachers and school nurses, the children played outdoors. Seeing their sons and daughters interact, parents began to take note of the fact that their girls and boys rarely split up along gender lines to play, and the parents of girls became interested in how similar their little "tomboys" were to the other little girls. Emboldened by her observations of the other children and understanding, for the first time, that she was not alone, Ruby started to raise questions. "*Why,*" Ruby remembers insistently asking the doctors, "do my girls behave this way? And what can I do to help them be more like girls?" Most of the doctors at the hospital had no answers to her questions. One impatiently cut her short: "They're girls. What's the problem?" It is tempting to speculate that the repeated failures to respond meaningfully to Ruby's questions might be symptomatic of doctors' own anxiety over whether they had made the right decisions in the management of Ruby's daughters. Ruby herself suspected then that it was the questions parents were beginning to raise that prompted doctors to withdraw their authorization of the support group and to take measures to ensure that it no longer met.

Vulnerability and trust. As a parent, Ruby made decisions on behalf of her young children. Such is the responsibility of those who must meet the needs of one who cannot meet them for herself. Where Ruby's own experience fell short of her ability to discern her children's needs, she learned what was necessary to identify them. More than thirty years later, she remains an expert on her daughters' CAH symptoms, identifying imminent crises before her daughters themselves recognize them. And yet, her connection to her daughters, and particularly her younger daughter, was strained for many years—the result, all agree, of the treatment of their ambiguous genitalia. It was not Ruby who performed surgery or conducted the exams. But it was Ruby who, willing or not, witting or not, sanctioned these actions. The tragic paradox of Ruby's situation is precisely this: her caring and concerned attempts to fulfill her responsibility to her daughters' well-being led her to consent to actions that resulted in harm to her daughters, and eventually, to an erosion of her connection with them.

Trust is one of the factors crucial to the success of the relationship between a parent and child. The fraying of trust between Ruby and her daughters is not owing to any questionable intentions on Ruby's part. Rather, it is Ruby's own vulnerability to her children's doctors that renders fragile, in turn, Ruby's relationship with her daughters. Her complicity in making decisions and maintaining secrets that effected so much harm in the lives of her daughters drove a wedge between her and the daughters for whom, and about whom, she cares so fiercely. Ruby's children experienced pain, momentary and enduring, physical and emotional, as a result of decisions in which she participated. And yet, isolated by doctors and herself subject to the secrecy of her children's treatment in which she was forced to collude, Ruby's own vulnerability was exploited, and so exacerbated.

It is precisely because inequality characterizes the relationship between parent and child that trust is essential to the success of that relationship (Kittay 1999, 35; Nelson and Mouradian, this volume). If trust that an abuse of power will not occur is essential to this relationship, the illegitimate exercise of power—domination—is anathema to it (Kittay 1999, 34). At several points, Ruby's story speaks to the illegitimate exercise of power. Domination manifests itself in the physical scars on her daughters' bodies; it reveals itself in her younger daughter's difficulty in forming intimate relationships, and it is evident in the emotional rift between Ruby and her younger daughter. At the same time, however, it is difficult to apply the term *domination* to a situation such as Ruby's. Domination, as most understand it, is associated with a willful agent of power, and while the illegitimate exercise of power has left its mark, it is nonetheless difficult to locate the agent who left those marks. Ruby, who went to such lengths to ensure her children's well-being, is an unlikely agent of domination. As Ruby tells it, the doctors, too, make for poor culprits. Those recommending and performing genital surgeries do not intend harm; on the contrary, it is their firm belief that genital surgeries are essential to the healthy psychosexual development of a child born with ambiguous genitalia. Doctors who ask that patients make themselves available to colleagues and medical residents for repeated examination by medical personnel do not mean for patients to experience violation; rather, they understand themselves to be engaged in important educational work that advances medical progress. And yet, the injury suffered by Ruby's daughters, by Ruby herself, and by the many others who have recently spoken out against cosmetic genital surgeries, points to the exercise of power absent "moral legitimacy" (Kittay 1999, 34).

Mary's Story

Twenty-five years after Ruby's first child was born, a young mother named Mary brought her 12-year-old daughter Jessica to the pediatrician. The day before, Jessica had just come out of the shower after a ballet lesson when Mary noticed, out of the corner of her eye, a "growth" emerging from her daughter's labia. Mary had called the doctor, who agreed that Mary should bring Jessica in the following morning. Her daughter did not question why they would be going to the doctor. "Jessica was the type of child who never questioned me. She never spoke back. Never. Because she wanted to make me—us, her parents—happy, and not displease us."

That same day, Jessica's pediatrician sent her to a pediatric endocrinologist. A sonogram revealed that Jessica did not have a uterus, but undescended testes.[8]

> The pediatric endocrinologist asked to speak with me alone. Jessica was in a different room. The doctor and I then sat and she explained to me that Jessica had XY chromosomes and Jessica would not be able to bear children. She also explained to me that this was something I should never, ever bring up with Jessica. I should never talk about it with Jessica. We should just take care of it as quickly as possible so that Jessica could live a normal life. I agreed to this because it was what she asked me to do. I was very young at the time. I was just in my late 20s.
>
> Naturally I was shocked; I was stunned, I was saddened. I went home and told my husband, who had just come back from work. I told him all about it, what the pediatric endocrinologist said. I had never seen him cry before but he just broke down and sobbed in my arms. That's when it impacted me the most

. . . There were a lot of tears, a lot of feeling bad for Jessica, knowing that she couldn't have children naturally.

Mary was instructed to tell Jessica that "her ovaries hadn't developed properly and they would have to come out." Jessica was not told that her testes would be removed because doctors feared they would become cancerous. Nor was she informed of the clitorectomy[9] that would be performed at the same time.

Just a month later, Jessica was in the recovery room of the children's hospital. Mary remembers finding her daughter moaning in bed as she recovered from the anesthesia. She thought it was only from the pain, but Jessica has since told her that, having reached down, she realized that "a piece of her was gone." In the week that Jessica spent in the hospital, nothing was said about the clitorectomy. Doctors did inform her, however, that she would have to return to the hospital in a week to evaluate the effects of what they called "the plastic surgery."

Mary remembers that before the surgery, immediately after, and in the follow-up evaluation, "scores of male residents would come in to examine" her daughter. Mary had consented to the examinations because she knew that her daughter was being treated in a teaching hospital. It was not until years later when Jessica had obtained her medical records and confronted her parents with what she had learned that Mary would hear from her daughter's mouth, the terrible effects, not only of the surgery and the deception, but of the repeated examinations.

Looking back, it seems obvious to Mary that her daughter, who regarded her enlarged clitoris as perfectly normal, would have experienced the surgery and the examinations as painful violations. But if at the time she entertained such thoughts, she put them out of her mind. She remembers asking whether she should seek counseling for Jessica, and in response was told the story of another girl with AIS who, as a teenager, had stolen a look at her records when the doctor was called out of the examination room. That girl, the doctors informed Mary, had had to be placed in a psychiatric institution as a result of learning "the truth." The surgery had taken care of the problem, Mary was told, and further discussion would only raise potentially damaging questions for Jessica. What was important was that Jessica look normal. If she looked normal, she would be able "to live her life as a normal girl."

A failure of identification. When Mary speaks of the importance of the "normal appearance" of her daughter's genitals, it is difficult to discern whether her remarks reflect her own concerns or those of the doctors. Appearance, as opposed to sensation, is the governing criterion that determines whether genital surgery (and, in some cases, a change in gender assignment) is indicated.[10] Perhaps it should not be surprising that parents of children with ambiguous genitalia follow the lead of doctors when it comes to making sense of a condition they have most likely encountered for the first time. Mary's response, as well as Ruby's, reflects the experiences of many other parents.[11] But in focusing on genital appearance, rather than the experience of the child, a parent puts both her child and her relationship to her child at risk.

Mary's story underscores one of the recurrent themes implicit in Ruby's narrative, namely, what might be described as a *failure of identification* with her child. Parents, and particularly mothers, are widely taken to have a kind of privileged knowledge of their children. Psychologists and other specialists in child development speak of the special kind of attentiveness or attunement that a mother must cultivate to meet the needs an infant and young child can express only imperfectly. Cultivation of this special connection is a necessary function of the child's development, and as a normal part of development it is also expected to diminish as the child grows and is capable of increasing self-sufficiency.[12] In the case of children with genital ambiguity, it appears that a parent may be forced to forsake this attunement to a child's needs or desires, and to put aside what her own common sense would tell her about her own desires, her own bodily experience, in exchange for the promise of a child who will "look normal."

It may be discomfiting for parents—or even, in the case of the students queried in Kessler's study, those simply imagining themselves in the position of parents—to focus on the feeling in a child's genitals; many parents may understandably resist what could appear as a kind of sexualization of their child. However, the case of children with ambiguous genitalia demands that parents take account of just those feelings in order to make an informed decision and fulfill their obligations as parents. To do that, parents require the assistance of the experts on whom they have come to rely when their own knowledge proves insufficient. It would have been interesting if the researchers on Kessler's team had asked the students participating in the first study— the study asking whether they would have wanted their parents to consent to surgery—what they would have done if faced with the decision of whether to consent to surgery for their children. If such questions had been included, it is possible that students in the first group would have been more disposed to identify with the children and to be more cautious about making cosmetic surgical decisions.

The juxtaposition of Kessler's studies suggests a conflict between the needs of an individual child and the norms and expectations that govern society. A parent's obligation to her child is complicated by the fact that socialization is also constitutive of her child's needs. But socialization, or the necessity to adjust one's behavior or person to the culture to which one belongs, is not generally taken to be a parent's primary obligation (Kittay 1999, 71). When parents are presented with situations for which they can provide no context and so are unable to make judgments concerning what is right for their children, they must rely on doctors to provide direction and advice. In place of the parent who has shared such a close relationship to her child, the parent becomes an agent of her daughter's violation. But parents who act as agents of violation are at the same time objects of domination. Their relationship with their child is compromised, and the parent, as a parent, is compromised, by virtue of her inability to identify with her child.

Normality by Other Means
Sarah's Story

From my first interview with Ruby to one of the last—with the mother of 4-month-old identical twin girls who were still recovering from surgery—there was a notable consistency in the experience they shared. All of their children had received surgery,[13] and all, including those who had recently consented to surgery and believed that they had done the right thing, expressed some degree of ambivalence. Among the parents I interviewed there was nevertheless one story that was exceptional. Sarah's is a story that begins in the early 1990s, after an uneventful pregnancy, a natural childbirth, and a child pronounced a "girl." But, Sarah recounts,

> it was funny because I had an immediate intuition that told me they had gotten it wrong as they announced "it's a girl." And I remember after he was born that there was a little bit of hesitancy with the nurses as they weighed and checked him. That morning [my son] returned from the nursery . . . and I could see from the pediatrician's face that something was wrong. But I kept thinking, I was prepared for everything! I had a birth plan with everything that I wanted to happen, accounting for every possibility . . . but this. Because I'd never heard of this.
>
> Gender is supposed to be a given. You have either a boy or a girl. But they said,
>
> "We have a problem: We're not sure your baby is a girl."
>
> "What do you mean, how can you not tell if a baby is a boy or girl? What's the problem?"
>
> "Well," the doctor said, he "couldn't find a vaginal opening." And I immediately began to think about all these terrible talk shows, because that's the thing you have a reference to. . . . They said, "We have to do more tests."

The prospect of a newborn fit for the likes of daytime talk shows was chilling. The small hospital in which delivery had taken place was ill-equipped to deal with anomalies such as genital ambiguity, but having had a case several years earlier the doctors knew to summon experts, and to maintain the privacy of the mother and child, "to protect us from other parents, who might be inquisitive about what was happening in the nursery." The secrecy and heavy mood of the hospital staff, together with Sarah's ignorance in the face of an unexpected—even unfathomable—event, cast a pall over the birth of her child. Her outlook quickly improved, Sarah remembers, with the thoughtful intervention of a labor nurse, who "knew someone who knew someone with a daughter with CAH." This woman came to the hospital the very next day, and helped ease the anxiety and worry that a first-time, single mother faced at the frightening news of a child born with genital ambiguity. Another important source of support came from her own mother, a retired La Leche League leader[14] who had raised Sarah to understand that while doctors had an unmistakable expertise, there were nevertheless certain things that physicians, historically, had gotten wrong, particularly where a paternalistic approach to medical care of infants was concerned. Sarah's own attendance of La Leche League meetings during pregnancy had equipped her for the birth and early raising of her child in a way, she now reflects, that gave her the resources to advocate for and raise questions about the care of her child.

Sarah hadn't wanted to name her child until she saw the baby. She had prepared, on a single sheet of paper, a list of possible girls' names on one side, and a list of possible boys' names on the other. On both sides of the sheet appeared the name "Robin," which was, as Sarah saw it, the natural choice for her new son.

Seeing that Robin was thriving, and tremendously relieved after having spoken with the mother raising a daughter with CAH, Sarah was able to dispel the frightening images that accompanied the announcement that her child might not be a girl. When they shopped for diapers that week, she and her mother wondered together whether it would make sense to buy those marked "boys" or whether the "girls" diapers were more practical, laughing when they caught the confused stare of an eavesdropping shopper. Sarah and her mother went to the doctor for a first consultation with light hearts. They were singing, finally celebrating the arrival of the baby. They had brought a recording of a favorite song by the children's folk singer and educational psychologist Peter Alsop, entitled "It's Only a Wee Wee," and played it for the doctors and nurses during the visit, wanting to communicate that what had been presented (and initially received) as such terrible news might not warrant such gravity. While the song is intended to make light of gender difference, Sarah reheard the song in more literal terms after Robin's birth:

> As soon as you're born, grownups check where you pee
> And then they decide just how you're s'posed to be
> Girls pink and quiet, boys noisy and blue
> seems like a dumb way to choose what you'll do
> [chorus]

Well it's only a wee wee, so what's the big deal?
It's only a wee wee, so what's all the fuss?
It's only a wee wee and everyone's got one
There's better things to discuss!
Now girls must use makeup, girl's names and girl's clothes
And boys must use sneakers, but not pantyhose
The grownups will teach you the rules to their dance
And if you get confused, they'll say "Look in your pants"

. . . .

Now grownups watch closely each move that we make
Boys must not cry, and girls must make cake
It's all very formal and I think it smells
Let's all be abnormal and act like ourselves

For all her open-mindedness concerning gender roles, however, Sarah also understood that her initial distress on hearing the news of Robin's difference was not aberrant: this was how the world would see her child, and, she believed, there was little hope for change. After a series of tests to determine whether Robin's body would respond to testosterone,[15] she agreed, on her doctors' strong recommendation, to an initial series of surgeries, including primary hypospadias[16] repair, cosmetic surgery of his scrotum, and relocation of his testes, which had not descended *in utero:*

> At the time it seemed like the right thing to do, but I should have done more research *then;* by now I've talked to people who've had hypospadias repair, and they've gone through hell. It's all about peeing standing up, but the body has ways of undoing these surgeries. He's developed a leak. . . . If I knew then what I know now . . .

Sarah's understanding has undergone a transformation since the birth of Robin. She has sought out adults with conditions like her son's, and has heard the tragic stories of men and women who have undergone any number of surgeries (see, for example, Devore 1999). When first presented with the "problem" of her son's difference, Sarah could imagine only the alternatives proposed by the doctors. From the adults with intersex conditions with whom she is now acquainted she knows that the poor surgical outcomes are only a small part of the pain they endure. They were robbed, she believes, of the signature experiences—the "normal kid stuff"—that she regards as crucial in a child's life: they didn't take baths with other kids, didn't run around naked in sprinklers in hot summers. Children with conditions like Robin's, she learned, often made repeated visits to the hospital, spending school breaks at home recovering from surgeries rather than going to summer camp. While daunted, at first, by the prospect of preparing her child for a world hostile to his physical difference, Sarah came to believe that she doesn't have to take on the world to care for her child, that is, to make him feel safe and to feel normal. Rather than focusing her energies on promoting a sense of normalcy through concealing Robin's difference by making it a secret, Sarah aims instead to facilitate the life experience that would normalize this difference:

> I developed friendships where [people] were supportive and knew about Robin, and then he did have kids to run around naked in sprinklers with, and he did have kids to take baths with, and he did all that normal stuff. . . . Kids knew he was different, but that was okay, and he learned that everyone, really, looks different from everyone else no matter what mold they come from.

If Sarah's story is remarkable, it is not because her commitment to her child's well-being rivals that of other parents. But even as it stands apart from others' experiences—flying in the face of prevailing management of ambiguous genitalia, resisting what Lisa Hedley calls (in this volume) the "seduction of the surgical fix"—it is, at the same time, an approach to raising her child that exemplifies the same principles of common sense that informed the acceptance of the recommendations made to other parents. This fact may explain the intensity of the anger that adults who have undergone surgery demonstrate: the often unmitigated betrayal they experience is a measure of the distance they feel from their parents, itself a product of their competing conceptions of what "common sense" would dictate in these cases.

Perhaps the hardest lesson that the experience of parents of children with atypical genitalia teaches is that there can be a conflict between caring for your child in the sense of being attuned to a child's needs and wanting what's best for your child. The conventional wisdom of "what's best" tells parents that their child should be spared the mark of difference. While genital surgery promises the erasure of that mark, parents and their children are faced with a lifetime of concealment of that difference, and with the shame and guilt that that concealment entails.

For Whose Sake?

Neither the doctors nor parents of children with ambiguous genitalia can take for granted the fact of sexual difference; and yet they can, and by and large do, continue to abide by its rules. Doctors and parents together maintain the secret of intersex because others' ignorance or cruelty could harm children with ambiguous genitalia. But do they do so for the children's sake? The silence that parents maintain to protect their children, protects parents, too, from a kind of guilt by association: as one parent of an intersexed girl remembers thinking before her daughter's birth, "What sort of people would give birth to a hermaphrodite?" But, as the doctors made clear to all the parents with whom I spoke: What sort of *parents* would subject their child to life as a hermaphrodite? The challenge for Ruby, Mary, and Sarah—the job of any parent—is not only to protect one's child, but also to accommodate her to the world in which she lives. If, in the case of intersexed children, cosmetic genital surgery is presented to parents as a necessary adjustment, it is only too easy to understand why parents would consent to its performance.

While parents are expected to be attuned to their children, such identification is discouraged in parents of children with intersex. Parents are not given the chance to imagine their children's lives in any way except as in need of immediate correction. Despite the fact that doctors know, for instance, that later surgeries are less dangerous and more likely to produce desirable results—both with respect to appearance and the preservation of sensation—they nevertheless promote early surgery. Children, they claim, will experience less trauma if they are spared memories of removal of gonads or the excision of phallic tissue. Doctors understate the eventual necessity of painful vaginal dilation in the case of the (majority of) children assigned female. The likely prospect of additional surgeries or other traumatic procedures in subsequent years generally also goes unmentioned, as does the option of delaying surgery until the child is older. If, as the experiences of the parents I interviewed suggest, decisions were not made *for* parents, they could be understood to have been made *through* them: parents are not simple instruments of doctors' agendas; at the same time, their decisions cannot be regarded as products of an uncompromised agency. Similarly, doctors' failure to present a complete picture to parents may be seen, not as a conscious and deliberate effort to mislead parents for the sake of the maintenance of the binary structure of gender, but as a function of *habitus* that functions, as Bourdieu understands it, to reproduce itself.

The very fact of intersex, that is, the material evidence that sex is not an either/or proposition, but rather exists on a continuum, poses a threat to the current construction of *habitus*—a threat that is managed by the prevention of the very possibility of posing questions about it:

> The *habitus* is a principle of the selective perception of indices tending to confirm and reinforce it rather than transform it, a matrix generating responses adapted in advance to all objective conditions identical to or homologous with the (past) conditions of its production; it adjusts itself to a probable future which it anticipates and helps to bring about because it reads it directly in the present of the presumed world, the only one it can even know. (Bourdieu 1990, 64)

The dispositions that motivate the practices associated with corrective genital surgery must be very narrowly concerned with the reinforcement of "the present of the presumed world." Consider doctors' resistance to reconsidering standard practices despite the revelation of the "true story" of John/Joan and the increasing publication of critical narratives by intersexed adults (Colapinto 1997; see also, for example, essays by Coventry, Devore, Cameron, Kim, Hawbecker, and Moreno collected in Dreger 1999). Consider the insistence with which doctors promote surgical treatments that are similar to many of the practices known in developing countries as female circumcision, or clitorectomy.[17] In a statement published in 2000, the American Academy of Pediatrics declared that "the birth of a child with ambiguous genitalia constitutes a social emergency" (American Academy of Pediatrics 2000, 138). If the American Academy of Pediatrics declines to elaborate on the nature of this emergency, it is perhaps because there is little question of the grave threat that the revelation of intersex poses to the existing social order.

Kessler's paired studies point to a contradiction between what individuals would wish for themselves and what they would feel was right for their children. In the space of this contradiction, we may, or perhaps we must ask: *What if* parents identified with their children as Sarah has done? *What if* parents opted to understand the decision to perform cosmetic genital surgery as the child's, that is, to forgo immediate corrective surgery? Understanding the current management of intersex as a function of *habitus* suggests the radical potential of normalizing ambiguous genitalia. If parents of intersexed children were to work to identify with their children as intersexed individuals, if doctors were to use their considerable authority to promote acceptance of genital variation instead of erasure, the prevailing *habitus* would undergo genuine transformation. Not only would such a positive identification lead to improved relationships between parents and children, it would also work against the conservative principles of *habitus* to effect social change.

NOTES

1. This prediction is borne out by the fact that there is no published evidence suggesting any "hazards, biological or otherwise, of having a large clitoris." While men with small penises have suffered some indignity, published studies have found that, "contrary to conventional wisdom, it is not inevitable that such [men] must 'recognize that [they] are incomplete, physically defective and . . . must live apart'" (Kipnis and Diamond 1999, 181).

2. In chapter 5 of this volume, James Edwards explores Heidegger's conception of technology (*die Technik*), which complements Bourdieu's conception of *habitus.*

3. One might object that medical professionals, most notably, John Money, were in fact pre-

scribing rules concerning gender. But it does not appear that Money prescribed new rules of gender; rather, he formulated medical protocols that would be consistent with the rules of gender that were already in place. It was not Money who made the rule that there were "only two" sexes, "only two" ways to express or experience gender identity. To say that Money did not invent the rules of sex and gender is not, however, to excuse him for the grossly unethical practices and the deception he perpetrated on the scientific community and the public at large; nor does it absolve the physicians who continue to be faithful to his protocol despite the shocking revelations of the deceptions Money engineered and promoted (see, for example, Colapinto 1997). Bourdieu's analysis goes far, however, to suggest why Money's theories were eagerly taken up by the medical community, and why, despite the publication of the truth about Money's work, doctors continue—without explicit justification—to embrace his protocols.

4. There is a single exception, published in 1970. See Bing and Rudikoff (1970).

5. Congenital adrenal hyperplasia (CAH) is a genetic condition associated with a deficiency in the enzyme 21-hydroxylase, involved in making the steroid hormones cortisol and aldosterone. Girls and boys with the "salt-losing variety" of CAH (such as Ruby's daughters) require regular doses of the steroid cortisol, which they cannot produce on their own, as well as of a salt-retaining hormone. Without such treatment, children will experience crises similar to the one that brought both of Ruby's daughters so close to death. For discussion of a variety of intersex conditions, as well as data concerning the frequency with which they occur, see Fausto-Sterling (2000, 51–54). See also the website of the Intersex Society of North America at www.isna.org.

6. The names of parents and their children have been changed to protect their privacy. The parents from the eight families I interviewed live in nearly every region of the United States, with the exception of one mother, who lives in a Westernized country outside the United States. All uncited quotations are taken from transcripts of interviews.

7. Perhaps for this reason, many parents of children with ambiguous genitalia, including many of those with girl children with CAH, resist the association of the term *intersex* with their children (see postings at www.congenitaladrenalhyperplasia.org). As used in the medical literature, however, the term *intersex* designates any "defect in the normal processes of sexual maturation that results in abnormality in . . . the karyotype, the internal and external sexual organs, the gonads and the secondary sex characteristics which appear at puberty." See Creighton (2002, 218). Resistance to the term *intersex* can also be understood as an effort, made by parents and individuals with intersex alike, to deny their difference and fit into the categories given by society. Bourdieu's analysis of *habitus* makes sense of this resistance.

8. Jessica had a form of androgen insensitivity syndrome (AIS), a condition in which a fetus with a normal (46XY) male karyotype is unable to absorb androgens *in utero*. In its complete form, AIS would result in a child with typical feminine external genitalia and undescended testicles. In its partial form, the body can absorb some androgens, and at puberty an enlargement of the clitoris can result.

9. The use of the term *clitorectomy* is controversial. Western doctors today do not refer to clitorectomy, but instead to clitoral recession, apparently to distinguish current practices from those that are now decades old. However, review of the older literature reveals that concern for the retention of erotic sensation was not absent, as some practitioners now suggest. In a chapter published in 1956, Hampson, Money, and Hampson write that "partial amputation of an en-

larged phallus in a girl is an operation approached with hesitation by many surgeons, in the fear that serious loss of sensitivity may ensue. Studies . . . indicate that these women have subsequently been erotically responsive and able to experience orgasm." See Hampson et al. (1956, 551).

Insistence on the more euphemistic term *clitoral recession* appears calculated not only to place distance between past and current practices, but also to distinguish "medical" (beneficent, scientific, modern) practices from "cultural" (ignorant, primitive, uncivilized) practices that occur in "other countries." On interrogation, the distinction is credible neither linguistically nor practically. -*ectomy* simply means "to cut," not to completely excise. Primitive genital surgeries are not able to remove the clitoris in its entirety, because the structure is too deep, and thereby inaccessible to the instruments used. Philosopher Diana Meyers proposes the term *genital cutting* to circumvent the euphemistic terminology used to characterize both medical and cultural practices. See Meyers (2000).

10. See Kessler (1998, 25–27). It is also noteworthy that penises are deemed unworthy if they are not of sufficient length to penetrate a vagina. Surgery is also indicated if the position of the urinary meatus will not permit a boy to urinate in a standing position. Genital surgery is conducted on those assigned female with an eye, not to performance, but to appearance. While neither is concerned with the sensate experience of the individuals, the emphasis on masculine performance (in sexual intercourse and in urination) and on feminine appearance is consonant with conventional conceptions of proper gender roles.

11. Of her examination of approximately 100 letters written by mothers of children with ambiguous genitalia, Suzanne Kessler notes that parents' accounts of their children's surgery focus "disproportionately on how the genitals look rather than on what the child might be experiencing or how her genitals might function in the future" (Kessler 1998, 98). The most recent accounts produced over the course of a year from a web forum of parents of children with CAH (www.congenitaladrenalhyperplasia.org) manifest a similar concern with the appearance of the genitals, rather than the experience of the child.

12. See, for example, Winnicot's discussion of the "good enough" mother (1971, 10–14). There is a strong resonance between the kind of attunement necessary to meeting an infant's needs with Kittay's discussion of the "transparent self" in *Love's Labor*. Kittay defines a "transparent self" as a "self through whom the needs of another are discerned." See Kittay (1999, 51).

13. All but one of the parents I interviewed had consented to the surgery. One family had adopted a child whose surgery had taken place while she was a ward of the state.

14. La Leche League is an organization whose stated mission is "to help mothers worldwide to breastfeed through mother-to-mother support, encouragement, information, and education and to promote a better understanding of breastfeeding as an important element in the healthy development of the baby and mother." See www.lalecheleague.org.

15. If Robin's body had not responded to testosterone, he would have been assigned female, and been castrated, his penis refashioned to resemble a clitoris, and a vaginal opening created then or at some projected point. One doctor told Sarah that he thought it best to reassign Robin in any case, but the idea seemed too preposterous to her to consider seriously.

16. Hypospadias is an unusual placing of the meatus, the opening through which urine passes.

17. Indeed, these practices are prohibited by federal law in the United States. It would ap-

pear that 18 U.S.C. § 116, entitled "Female Genital Mutilation" (1996), would apply to surgeries performed on intersexed children. The law states that "whoever knowingly circumcises, excises, or infibulates the whole or any part of the labia majora or labia minora or clitoris of another person who has not attained the age of 18 years shall be fined under this title or imprisoned not more than 5 years, or both." An exception is noted, however: "A surgical operation is not a violation of this section if the operation is . . . *necessary to the health of the person on whom it is performed,* and is performed by a person licensed in the place of its performance as a medical practitioner." In applying this exception, a subsection of the law clarifies that "no account shall be taken of the effect on the person on whom the operation is to be performed of any *belief on the part of that person, or any other person, that the operation is required as a matter of custom or ritual*" (emphases added). That the very conventions of gender (as understood by Money and his colleagues) which explicitly motivate the surgeries could themselves be understood as "a matter of custom or ritual" is elided by the health exception written into the law.

REFERENCES

American Academy of Pediatrics. 2000. Evaluation of the newborn with developmental anomalies of the external genitalia. *Pediatrics* 106 (1): 138–42.

Bing, E., and E. Rudikoff. 1970. Divergent ways of coping with hermaphrodite children. *Medical Aspects of Human Sexuality* (December):73–88.

Bourdieu, P. 1990. *Logic of Practice.* Translated by Richard Nice. Stanford: Stanford University Press.

Colapinto, J. 1997. The true story of John/Joan. *Rolling Stone,* December 11.

Creighton, S. 2002. Surgery for intersex. *Journal of the Royal Society of Medicine* 94:218–20.

Devore, H. 1999. Growing up in the surgical maelstrom. In *Intersex in the Age of Ethics,* edited by A. D. Dreger, 79–82. Hagerstown, MD: University Publishing Group.

Dreger, A. D. 2000. Jarring bodies: Thoughts on the display of unusual anatomies. *Perspectives on Biology and Medicine* 43 (2):161–72.

Dreger, A. D., ed. 1999. *Intersex in the Age of Ethics.* Hagerstown, MD: University Publishing Group.

Fausto-Sterling, A. 2000. *Sexing the Body: Gender Politics and the Construction of Sexuality.* New York: Basic.

Hampson, J. G., J. Money, and J. L. Hampson. 1956. Hermaphrodism: Recommendations concerning case management. *Journal of Clinical Endocrinology and Metabolism* 4:547–56.

Kessler, S. 1998. *Lessons from the Intersexed.* New Brunswick, NJ: Rutgers University Press.

Kipnis, K., and M. Diamond. 1999. Pediatric ethics and the surgical assessment of sex. In *Ethics in the Age of Intersex,* edited by A. D. Dreger, 173–93. Hagerstown, MD: University Publishing Group.

Kittay, E. F. 1999. *Love's Labor: Essays on Women, Equality, and Dependency.* New York: Routledge.

Meyers, D. 2000. Feminism and women's autonomy: The challenge of female genital cutting. *Metaphilosophy* 31 (5):469–91.

Money, J., and A. A. Erhardt. 1982. *Man and Woman, Boy and Girl.* Baltimore: Johns Hopkins University Press.

Ruddick, S. 1989. *Maternal Thinking.* Boston: Beacon.

Winnicot, D. W. 1971. Transitional objects and transitional phenomena. In *Playing and Reality.* New York: Routledge.

CHAPTER FOURTEEN

Toward Truly Informed Decisions about Appearance-Normalizing Surgeries

Paul Steven Miller, J.D.

> I thought that after talking to me he would decide that I was normal
> and leave me alone. But I was beginning to understand something
> about normality. Normality wasn't normal. It couldn't be. If normal
> were normal, everybody could leave it alone. They could sit back and
> let normality manifest itself. But people—and especially doctors—had
> doubts about normality. They weren't sure normality was up to the
> job. And so they felt inclined to give it a boost.
>
> *Jeffrey Eugenides, Middlesex*

Growing up a dwarf, I was not a shy or retiring kid. Being different, I experienced a good deal of attention, both negative and positive. I recall that sometimes adults would ask me, "If there was a pill that would make you tall, would you take it?" As a 10-year-old boy, I knew that I wanted the teasing to stop. As a 15-year-old boy, I just wanted the girls to kiss me.

And yet, even as a child, I recognized that my entire identity was connected to being a dwarf. I did not view that fact as either good or bad. I could only imagine my life as a dwarf—it was integral to my being, it was how I related to everything, including other people and the world around me. It was not limiting, it just was. I did not constantly think, "Oh no, I am a dwarf, and I cannot reach the faucet in the washroom." Nor did I notice every time that people stared at me when I walked down the street. These were simply facts in the background of my life. It made little sense to me at the time to imagine myself *not a dwarf*. It was not my wish. I can imagine the same perspective from African Americans who experience their lives in a predominately white society. Most do not daydream about what their lives would be like if they were white, nor do they yearn to be white.

Adults were always curious about my answer to the magic-pill question: If I could take a pill to make me average-sized, would I? The issue intrigued and concerned average-sized parents. Most of them expected me to want to take the pill. As a boy, I never spent much energy on the issue because it was a hypothetical; there was no pill. Today is different because surgical options are available to normalize people like me who are different.

This chapter explores the decision-making process for surgeries that seek to make children appear more normal and less disabled. Surgeries, such as limb-lengthening, cochlear implants, and gender assignations, are becoming increasingly available to young children and their parents. These surgeries are not performed for medically necessary reasons, such as to save or to prolong the life of the child. Rather, the surgeries aim to make the child appear less different or disabled, with the goal of reducing the societal stigma or environmental inconveniences associated with norm-challenging anatomical differences. Due to the elective nature of these surgeries and the fact that such surgeries alter the natural identity of the child, traditional consent procedures may not be sufficient to protect the best interests of the child.

The Legal Standard

Broad parental decision-making authority with respect to raising children is a long-held principle of law.[1] As part of that broad discretionary authority, courts have determined that parents have the obligation to look after their child's medical needs.[2] Parents act as surrogates for children who are not in a position to decide for themselves regarding issues of medical treatment.[3] It is presumed that the "natural bonds of affection" lead parents to act in the best interest of their children.[4] Furthermore, the consent of a parent is necessary for medical treatment, including surgery, involving a child.[5]

Courts have also, however, recognized the state's ability to exercise discretion over parental choices in child rearing, including health care decisions, when the physical or mental health of the minor is in jeopardy.[6] Generally the state has the burden of proving by clear and convincing evidence that intervening in the parent-child relationship is necessary for the safety or health of the child, or to protect public at large.[7]

Overall, decisions about the medical care and treatment of children involve the rights and interests of three parties: the child, the parent, and the state.[8] Parents are given primary responsibility in making medical decisions for their children, who do not have the capacity or maturity to make decisions for themselves, because courts have determined that parents are in a better position to make certain decisions than any other third party.[9] Traditionally, lawyers and other professionals involved in the medical care of children speak of parents giving "informed consent" for their children to get a procedure. Parental decision making derived from a process of informed consent has been meant to help the parent determine the child's best interest. After providing parents with all relevant information about a proposed medical procedure or treatment before its commencement, physicians must obtain a voluntary informed consent.

More recently, however, the 1995 policy statement by the American Academy of Pediatrics (AAP) recognizes that "the doctrine of 'informed consent' has only limited *direct* application in pediatrics." According to the AAP statement, "Only *patients* who have appropriate decisional capacity and legal empowerment can give their *informed consent* to medical care. In all other situations, parents or surrogates provide *informed permission* for diagnosis and treatment of children with the *assent* of the child whenever appropriate."[10] If people are to make truly informed decisions, whether it is parents alone, children alone, or parents and children together, they have a right to receive the information relevant to the decision they face. In the end, I speak to the type of information I think parents and children need to give truly informed permission, assent, or consent, but first, I want the reader to understand the legal history of the debate about the limits of parental discretion in cases involving appearance-normalizing surgeries.

Medical Informed Consent for Children

The doctrine of informed consent serves to protect a patient's body, including a child's, from an unauthorized invasion. Three requirements are needed to satisfy the doctrine for a child.[11] First, the physician must describe the nature of the procedure so that the parent has adequate information about the proposed treatment, including the risks, benefits, and alternatives.[12] Second, the consent must be voluntary, and the physician may not coerce or otherwise improperly influence the parent's decision.[13] Third, the consent must be competent, which requires that the parent possess an appreciation of the nature, extent, and probable consequences of the medical treatment.[14] However, the informed consent doctrine is mostly concerned with parental understanding of the health and safety of the surgical procedure, and not necessarily with the outcome for the child.[15]

Some scholars, such as Priscilla Alderson (see her chapter in this volume), have been arguing for some time now that children should have a direct role in health care decision making, including the issue of whether to undergo surgery. Again, the AAP

"Policy Statement on Informed Consent, Parental Permission and Assent in Pediatric Practice" states that patients, including children, should participate in the decision-making process regarding their medical care commensurate with their development. "Parents and physicians should not exclude children and adolescents from decision-making without persuasive reasons."

When parents fail to provide adequate medical care to their children due to neglect, poor judgment, or even religious beliefs, the state can intervene as *parens patriae* to protect a child's general health and welfare.[16] Generally, though, the court considers the parent to be the individual who will make decisions in the best interest of her child.

Giving Informed Consent to Surgeries for Non-Life-Threatening Conditions

How should parents, physicians, or courts, for that matter, respond when presented with a surgical option to correct a physical anomaly that does not threaten the child's life or health? The question is particularly pressing when surgery must be performed before the child reaches the age of assent, which the AAP states is "older school-age children."

Throughout the years, courts have grappled with developing appropriate standards of parental rights to elect or not elect surgery for their children. Consistently, courts have looked to conceptions of a "normal childhood," balanced against the interests of the parents and state.

Almost a century ago, a county court in Pennsylvania assessed conceptions of a "normal childhood" when deciding whether or not to allow surgery on a child, and determined that it could not interfere with parental rights. In that case, a boy was born with rachitis, a non-life-threatening illness that can lead to reduced mobility. Because the parents had already lost seven of their ten children to other illnesses, they feared surgery could lead to the death of their child. Medical experts countered and testified that the child had a high chance of being cured of rachitis through surgery. In reaching its decision, the court evaluated the benefit of the surgery by determining whether a "normal life" could result for the child. The court also evaluated whether the rachitis was serious enough to warrant an intrusion into the parents' interests, and concluded the condition was not life-threatening. The court asserted that because a child with rachitis would still be capable of a reasonable amount of activity in normal affairs, it could not displace the natural guardians' decision.[17]

Years later in the State of Washington, the court in *In re Hudson* ruled for parents who argued against surgery on their child. In opposition, the state testified that a child with an abnormally large arm would be unable to lead a normal life without treatment to correct the impairment. The girl's siblings argued that the deformity was a handicap in her associations" with other people. Furthermore, physicians testified that the girl's exceptionally large arm would lead to her inability to live normally in society. The physicians also argued that the impairment would physically burden the child because of a greater need for blood. Despite arguments by the state, family, and physicians surrounding a "normal childhood," the state supreme court relied on the assumption that parents traditionally have the best interest of the child in mind. The court determined that it was necessary to respect the parents' interests, and in this case, the parents feared for the child's possible death as a result of surgery. Furthermore, the court reasoned that the girl could make the decision for amputation later in life.[18]

Although infrequent, courts have ruled for the state over parental objections in the case of elective surgery on children by asserting the doctrine of *parens patriae*. Specifically, the state will prevail in instances where the court determines the child's deprivation of a "normal childhood" outweighs the parental interests. In New York, the court of appeals affirmed a family court decision and ordered surgery on a 15-year-old boy born with neurofibromatosis, a condition that caused a disfigurement to his face and neck. The mother, a Jehovah's Witness, objected to the use of blood transfusions to treat her son. The state posited that the child would be deprived of a normal life without surgery. The court found that the child's deformity, though not life-threatening, severely retarded his social and psychological growth. The court ruled that the child's and state's interests outweighed the mother's religious objections, and decided the child would submit to transfusions.[19]

In another instance, the court of appeals of Oregon applied its conceptions of "normal childhood" in *In re Jensen*.[20] The court held that the state could intervene in the general health care of a 15-month-old girl born with hydrocephalus, a condition that caused an enlargement of her head. The child was born to parents who were members of a religious sect that believed that only prayer by church elders could be treatment for illness or impairment. The court determined that the child was unable to make a reasoned personal decision of what was in her own best interest because she was only 15 months of age. The court then balanced the state's *parens patriae* role with parental interests in reaching its decision. Reasoning that without surgery the child would be unable to live "some semblance of a normal life," the court found that the possible chance of retardation outweighed the parents' religious rights.[21]

The tension between the actual standards and rights when a court grapples with whether a state may interfere in a parent's right to choose elective surgery for a child still exists and is just as difficult to resolve, even with modern-day medical advances.

For example, the following unpublished case from the Midwest explores the legal standards and reasoning to be applied in cochlear implant surgery of children.[22]

In Michigan, for reasons of neglect, a deaf mother temporarily lost custody of her two deaf sons, ages 3 and 4.[23] Public school officials suggested the children receive cochlear implants, and the children's court-appointed attorney petitioned the court to order cochlear implant surgery for the boys. Both the mother and the father, who was also deaf, vigorously opposed the surgery. The children's lawyer argued the implants were necessary to allow the brain to develop normally, and should not be considered elective surgery.

The court ruled that pursuant to Michigan statutory law and constitutional precedent, a parent, unless permanently deprived of custody over his child, has the final authority to determine whether or not the child will undergo elective surgery for a non-life-threatening condition. Thus, the court did not order the surgery. Still, the judge herself stated that she personally believed the cochlear implants were in the best interest of the children, and stated she would revisit the issue if the mother permanently lost custody of the children. The deaf community had actively supported the mother's decision by protesting outside the courtroom, attracting media attention, and raising funds for an expert witness to testify at trial on the mother's behalf. Deaf activists were outraged at the judge's suggestion that "deaf children need fixing" and at the fact that she would consider ordering the procedure over the objection of the children's deaf mother.[24]

A non-U.S. court, however, took a very different stance toward childhood elective surgery, and has precluded appearance-normalizing surgery for children with atypical genitalia. The constitutional court of Colombia dramatically limited the ability of doctors and parents to conduct genital surgery on intersexed children.[25] In a series of two landmark cases, one involving a 2-year-old child[26] and the other involving an 8-year-old child,[27] the court ruled that the consent given by parents for genital surgery was invalid. The court concluded that the surgery may be a violation of children's autonomy and bodily integrity that is motivated by their parents' intolerance of their own children's sexual difference. The court considered that the parents' authority to consent to medical procedures on behalf of children who are too young to consent for themselves depends on the exigency and urgency of the procedure; how invasive and risky the procedure is; and the age and degree of autonomy of the child. In the court's opinion, these factors weighed against authorizing the parents to consent on behalf of their children in these instances. In the case of intersexed infants, the court found that parents are likely to make decisions based on their own fears and concerns rather than what is best for the child, especially if they are pressed to decide quickly. The court further held that criticism of the surgical procedures by intersexed people themselves, expressed in an *amicus* brief filed with the court, was of "decisive importance."

Determining the Best Interests of a Child

Generally, acting in the best interests of a child means protecting her health and safety, and creating an environment in which she can achieve her full potential. For children who are born with norm-challenging anatomical differences, the question arises over how to determine what is in the best interest of that child. Is it to leave the child alone, and let her be potentially subjected to teasing, ridicule, and inconvenience because of the difference? Or is it to allow surgery to normalize the difference and alter forever the body and, thus in significant ways, the identity the child was born with, while potentially reducing psychosocial trauma? If the surgery is such that it should be done while the child is too young to participate in the conversation, the predicament can be terribly difficult. (See the chapters by Hedley and Aspinall in this volume.) The predicament is especially difficult and confusing as it is impossible to determine the child's preference.

To reflect on how complex that predicament is, it may help to consider three different scenarios. The first involves a child with an anatomical difference, whose parents do not have the same difference. The second scenario involves an affected child born to an affected parent, but a third party, such as a judge or court, acts on behalf of the child, evaluating the appropriateness of the surgery. In both of these instances, an individual without the condition in question is substituting her point of view for the child's.

A third scenario is when an affected child is born to affected parents, and no third-party decision maker intervenes. I am less concerned about the scenario where an affected parent must make a surgical decision before the child can participate. Why? Because an adult with the condition in question has personal life experience and is better informed about the challenges of living with the condition. Regardless of whether she chooses the surgery for the child, that parent is not making the decision in a vacuum. Because of her own experience with the condition, she is aware of the benefits and detriments of being different, and thus, can better evaluate the potential psychosocial impact.

Parental Discovery of Disability

Deciding whether a child should undergo surgery to normalize a disabling trait can be complex because of the alarm, confusion, and anxiety that parents sometimes experience on the birth of a child with an anatomical difference. Even though the law presumes that a parent will act in the best interest of a child, this presumption may not always be true in the case of a child, born to able-bodied parents, who is disabled and different from the norm. The issue has little to do with the amount of love and care that the parent showers on such a child.

The birth of a disabled child to able-bodied parents is often met with disappointment, or even anger, due to the loss of the idealized child. Where the birth of a newborn is usually anticipated with excitement and great expectation, this joy may become muted with the birth of a disabled infant. The birth of the disabled child often leads to a period of grief.[28]

Parents, no matter how much they love the child, may thus harbor fears, myths, and stereotypes about their child with a disability. They may not understand the disability, or have any personal experience with others who have the same condition. They mourn the loss of their "normal" child. For example, Joan Ablon's case studies of parental response to the birth of a dwarf child typically centered around a fear of the unknown. "When he came in I said, 'Dwarf? Are you saying my child is a dwarf?' What dwarf meant to me was a leprechaun. What would that mean? Would we have to send her to the circus? What kind of life would she have?"[29] Often, doctors reinforced parental fear by either avoiding parents altogether or not providing them with adequate information while at the same time isolating the new parents from their child. Ablon describes one of these situations:

> Ed knew something was up because, when he went into the nursery to look, our baby wasn't there, and there were a group of doctors in the back. Still I hadn't gotten the baby, and they didn't say anything . . . I said, "Something is wrong." They would say, "I'll go see," and then I'd never see them again. They just avoided me, and every time I'd ring, the nurses would say, "Oh, I don't know," and they'd leave.[30]

It is within this context that the solution of normalizing the child by surgery is presented to the parents.

In her chapter in this volume, Lisa Hedley describes, from the perspective of a parent of a child who is a dwarf, the desire for surgery to attain the appearance of normalcy. That desire is alluring—and potentially sends a very mixed message. Hedley wonders if, in choosing an appearance-normalizing surgery, she and her husband would be sending their daughter the message: "We love you, you're perfect the way you are. Now change." Though Hedley and her husband resist the desire to try to equalize their daughter's opportunities by normalizing her appearance, they attest to how strong that desire can be. They decide to wait until their daughter is old enough to participate in the conversation about whether to undergo appearance-normalizing operations.

That is, they can imagine both that their daughter might decide to get such surgeries—and that she might not. On the one hand, their daughter might meet Emily Sullivan Sanford or read her essay in this volume and decide that surgery is for her. On the other hand, given the growing strength of the disability rights movement, it is much easier than it once was to imagine that a person might decide not to have such surgeries.

Disability is, after all, a socially constructed concept, which rests on an unstated norm.[31] But, societal norms about disability are changing. For example, the Americans with Disabilities Act provides disabled people with substantive civil rights, and as a result, they are becoming more integrated into society.[32] People are becoming more accepting. Disability stigma is on the decline. And yet, what young adolescent, disabled or not, does not yearn to conform, fit in, and be like everyone else? When parents discuss the surgical option with their children, they should remember just how normal it is for teenagers to be anxious about being abnormal.

Incorporating the Perspective of Affected Adults

While it may be perfectly true that parents feel large internal or external pressures to choose appearance-normalizing surgeries for their children, I believe the general rule should be that, in the absence of a strong consensus that an appearance-normalizing surgery is in the child's best interest, as exists in the case of cleft lip and palate surgeries, parents should wait until their children are old enough to participate in the decision-making process. Numerous studies have indicated that adults born with ambiguous genitalia have expressed regret and anger about the genital surgeries they experienced as children.[33] For example, one intersex woman, in discussing the pain she has struggled with since her genital surgery, describes her depression and her struggles to "express the fear, shame, rage, and intense body-hatred that I have felt as a result of the—until now—unspeakable assault that I experienced under the guise of medical treatment . . . I am horrified by what has been done to me and by the conspiracy of silence and lies. I am filled with grief and rage, but also relief finally to believe that maybe I am not the only one."[34]

Another adult who, at age 40, had undergone sixteen surgeries on his genitals stated: "A lot of defeat and depression that I felt growing up left me when I realized that doctors and parents were wrong. They believed that I could not be happy without normal genitals. When I understood that wasn't true, my life completely changed."[35] In addition, historical and anecdotal evidence demonstrates that, given the opportunity to grow up and decide for themselves, most people who are conjoined twins would *not* choose normalizing surgeries for themselves.[36] Alice Dreger found that even conjoined twins who were separated as children felt that they did not need to be separated as they were not trapped by their conjoinment.[37] Little People of America, a national advocacy organization of and for people of short stature, have taken the position that limb-lengthening is an unnecessary surgery, with unknown long-term results, and that it is far more useful to build a dwarf child's self-esteem with nonsurgical means (www.lpaonline.org/resources_faq.html).

The problem of a third party choosing a surgery for a child, who is too young to decide for herself, is clear. As Alice Dreger writes, "We must not forget that the decision maker in virtually all these cases is a person who lacks first-hand knowledge of the condition, who will not undergo the procedure, who will not suffer the costs and bear the risks. We must not forget that although normalizations *may* sometimes be wise—may even be the best choice—they are not the only option, and should not be chosen hastily."[38]

Currently, the responsible parent, or in the rare instances in which a court is involved, the judge, has the sole discretion to decide on behalf of child who is too young to participate in the decision or decide for herself. To increase the quality of the informed permission, or assent or consent, the life experiences, perspectives, and independent judgment of the community of affected adult individuals must be considered.[39] In this way, parents will be more fully and broadly educated about the psychosocial impact of the disability.[40]

Involving affected adult individuals as a resource of information for the decision maker addresses the problem of stereotypes about the child's difference that the parents may harbor. The purpose of the affected community voice is to pierce through the myths and fears about the condition. There should be a counterbalance to any stereotype that a parent or physician may have about a child born with a physical difference or anomaly. As Cassandra Aspinall makes plain in her chapter in this book, even people who love and care about the child born with a physical anomaly can harbor fears about the child being subjected to a life of alienation, loneliness, discrimination, and freakishness. Different from physicians and nonaffected family members, affected individuals can help to ally such fears—or at least can help to put them into better perspective.[41] As Adrienne Asch has written, "Doctors and bioethicists shape decisions of individual patients and families, and they cannot help others make genuinely informed decisions about how to handle life with a disability if they themselves continue to be disbelieving or astonished that people with a variety of impairments can pursue life plans they find satisfying."[42]

Normalcy may be an important value, but it is not the only or highest value. Affirming difference is another important value. Pursuing normalcy and affirming difference are both social activities that, in the future, we can engage in differently than we have in the past. One should not be dismissive of the psychosocial issues that disabling traits can create for affected children, but neither should one overemphasize them. Life with a disability is no more often a tragedy than is life without a disability.[43] The more information parents have about what life with the trait really is—and is not—like, the better they or another proxy will be able to decide for their child, if their child is too young to participate in the decision or decide for herself.

I acknowledge that the best approach to getting input from the affected community is not obvious. Communities of affected individuals are heterogeneous and opinions vary. Moreover, it is unclear whose perspectives in the community should be considered. Should it be affected individuals, parents of affected individuals, siblings, or others?

Again, the purpose of gathering insight and information from the community of affected individuals is to provide a perspective that will complement the perspective of the medical community. With a broad range of perspectives, parents and children can choose the alternative that best suits their conceptions of what is good for them. While it might also be important and relevant to hear from affected adults who support the recommendation of the medical professional, the primary goal here should be a validation of multiple alternatives, rather than uniform support for one. Rarely is there unanimity of opinion regarding which alternative is best; thus, an emphasis should be placed on providing the decision makers with a full range of options.

There may be as many reasons for not performing normalizing surgery on a child as there are for doing the surgery. And the argument against surgery may be counterintuitive to a parent who does not fully understand the psychosocial implications of the disability. Involvement by members of the affected community gives the parent or other decision maker greater context for making an informed choice.

In an effort to normalize a child through surgery, it is important to recognize then that there are both risks and benefits. Some of those risks and benefits are physical. But because the purpose of these surgeries is to change an individual's identity, the risks and benefits are also psychological. If those risks and benefits are to be weighed carefully, if the decisions made with or for children are to be truly informed, then it will be essential to seek out the perspectives of those who live with the trait that the surgery seeks to change.

ACKNOWLEDGMENTS

The author would like to thank Dipal Shah and Mona Papillon for their valuable research assistance.

NOTES

Epigraph: Eugenides (2002, 446).

1. See *Prince v. Commonwealth*, 321 U.S. 158, 166 (1943) (holding that a parent generally has the ability to make decisions surrounding the custody, care, and nurture of her child).

2. See *Parham v. J.R.*, 442 U.S. 584, 602 (1979) (determining that in almost all cases, a parent has broad discretion in the physical and mental health of his child, even if there is risk involved).

3. See, for example, *Bonner v. Moran*, 126 F.2d 121, 122 (D.C. Cir. 1941). (Children are usually incapable of important decisions regarding their rights. In this case a 15-year-old boy requested a surgeon to remove some of his tissue and transplant it into his cousin. The court determined that in this instance, the boy's age precluded an intelligent decision in the matter, and the situation necessitated parental guidance and consent.)

4. See *Parham*, 442 U.S. at 602. (Due to an inherent love for their children, parents are presumed to act in their best interest. In this case, the court readily acknowledged that parents who wanted their child committed to a mental hospital did so believing it was in the child's best interest.)

5. See *Bonner*, 126 F.2d at 122 (acknowledging that a physician must have the consent of a minor's parent to operate on the minor).

6. Compare *Parham*, 442 U.S. at 619 (The court held that a parent's capacity to make medically related decisions for her child may lead to error and may not always be in the child's best interest. It is occasionally necessary for a neutral decision maker to consider and decide what is truly in the best interests of the child. Finally, the court reasoned a state agency could decide whether or not to release a child even though his parents claimed he needed to be further institutionalized based on mental illness.) with *Wisconsin v. Yoder*, 406 U.S. 205, 234 (1972) (The state may intervene in situations where parental rights interfere in the objectives of the state. Here, the state argued defendants were in violation of a compulsory education law because defendants refused to send children to school after eighth grade, claiming it violated principles of their Amish heritage. The court, after balancing interests of both parents and state, determined that the state's desire to compel Amish children to attend school would violate First and Fourteenth Amendment rights of parents.).

7. See, for example, *Newmark v. Williams*, 588 A.2d 1108, 1110 (Del. 1991). (Under the standard of *parens patriae*, the state has a duty to protect its youngest citizens, children. This case involved invasive medical treatment of a child of two Christian Scientists. The court held, after weighing both the parents' interests and the state's interest in protecting the child, that the projected success rate of the treatment did not outweigh the parents' right to reject surgery based on religious beliefs.)

8. See *Parham*, 442 U.S. at 584–85 (discussing the fundamental tensions inherent in situations of medical treatment and elective surgery for children). See also *In re Green*, 292 A.2d 387 (Pa. 1972). (The state's interest does not outweigh a parent's religious beliefs that preclude medical treatment, when the child's life is not immediately imperiled by her condition. In the instant case, the minor was impaired by paralytic scoliosis, requiring him to sit and precluding him from standing or upright movement. Here, a mother's religious beliefs precluded her son from receiving blood transfusions necessary for surgery to treat the condition. In this rare in-

stance, the court remanded the issue for an evidentiary hearing to discover what the 16-year-old minor felt, particularly if his own religious beliefs precluded treatment.) See also Amy Elizabeth Brusky, Note, *Making Decisions for Deaf Children regarding Implants: The Legal Ramifications of Recognizing Deafness as a Culture Rather than a Disability,* 1995 Wis. L. Rev. 235, 243 (1995).

9. See *Parham,* 442 U.S. at 604 (arguing that based on legal standards, courts will usually consider a parent to be the best advocate of the rights of his child).

10. American Academy of Pediatrics Committee on Bioethics (1995). Further, "Usually parental permission articulates what most agree represents the 'best interests of the child.' However, the Academy acknowledges that this standard of decision making does not always prove easy to define." The statement indicates that nonessential surgery should be deferred until the child is able to provide consent on her own behalf.

11. See J. D. Lee and Barry Lindhal, *Modern Tort Law: Liability and Litigation* 3 § 25:34 (2 ed., 2003) (defining the concept of informed consent as it applies to children, infants, and the mentally incompetent).

12. See *Hart v. Brown,* 289 A.2d 386, 391 (Conn. 1972). (The court upheld a parent's consent to a 7-year-old girl's donation of a kidney to her twin sister only after the parents could establish the independent psychological and emotional benefit to the girl. The parents successfully argued, using information gained through the informed consent process, that the girl would be less harmed by the loss of her kidney than by the loss of her twin sister.)

13. See *Bailey v. Lally,* 481 F.Supp. 203, 220 (D. Md. 1979). (The court determined that under the doctrine of informed consent, participation in medical research and treatment must be voluntary and may not be coerced.)

14. See *Dunham v. Wright,* 423 F.2d 940, 945–46 (3rd Cir. 1970). (A patient must have complete knowledge and a true understanding of the consequences of the medical treatment or surgery, the seriousness of it, the organs involved, and the possible results to satisfy informed consent.)

15. See J. D. Lee and Barry Lindhal, *Modern Tort Law: Liability and Litigation* 3 § 25:34 (2 ed., 2003) (emphasizing the importance of the process behind informed consent rather than its effectiveness in producing a beneficial outcome for a patient).

16. See, for example, *Jehovah's Witnesses v. King Count Hosp No. 1,* 278 F. Supp. 488 (W.D. Wash 1967) (declaring under *parens patriae* that parents neglected a child by refusing lifesaving medical treatment). See also *Ginsberg v. New York,* 390 U.S. 629, 641 (1968). (The state exercises a *parens patriae* function by protecting those who cannot make decisions for themselves. This includes children or minors.)

17. *In re Tuttendario,* 212 Pa.D. 561, 1912 WL 3920 (Pa.Quar.Sess 1912). (The court applied the testimony of a state physician to determine whether or not the boy could lead a "normal life." The physician indicated that the condition could interfere with a person making a livelihood in anything that requires standing or walking, but that any occupation that he could perform to sitting down would not be interfered with. The disease would not in any manner shorten the boy's life.)

18. *Accord, In re Hudson* 126 P.2d 765 (Wash. 1942).

19. *In re Sampson* 29 N.Y.2d 900, N.Y.S.2d 686 (N.Y. 1972). Cf. *In re Seiferth,* 127 N.E.2d 821–23 (N.Y. 1955). (The court of appeals affirmed the lower court's ruling, deciding that the state could not force a child to submit to surgery over parents' religious interests. The 14-year-old boy

in the instant case had a cleft palate and his father refused treatment based on personal healing beliefs. The boy's father attempted to use a form of mental healing to cure boy. The court decided that the father inculcated his son with such a fear of surgery that the boy would be uncooperative after operation and would be unable to benefit from treatment. Supporting its conclusion, the court described the boy as likeable and not socially stigmatized, attempting to make him sound as "normal" as possible. The court finally argued that allowing the boy to decide on the issue of surgery when he reached the age of majority would be in the boy's best interests.)

20. 633 P.2d. 1302 (Or. Ct. App. 1981).

21. *Jensen*, 633 P.2d at 1303.

22. Jon Hall, *Update on case in Grand Rapids, Michigan: Judge's ruling* (2002), available at http://deafbase.com/article280.html (asserting the implications of an adverse ruling for deaf advocates, and the position of the major parties in the case).

23. Ibid.

24. Ibid.

25. See Julie A. Greenberg and Cheryl Chase, "Colombia High Court Limits Surgery on Intersexed Infants," Intersex Society of North America http://www.isna.org/colombia/background .html referring to Sentencia SU-337/99, Bogota, May 12, 1999, and Sentencia T-551/99, Bogota, August 2, 1999.

26. Sentencia T-551/99, Bogota, August 2, 1999.

27. Sentencia SU-337/99, Bogota, May 12, 1999.

28. Linda Murphy, *National Down Syndrome Society: Grandparent's Role* (2003), available at http://www.ndss.org (explaining the stages in a parent's reaction to the birth of their disabled child).

29. Ablon (1988, 13).

30. Ibid., 15.

31. Theresa Glannon, *Race Education, and the Construction of a Disabled Class,* 1995 Wis. L. Rev. 1237, 1304 (1995) (detailing the different processes by which culture creates a disability from its own standards and conceptions. For example, deafness was normalized by heredity in Martha's Vineyard, where over the course of three centuries a large group of deaf individuals raised families there. Deafness was simply the status quo, and Martha's Vineyard was a place where everyone knew sign language, accepting what we consider today an impairment as the norm). See also Harris (1997) (revealing the media's and mass culture's effect on the perception of what is normal and abnormal with regards to appearance. Additionally, what society conceives as abnormal appearance due to ambiguous genitalia or achondroplasia is an appearance that deviates from an individual's concept of "normal appearance." The process by which we establish a concept of normal appearance is influenced by the cultural environments in which we live, and what different forms of media and culture present to us as perfect or the standard.).

32. Pub. L. No. 101–336, 104 Stat. 327–33 (codified at 42 U.S.C. §§ 12101–13 (1990)).

33. See Dreger (1999, 138–39). See also Presentation of Joan Whelan at the Robert Wood Johnson Medical School (January 2002) available at http://isna.org/library/whelanjan2002 .html.

34. Dreger (1999, 138–39).

35. Ibid., 79.

36. Dreger (2004, 67).

37. Ibid., 67–68.

38. Ibid., 59.

39. Such involvement is not unprecedented, as parents often seek input in such decision making, for example, from doctors offering a second opinion, social workers, family members, religious leaders, other parents, and written materials from the library or the Internet. See *Seiferth*, 127 N.E.2d at 822. (The parent of a child born with a cleft palate consulted with a field of plastic surgeons and orthodontists, workers at a corrective speech school, and children affected by cleft palate before deciding whether or not to opt for surgery for his child.) Moreover, in instances of court involvement, judges may seek input from outside experts. See generally *Letoski v. U.S. Food and Drug Admin.*, 488 F.Supp. 952 (M. D. Pa. 1979). (The court appointed its own medical expert to assist in adjudication. This expert supplied the court with neutral scientific and medical information.)

40. Dreger (2004, 78).

41. See NAD Cochlear Implant Committee, *NAD Position Statement on Cochlear Implants* (2000) available at http://www.nad.org/infocenter/newsroom/positions/CochlearImplants.html (urging physicians, audiologists, and allied professionals to refer parents to qualified experts in deafness and to other appropriate resources in order to make fully informed decisions. Additionally, the paper emphasizes the myths of implants, and possible complete destruction of hearing because of surgery.). See also LPA Medical Advisory Board, Extended Limb-Lengthening Position Paper (year omitted), available at http://www.lpaonline.org/library_ellmedboard .html. (Because complications are numerous and substantial, potential candidates for limb-lengthening should only choose this surgery after adequate discussion of benefits and risks. Individuals should choose treatment only in an institution that can offer a thorough, multidisciplinary approach, including image and psychological evaluation.) See also Dreger (1998, 35) (parents must consider and solicit the experiences and advice of adult intersexuals before opting for surgery, as the correction of genitalia is often unnecessary and parents are usually uninformed regarding the overwhelming number of risks).

42. Asch (1998, 80).

43. For example, Dreger (1999, 88–89) describes the case of an intersexed woman whose mother chose not to opt for normalization surgery for her child. When asked whether she had any regrets about her mother's choice, the woman stated, "'A', I'm not ashamed of my physiology, my anatomy; 'B', it has not been a detriment at all to any aspect of my development—social, psychological, sexual, or otherwise—and I have no regrets, and no misgivings about how I am. I wouldn't rather be any other way, to tell you the truth. You know, even if I could completely dial in what I wanted to be like, or look like, that would be pretty low on the list of things I'd want to change." See also Ferguson et al. (2000).

REFERENCES

Ablon, J. 1988. *Living with Difference: Families with Dwarf Children.* New York: Praeger.

American Academy of Pediatrics Committee on Bioethics. 1995. Informed consent, parental permission, and assent in pediatric practice. *Pediatrics* 95 (2):314–17.

Asch, A. 1998. Distracted by disability: The "difference" of disability in the medical setting. *Cambridge Quarterly of Healthcare Ethics* 7:77–87.

Dreger, Alice Domurat. 1998. Ambiguous sex—or ambivalent medicine. *The Hastings Center Report* May–June.

———, ed. 1999. *Intersex in the Age of Ethics.* Hagerstown, MD: University Publishing Group.

———.*One of Us: Conjoined Twins and the Future of Normal.* Cambridge, MA: Harvard University Press.

Eugenides, E. 2002. *Middlesex.* New York: Farrar, Strauss and Giroux.

Ferguson, P. M., A. Gartner, and D. K. Lipsky. The experience of disability in families: A synthesis of research and parent narratives. In *Prenatal Testing and Disability Rights,* edited by E. Parens and A. Asch, 72–94. Washington, DC: Georgetown University Press.

Harris, David. 1997. Types, causes and physical treatment of physical differences. In *Visibly Different: Coping with Disfigurement,* edited by E. Bradbury, T. Carr, R. Lansdown, J. Partridge, and N. Rumsey, 79–90. London: Holder Arnold.

CHAPTER FIFTEEN

Appearance-Altering Surgery, Children's Sense of Self, and Parental Love

Adrienne Asch, Ph.D.

I am finishing this chapter while on a group tour in another country. During dinner one evening, a member of our group turns to ask whether she is possibly breaching the etiquette of the country we are visiting. She does not expect to become a full-fledged member of the culture and will be returning to the United States in a few weeks, but she would like to make sure she does not needlessly give offense to others.

Most observers of this transaction probably would believe that she is trying to be a good guest in a country but would not claim that she is "going native" or trying to "pass"; she is instead trying to learn enough of the rules to make others comfortable with her. Life in any family, group, or society requires ongoing negotiation, compromise, and at times the willingness to change in various ways to accommodate to others' preferences. Some changes or accommodations, however, raise disturbing questions that my traveling companion's willing modifications of her behavior do not.

In our project we have wrestled with how to assess whether parents and professionals should choose appearance-normalizing, perhaps better thought of as appearance-altering, surgery on behalf of children with atypical bodies. Here I consider many analogies and arguments that have emerged during our deliberations as I articulate my constantly evolving views about these surgeries.

These surgeries are considered for people with conditions that often require non-appearance-related medical care. For people with such conditions as achondroplasia, should appearance-altering surgery be thought of as akin to other nonemergency therapeutic interventions that ameliorate the physiologic effects of impairment (e.g., surgery that might help LilyClaire "to avoid damaging misalignment and wear and tear on cartilage")? (Hedley, this volume). Moving from interventions specific to people with impairments, is such surgery for children with atypical bodies analogous to what people with more-or-less typical bodies do when they use nonsurgical techniques (orthodonture, hair dyeing, acne medication) to make their appearance more acceptable to others?

If adults can decide to undertake all sorts of medical and surgical interventions on behalf of their own appearance, is there any reason why parents should not make such decisions on behalf of their children's futures? After all, Lindemann (this volume) reminds us that all parents directly and indirectly influence their children. Children's lives are affected by their parents' jobs and friends, as well as by decisions made specifically on behalf of their children. If they have the financial and social resources, parents select neighborhoods, schools, or daycare options based on how they assess their children's needs and also what they want for their children. Parents encourage some of their children's friendships and discourage others. If parents choose surgeries as a means of helping their children with atypical bodies better fit into the world around them, are they doing anything different from what they do when they teach those same children to say "please" and "thank you," to wear clothes that match, or to learn how to behave at meals?

Having wavered, struggled, and searched my life and my soul throughout the years of this project, I can finally comment on these analogies and arguments and can offer professionals, parents, and their children something beyond ambivalence. In what follows, I question some of the assumptions leading well-intentioned people to believe that surgery for children with atypical bodies is a good solution to the difficulties children may face because of their atypicality. For many of the reasons offered in our project's statement on delaying surgery for children with intersex conditions (Frader et al. 2004), I urge delaying all appearance-altering surgery until children can participate in the deliberations. Parents and professionals should recognize that although they may find pleasing appearances desirable, they should not overestimate the relationship between good looks and a good life. They should also consider that routine surgery may exacerbate the societal values that make them propose changing the child's body in the first place: an intolerance of what seems different, and an erroneous belief a child's unusual features will render her different and inferior in all ways. No matter how many of the child's physical features differ from what is viewed as typical, there are going to be many ways in which the child is similar to the typical child the parents were expecting.

As long as appearance-altering surgery will not erase all of the child's physical differences from species-typicality, they, their child, and the society will have to learn to appreciate and to destigmatize difference. Moreover, what seems like a "fix" to the parents and the professionals may not feel like a "fix" to the child whose body has been changed. By undertaking the surgery before children can voice feelings about their bodies and their lives, the most loving parent can unwittingly undermine the child's confidence that she is lovable and loved. It is confidence in that love and lovableness that provides the foundation for dealing with what life brings.

However, I think parents and children together may decide that appearance-altering surgeries will improve social relationships and consequently, psychological functioning; when they arrive at that decision, the surgeries should be available as other medical services are available. Along with Priscilla Alderson (this volume), and the American Academy of Pediatrics (1995), I would involve children in such conversation and decision making when they are very young and would urge parents to decline non-emergency surgery if their children do not see it as a solution to social difficulties or psychological distress. During their child's early life, the adults need not be passive and feel that their options during this time are limited to railing at societal cruelty. Whether or not the children ever choose surgery, how their parents and doctors behave toward them can give children tools for dealing with decisions about surgery and life.

Appearance: Means to an End, or End in Itself?

Two contradictory strands run in most people's heads about physical appearance. One strand of thought downplays its importance in life. Beauty is only skin deep; beauty is in the eye of the beholder; looks can be deceiving, so don't judge books (or people) by their covers. The other strand is virtually opposite: appearance does matter and should matter. First impressions say a lot about you; how you look and present yourself tells others how you think about yourself; you will be judged by your looks, and so if you want to get anywhere in the world, you should always be appropriate. The better-looking you are, the better your life will go because social and economic rewards flow to good-looking people.

Note how the "looks do and should matter" strand combines esthetic and psychological satisfactions with a much more utilitarian approach, which assumes that looks influence life outcomes. The raison d'etre of appearance-altering surgery for children with atypical bodies is that children and adults who don't look good, or at least typical, will not have good or typical lives. Two versions of this "looks matter to life outcomes" justification for surgery emerged during our working group deliberations.

One version went something like this:

The simplest argument for doing normalizing surgeries is that, like departures from species-typical physiological functioning, departures from species-typical form can compromise a person's ("equal") opportunity to pursue her life projects. This version of the medical model of disability assumes that damage to physiological and psychosocial functioning can both compromise equal opportunity—and that both equally deserve "repair." We think insurance should pay for cleft lip surgery because we think making the child look "more normal" will improve her psychosocial functioning; without the surgery, she will not enjoy "equal opportunity."

Another version of the "looks-matter-to-life-outcomes" argument took a social model approach to disability:

> When a technological fix is effective and relatively within reach of most people, and the social accommodation is much more substantial, it is easier on everyone to go with the fix. It is one way to see to it that the person's life does not go badly because of the impairment given the limitations of physical accommodation and psychological openness.

According to both formulations, surgical change is perceived to be the easiest way to give the person with the atypical body a chance at participating in the neighborhood, the classroom, the team, and the dance. The formulations see appearance change as a means of achieving inclusion, social acceptance, belonging, and love. If we are really only after these psychological and social rewards, I suggest later that we might find strategies for helping children achieve them without appearance change. I think, though, that appearance matters to us for reasons that are not entirely covered by saying it is a means to these rewards.

Even if we didn't suspect that physical attractiveness influenced quality of life, we might still value it in people, just as we take esthetic pleasure in nature and the arts. People do not live in the world as disembodied minds, souls, or spirits. We meet the external world in our bodies, and each meeting is an encounter with people's physical characteristics.

Exactly which physical features count in a given era or culture may vary, and not everyone adopts the culture's preferences. In some fundamental way though, we want our bodies, as well as our minds and hearts, to be pleasing to ourselves and to others, and we surely do not want our physical selves to prevent other people from knowing the rest of us. We dress differently for picnics than for professional conferences, and in each setting, we select clothes that emphasize the parts of our bodies we like. I do mean "we" here, for neither my upbringing, which stressed the mental and the moral, nor my blindness, exempts me from being interested in how I and others appear. (Like other people I know who are not blind, I ask for feedback on whether I should change my hairstyle, or on what to wear to a certain meeting or social event; and I sometimes try to reduce impairment-related atypicality by learning the visual effects of different postures.)

In addition to the social or professional rewards that come from looking our best, we can enjoy presenting our best selves to the world. We needn't apologize for taking pleasure in our own and others' appearances any more than we should be embarrassed about enjoying good conversation, improving our swimming or skiing, or selecting comfortable and attractive furniture for our homes. We want our homes to reflect who we are, and we want people to like the home to which they have been invited. If our homes are personal to us, how much more personal are our own bodies? We want to be comfortable with our own bodies and to have them at least accepted by the world.

Although our desire for pleasing appearances may stem in part from seeing appearance as a means to another end, we can see that meeting whatever standard we have of appearance may be one of our ends as well. People like to look good, to themselves as well as to others. If we are clear that even people with more-or-less typical bodies often get pleasure from doing something to improve their appearances, we may be able to acknowledge that parents and physicians might consider appearance-altering surgery for very young children because they want to enjoy the esthetic and psychological rewards of the child's more customary, more pleasing appearance.

Appearance, Stigma, and Impairment as a Violation of a Suspect Norm

Of course, my means-end differentiation can be only partly successful, because people acquire their own internal standards of esthetics partly from the culture in which they live. Sometimes people will ignore cultural norms and friends' advice about dyeing their hair or discarding a sweater for nonappearance-related reasons. (They don't want to go through the time and expense of repeated beauty parlor appointments, or they find the sweater warm and comfortable, but in these instances they have let other values take precedence over their interest in being esthetically appealing.) I understand the satisfactions of doing appearance work and the pleasure that can come from others' favorable responses to pleasing appearances, but I want to challenge the notions that appearance does matter and should matter to life outcomes.

So let's leave the part of the "appearance matters" strand that enjoys the process and the product of appearance work and return to the underlying utilitarian assumptions of appearance-altering surgery put forward in our working group's ongoing conversation: appearance matters to life outcomes, and if we want people with atypical bodies to have a chance at social inclusion and a rewarding life, we should do whatever we can to make their appearances less atypical. Changing people's attitudes toward appearance is arguably far more difficult than changing laws and practices to require access to the built environment; laws that facilitate the inclusion of children with disabilities in the classroom do nothing to guarantee that teachers will pay attention to them or that students will become their friends.

What do we actually know about how physical attractiveness or unattractiveness affects life outcomes? Lindemann (this volume) cites data showing that appearance matters in school and at work: teachers punish "ugly" students more harshly and grade them less well than other students. People rated "ugly" earn less than workers rated better-looking. Some commentators would broaden antidiscrimination legislation to encompass denials of opportunity based upon physical appearance (Note 1987; Wasserman 2000). Yet the academic literature doesn't entirely support the "looks matter to life" stereotype. It yields several qualifications to the stereotype by showing that appearance influences some arenas of life but not all, and that looks by themselves don't account for the whole story in any area of life outcome. The research tells much more about how attractive people are *perceived by* others than it does about how they are treated or what their personalities are like. To the extent that the research supports the "looks matter" stereotype, it finds that personality and self-esteem factors also count in how others perceive and treat people.

The social-psychological literature indicates that people expect attractive people to have better lives and personalities than those considered less attractive. This expectation applies, however, only to the dimensions of social popularity and romantic life. In a 1991 review of work on the stereotypes of physically attractive people, the authors wrote:

> Although subjects in these studies ascribed more favorable personality traits and more successful life outcomes to attractive than unattractive targets, the average magnitude of this beauty-is-good effect was moderate . . . The differences in subjects' perception of attractive and unattractive targets were largest for indexes of social competence; intermediate for potency, adjustment, and intellectual competence; and near zero for integrity and concern for others. (Eagly et al. 1991, 109)

Another review of voluminous research on both perceptions of and personality correlates of physical attractiveness revealed that physical attractiveness affected some parts of life, but by no means all:

> The experimental literature found that physically attractive people were perceived as more sociable, dominant, sexually warm, mentally healthy, intelligent, and socially skilled than physically unattractive people. Yet, the correlational literature indicated generally trivial relationships between physical attractiveness and measures of personality and mental ability, although good-looking people were less lonely, less socially anxious, more popular, more socially skilled, and more sexually experienced than unattractive

people. *Self-ratings of physical attractiveness were positively correlated with a wider range of attributes than was actual physical attractiveness.* (Feingold 1992, 305, emphasis added)

Yes, people assume that attractive people will be more socially successful, popular, outgoing, and desired than people who are considered less attractive; and as stated in the Feingold review, attractiveness did correlate with these outcomes. I draw attention to the last sentence of the passage, however, to note that self-esteem and self-confidence were correlated with a larger group of positive qualities than attractiveness itself. At least in studies using people with typical bodies, how people feel about themselves is broadly more important to psychological well-being than the physical self one presents to the world, a point that bears on my conclusions and recommendations later in this essay.

So the psychological literature says that appearance does influence outcomes in some areas, but the influence is itself mediated by personality differences. The attractiveness literature doesn't consider children and adults with atypical bodies, but the stigma literature shows that their atypicality often negatively affects how others treat them. There is substantial information to support the claim that people with atypical bodies, especially people considered to have impairments or disabilities, are treated as inferior to those whose bodies are considered broadly acceptable (Gliedman and Roth 1980; Shapiro 1994; Francis and Silvers 2000; Heatherton et al. 2000).

Public law and policy has recognized that people with physical atypicalities experience adverse treatment and discrimination, and the populations we considered in this project all would come under the protection of the Americans with Disabilities Act as it was originally understood in 1990. People with achondroplasia, intersex conditions, and craniofacial anomalies are impaired or are regarded as being impaired in one or more substantial life activity. Notwithstanding later court decisions that may have weakened the power of the act, there can be no doubt that its passage signaled recognition of pervasive mistreatment and discrimination not unlike that to which other groups in the United States had been subjected.

Individuals with disabilities are a discrete and insular minority who have been . . . subjected to a history of purposeful unequal treatment, and relegated to a position of political powerlessness in our society . . . resulting from . . . assumptions not truly indicative of the . . . ability of such individuals to participate in, and contribute to, society. (Americans with Disabilities Act 1990)

Even without knowing the extent of legal discrimination they experience or report (Miller, this volume; Greenhouse 2003), parents and professionals have reason for concern about the life prospects of people with short stature, intersex conditions, and craniofacial differences. The goal of proposed appearance-altering surgery is to minimize the departure from species-typical form in the hopes of forestalling or lessening instances of mistreatment and social isolation so frequently featured in academic and autobiographical accounts of people with what Goffman (1963, 5) referred to as "abominations of the body."

Parents are undoubtedly concerned about the social, occupational, and personal lives of their children. Recalling that physical attractiveness is reported to correlate with popularity, social skill, and sexual experience (Feingold 1992), and noting the difficulty often reported by people with a range of disabilities in finding dates and mates (Shakespeare et al. 1996), it is surely tempting to endorse a surgical solution. In order to have confidence that altering a child's appearance would lessen cruelty, teasing, social rejection, or employment discrimination, we would have to believe that appearance, not the underlying impairment, elicits the aversive responses. If some, but not all indications of disability were removed, would there be less cruelty?

The available research and theory cannot yet answer these questions. Researchers propose that individuals will be subject to stigma if others suspect that their characteristics or their actions threaten effective group life (Neuberg et al. 2000; Stangor and Crandall 2000). Historically, people with visible impairments were thought to endanger group safety and survival if they could not perform necessary tasks and if they reproduced their abnormalities in the next generation.

Hahn (1983) posits that disability arouses both esthetic and existential anxiety in the nondisabled population. Scholars who have examined interactions between people with and without disabilities stress the existential as much as or more than the esthetic anxiety. They explain that nondisabled people fear what will occur in their dealings with someone who has an impairment: Will the nondisabled person be too helpful or not helpful enough? Will they offend by discussing activities that might be difficult or impossible because of the disability? And will they become entrapped, demanded of, or disappointed because the person with the impairment will need more than they offer (Davis 1961; Gliedman and Roth 1980; Stroman 1982; Harris 1997; Hebl and Kleck 2000)?

These scholars have not sought to tease out whether it is the visibility of the characteristic or its link to a functional impairment that arouses the difficulties. To add to the problem of sorting out the sources of discomfort and stigma, a large body of literature shows that when nondisabled people learn of the hidden impairments of acquaintances or friends, they often engage in cruel and stigmatizing behaviors (Goffman 1963; Schneider and Conrad 1980; Wright 1983). Many people with achondroplasia and craniofacial conditions have physical impairments that would remain after even the most successful surgery reduced the departures from typical form. Without being confident that appearance, and not underlying impairment, triggers the stigma the surgery is supposed to alleviate, parents, professionals, and policy makers may prescribe something that does little to alleviate the problem it is supposed to solve.

Although there is very little information available specifically about how people with achondroplasia, intersex conditions, and craniofacial abnormalities view their bodies or lives, the literature on the general disabled population reveals that people with disabilities judge their lives much more positively than nondisabled people—including medical professionals—expect (Albrecht and Devlieger 1999; Basnett 2001; Gill 2001). When they report disability-related dissatisfaction, they attribute the problems to how individuals and institutions respond to their impairments, not to unhappiness with their physical state (National Organization on Disability 1999). We don't know whether people with atypical bodies internalize the world's negative responses to their own bodies or whether they, like the larger disabled population, see stigma and discrimination—not their bodies—as their real problem. We also cannot cite empirical data concluding that life is better for the same person after surgery, or that surgically altered individuals fare better than those without the surgical fix.

We found no reviews of the social and psychological consequences o limb-lengthening surgeries, only testimony about negative consequences for people with intersex conditions, and little about responses to surgery for craniofacial disfigurements. In one of the few studies following children after surgery for craniofacial conditions, positive outcomes for the young people were attributed to increases in self-confidence whether or not the surgery had noticeably improved physical appearance (Lefebvre and Munro 1986). As with the findings that self-rated attractiveness was more related to positive ratings on personality attributes than was actual attractiveness measured by others (Feingold 1992), this finding about postsurgical self-confidence leads me to wonder whether the alteration could come in the self-confidence, and not the body, of the person described as disfigured or impaired. Nearly twenty years later, our working group experts on these craniofacial conditions concluded that surgeries were continuing to be offered without empirical evidence to demonstrate that they improved children's lives (Mouradian et al., this volume).

Whether others' dislike of atypical appearance or discomfort with impaired function is the principal source of stigma and discrimination, the negative response to people with disabilities leads me to urge that discussion of appearance-altering surgery for people with departures from typical form should be analyzed much as Margaret Little (1996) analyzed potential requests for alterations to women or to people of color that grow out of entrenched sexism and racism. She differentiated between the prejudice toward a boy with unusual-appearing ears and the history and contemporary social system of racism and sexism that might lead members of stigmatized groups to seek physical changes to their bodies. I understood her to be open to applying her racism-sexism analysis to people with Down syndrome, but not to everyone with an atypical body such as a boy whose ears stick out from his head.

The pervasiveness of stigma toward people with departures from species-typical form, and the fact that people with facial disfigurements are often "regarded as" having impairments even if they have no diminished physical function, convinces me that the people we are discussing are surgical candidates because their departures from typicality are seen as signs of disfavored impairment. Although atypical ears may evoke less stigma and ridicule than atypical faces, heights, or genitals, the history and contemporary record of mistreating people based on biology merits Little's eloquent description of the wish for surgical alteration as growing out of a "suspect norm."

> The cases of cosmetic surgery that raise special moral concern, then, are cases in which the dissatisfaction or distress that people ask medicine to alleviate results, not from morally innocuous preferences, but from practices or ideologies that are morally troubling—for instance, suffering that stems from cruel teasing, or distress that arises from trying to meet the pressures of a norm whose content is steeped in injustice. (Little 1996, 169)

The injustice at issue is in treating people with impairments, or those regarded as having impairments, as moral and social inferiors because they differ from and cannot meet certain typical norms of appearance and health. To many physicians, the appearance-altering surgeries are ways out of what was once the "given" of disfigurement, and presumably the procedures were developed as solutions to negatively perceived bodily difference. Rather than being distracted from the whole child by the disfigurement (Asch 1998), the surgery is a way to discover the whole of the child; surgery removes the distraction and lets the world find out what the personality of the child can be. But the very surgery to remove the different and unacceptable appearance legitimates, or is at least complicitous with, the idea that atypical appearances are reasons to avoid or mistreat people. If we want to create a society that judges others by their character and not by their height, facial features, or genitals, we must suggest that it could be acceptable to "let things be," and to let people be (Parens 2005). When physicians propose surgery to normalize a child in order to prevent other people from being distracted by disability, those physicians imply that it is permissible for difference/disability to be distracting.

The surgical "fix" of the person leaves unchallenged, and arguably endorses, the practice of isolating, rejecting, or denigrating people with atypical bodies. Using this "fix" accepts the idea that appearances can legitimately influence life outcomes and undermines the morality that character, not outward form, is what ought to count. Automatic appearance-altering surgery fails to promote the idea that disability and physical difference is a legitimate form of human variation that a just society can and should include (Scotch and Schriner 1997). Instead, routine endorsement and promotion of the surgery continues the historic practice of suggesting that the traits are mistakes of nature that ought to be changed. In something of the same spirit as Edwards (this volume), I suggest that the surgical technology is not neutral but is instead a professional and societal statement that certain anatomical variations should be eliminated or ameliorated. One need not be theologically or politically traditional to be wary of the idea that technological solutions will obviate the need to incorporate people into the community irrespective of physical difference. And, as Lennard Davis (1995) has pointed out, it is regrettable that many people deeply committed to respecting pluralism and family diversity endorse surgeries to achieve physical uniformity.

The Parent-Child Relationship and the Child's Sense of Self

Thus far I have contended that when physicians propose very early appearance-altering surgeries for the child with an atypical body, the proposal stems from the limited data but powerful stereotype that a person's appearance determines how well his or her life will turn out. The recommendation also inadvertently reinforces that strand in our heads that condones letting looks influence life. The physician's recommendation for surgery conveys the view that the child is different, the difference is bad, and the child's difference and badness must be fixed or reduced so that she can have a chance to fit into the world. The child is the problem, not others' mistreatment. The conversation about changing the child often comes very shortly after birth, before the parents know their child, before the child has had much chance to learn about his body or his parents, and years before he has met the dreaded bully on the playground.

Yet literature on child development for typical and atypical children overwhelmingly demonstrates that early relationships with caretakers provide the child a crucial foundation for dealing with the world. Caretakers must provide children with the sense that their needs will be met and must simultaneously convey that the child is enjoyed and valued (Karen 1994). Ornstein and Ornstein (1984, 96) argue that the task of caretaking adults "is the development of parental empathy in relationship to a particular child." According to them, parental empathy is "a capacity in which an adult man or woman can immerse him- or herself into the inner life of a child"; in that activity adults try to separate their needs and desires from those of the child. The child's atypical body, and an early discussion about surgical alteration of the child, can each disrupt developing parental empathy and the child's feeling of trust in others.

Caretakers, most often biological parents, are aided or thwarted in achieving a sense of empathy and effectiveness as parents by their interactions with the child. Ornstein and Ornstein (1984) and Stern (2004) demonstrate that infants influence the interactions by how they respond to caretaking behavior. Parents expect their infants to be comforted by their touch, their voice tones, and their facial expressions, by how parents play with them, and by how parents handle them during feeding, bathing, and diaper changing. If parents perceive their infants as inconsolable, or if parents don't get the smiles or looks they expect from their infants, they may feel ineffective and disappointed. If parents cannot read what the infant needs and respond appropriately, parents and infant are deprived.

Parental confusion, ambivalence, and apprehension are unfortunate for the child and the parents, but these responses do not indicate ill will or malice. They can result from an absence of expected cues or from failing to read what cues the infant gives. Without aid from medical or mental health professionals, or contact with others raising similarly atypical children, it is very likely that new parents would have trouble responding positively and warmly to their baby.

All parents don't love all children, and not all parents of children with disabilities learn to read their cues or otherwise come to love them. In a six-year study of more than 1,200 Israeli families whose children had atypical appearances, sociologist Meira Weiss (1994) found that 80 percent of the parents overtly rejected their children, either abandoning them altogether or isolating the children in the home away from the rest of the family. Literature about parents of disabled children in North America is not filled with such overtly rejecting behavior, even when it suggests initial stress and difficulty. Leaving aside for now the question of whether parents should have altered their children's appearances, the accounts on the Intersex Society of North America (ISNA) website demonstrate that many people with intersex conditions deal with pain and anguish resulting from less-than-empathic parental responses. Studies of parents of children with cleft palate, cleft lip, and other craniofacial differences also reveal that parents were much less involved in play, touch, smiling, laughing, and interacting with their impaired children as compared with parents of children who did not have impairments (Rogers-Salyer et al. 1987; Walters 1997).

Most parents become good enough at this business of attunement and empathy, and this statement holds for the parents who discover that their child has an atypical body. The research on parents raising children with disabilities reveals that by and large, parents learn to read the cues of a child with an atypical body, and they come to appreciate the child in front of them even though she may look very different from other children (Ferguson 2001; Klein and Schieve 2001).

When adults with childhood disabilities reflect on their lives, they attribute success in meeting schoolyard bullying, adolescent isolation, and adult discrimination to the acceptance and support they received from their parents; when they are asked their advice for parents of future children with disabilities, a consistent message runs through their accounts: "Love me and accept me as I am" (Klein and Kemp 2004).

Much recent narrative and qualitative research on the experiences of people who grew up with visible disabilities describes their confusion, anger, and pain at therapeutic regimens devised by professionals but implemented by parents (Gill 2001). Anthropologist Gelya Frank (1988) found that the people she interviewed felt more whole and more "normal" without the uncomfortable prosthetic limbs that were urged on them because the prostheses were alleged to make their bodies look more typical.

Writing in 1984 about her life with a disability, therapist Harilyn Rousso eloquently articulates a difficult episode in a family life that included warmth and encouragement:

> She [her mother] made numerous attempts over the years of my childhood to have me go for physical therapy and to practice walking more "normally" at home. I vehemently refused all her efforts. She could not understand why I would not walk straight . . . My disability, with my different walk and talk and my involuntary movements, having been with me all of my life, was part of me, part of my identity. With these disability features, I felt complete and whole. My mother's attempt to change my walk, strange as it may seem, felt like an assault on myself, an incomplete acceptance of all of me, an attempt to make me over. (9)

A psychoanalyst writing about his analysis of a 12-year-old boy born with short and deformed arms further underscores the point about the boy's sense of his body as intact and his need for parental acceptance and love. Lussier (1980) admits his own surprise at discovering that

> the boy seemed to have been much more in need of confidence of his mother in him than in need of normal arms . . . The body one cathects from birth on, as it is and as it is perceived by the child, not the body as it could or should be, is what matters psychologically. Any child is destined to invest, to cathect the body he has, as it is, which will soon become a basic part of what he is. And this is the body that the mother has to acknowledge, to incorporate, to fuse with, in order to grant it psychological existence for the child, a safe, secure, existence. Mental health grows on this soil. (181)

What does it mean for a parent to accept a child in the sense Lussier means, of accepting the child's body as it is? If an appearance-altering surgery will change that body in ways that are promised to give the child more social acceptance in the world later on, should the parent accept the existing body or change the child's body to make the child more acceptable to the world? Do physicians propose early appearance alteration not simply for easing the child's acceptance into to the world beyond the family, but to ease the parents' path to incorporating the child into the family? Given that the essence of early parenting is intense physical involvement with the child, medical professionals may see appearance alteration as a way to ensure that parents will take pleasure in their child's body, indeed will invest in it just as Lussier claims children need.

During our deliberations, we read of one surgery to change the appearance of a fatally ill infant to aid her parents to relate to and care for her (Frankel and Juengst 1991). In a study that compared the interactions of mothers and typical infants with those of mothers and their infants with craniofacial deformities, the authors noted marked and troubling differences that led them to believe that the mothers of the atypical children were not as comfortable, involved, or bonded with their children as were the other mothers (Rogers-Salyer et al. 1987). Interestingly, the study led to two recommendations: early surgery for facial differences to change the appearance in the hopes of changing the mother's behavior; and parent education about the potential disruptions of the parent-child relationship signaled by the less attentive parenting they observed.

I firmly believe that infants need to trust and become attached to the people who care for them, and I equally firmly believe that parents are deprived of one of the joys of raising children if they do not have the experience of delighting in their child and in the time they spend with their baby. The most compelling argument for early surgery is that by altering the child's appearance, the parent will more easily, naturally, and wholeheartedly invest in the child who looks more like what she envisioned. If parents themselves feel that they cannot wholeheartedly embrace, welcome, and love their child without such a surgical alteration, surgery may be an appropriate path, but I strongly recommend a path that delays the surgery until the child can be involved in the conversation about altering her body. Instead of surgery, I endorse the kind of parent education mentioned above, as well as other activities I discuss shortly. I am concerned that altering children before they can participate in the decisions made about their bodies can be seriously detrimental for parent-child relations throughout life. The surgically altered child may come to appreciate her parents' love, but she may also live with discomfort and anxiety that could come from suspecting that the parents needed her changed in order to love her. The surgery and the parental acceptance it achieved may damage the very self-esteem and self-confidence the surgery is intended to foster.

Earlier I asked whether appearance-altering surgery could be thought of as a means of socialization for living that resembled other socializing activities: toilet training, learning to use a fork, learning to say "please" and "thank you." I have concluded that the surgical alteration of an infant's or very young child's body differs from activities that parents undertake with their growing children to develop or to change behavior. Behaviors like learning to thank people or learning to use the bathroom are all activities, things people do; they are changes to particular ways a child acts in specified situations. They are not irreversible changes to one of the child's first pieces of knowledge—his sense of self, his own body. Infants and very young children know their bodies and are engaged in the process of differentiating themselves from other people and from the external world. Just as parents first know their children through their bodies, young infants know themselves in their bodies. They explore their own bodies and experience the world with and through their bodies. Infants touch their mouths, faces, and genitals. Long before they can speak or understand a lot of what others say to them, they look at themselves. Changing a child's body early in life alters one of the only things a child knows and experiences.

From the small child's point of view, the face with the cleft lip is the face she touches throughout the day. Waking up after an appearance-altering surgery, the child discovers that something has changed about her lip and face, but she cannot ask what it is or why it has occurred, and she cannot understand what her father or mother might want to tell her. Something confusing, probably frightening has happened to one of the only things the child knows and trusts in the world, her own body. What is sacred in medicine and bioethics may be important to infants and young children also: bodily integrity.

The parents who decide that their child's welfare will be jeopardized without immediate surgery should be helped to recognize that this action is likely to cause its own psychological problems for the child that will be resolved only with sensitivity and empathy from the parent. Remember that as yet there is no true surgical "fix" for the differences from typicality that the surgery is intended to eradicate. Existing surgeries leave physical scars and do not make the child's face look typical. After the surgery, the parents may be disappointed to find that the difference is less, but not gone. At some time the child will realize that her face is not quite like those of other children and adults she knows, and it isn't exactly like the face she had at birth. Both the residual difference, and the attempt to minimize it, are parts of life the parents will need to explain.

Can parents communicate their pleasure in and commitment to their child, their "acceptance" of their child, and simultaneously explain that they believed it necessary to change something about their child's body? Such a communication may not be logically impossible, but it is fraught with psychological difficulties. This is a very different sort of communication than asking a child to cover her mouth when she coughs, or to use a Kleenex after she sneezes, or to brush her teeth morning and night. Parents explain how these activities protect other people's health and welfare, as well as how they conform to social expectations. Her father and mother told the same thing to her older brother, and her playmate is getting the same instructions from her parents. These lessons happen to everyone; they are about things a child does, not about her body itself, and they are not unique to her, because her body is different and is somehow different in an undesirable way.

I go back to the messages of people with disabilities to their parents to be loved and accepted as they are, and to Lussier's discovery that his 12-year-old patient was comfortable with his arms and body and needed parental approval and affirmation. To the parents and physicians living in typical bodies, the surgery normalizes the child by making her body more like that of the people she knows, more like the statistical majority. To the child, though, her body is normal, it is the one she knows and accepts (Aspinall, this volume). The surgery changes her, her sense of the expected, the ordinary, the normal.

In most situations of appearance-altering surgery, the underlying medical condition, impairment, disability, difference is going to remain even after the most physically effective alteration. The parents are raising a child with some medical needs and some stigmatized observable differences. This is one of the givens of the parents' and child's lives at a particular time and for the foreseeable future, just as being the third child of the family is a given. Parents and children will find some givens positive, others neutral, others perhaps regrettable, but they are givens; one of the most important tasks of parenting and of life is figuring out how to live with those givens.

Philosopher Michael Sandel (2004), quoting ethicist William May, speaks of the two kinds of love children need: accepting love and transforming love. Accepting love affirms a child's being; transforming love promotes the child's well-being. Before the child needs transforming love, he needs accepting love. The child with a difference from the species-typical needs his parents to let him know that to them he is an acceptable, valuable, delighted-in, lovable being; he may differ in some way from other people around him, but he is valuable and valued by them. His body doesn't need to change for them to enjoy him.

Parental acceptance and affirmation of a child with a visible stigmatized difference that parents may find startling and disappointing may initially emerge as a psychological challenge, but family research and personal narrative demonstrates that most parents accomplish it (Darling 1979; Ferguson 2001; Klein and Schieve 2001; Klein and Kemp 2004). Such parental acceptance and affirmation can acknowledge that the child's difference may cause him problems down the road. When the child starts to ask about the difference, parents can say that they regret that their child is experiencing problems because of this difference. Such acknowledgment differs from parents believing and communicating that they see the child as flawed, disappointing, or imperfect. The work that the parent needs to do with himself, and then with the child, is work that says to the child, "No, not everyone looks like you, has this particular characteristic, but you do. You can live a good life." The parent does not have to feel or to say that this difference is a desirable feature of the child; the parent just has to communicate that the child is desirable, even if not every facet of his appearance or his behavior is what the parent hoped for or expected.

Along with Sandel (2004), I am urging that parents of all children, not only children who have stigmatized differences, go beyond Sara Ruddick's (1989) set of crucial tasks in child-raising. To the tasks of protection, fostering physical growth, and training for becoming a socially acceptable member of a community, the parent must affirm the child in her or his uniqueness, must appreciate who the child is, with that child's set of attributes, some of which may be strengths, others problems. Parents, physicians, and bioethicists should not confuse the work of accepting the unique child with the work of later helping that child become an accepted and appreciated member of a community. If fathers and mothers affirm, enjoy, and love the child with the unusual face, they give the child the foundation for believing that others can love her too. Parents usually love their children, even when those children don't look the ways that parents expect, just as they love children who choose politics, religion, lifestyles, and mates their parents don't like. The work of "adopting" (Ruddick 1989) the child with a stigmatized visible difference is the same work parents do with all their children; that work of adoption and commitment differs in degree, not in kind, from the work all parents must do to raise all their children.

A decision for appearance-altering surgery, made with the child's collaboration, can be an instance of the love that promotes the child's well-being, after accepting love is clear to that child. In the next section, I comment on how parents can demonstrate parental love before making the decision about surgery. I conclude this essay by discussing how parents and children together may approach decisions about appearance-altering surgery.

Demonstrating Parental Love

In much the same spirit as Alice Dreger (this volume), I offer parents whose children have atypical bodies some suggestions for how they can provide both accepting and transforming love. Here I am trying to operationalize a version of parental love that may help future parents escape the tragedy that befell the first two mothers Feder (this volume) describes and may promote parental behavior portrayed in Feder's last example. No one reading the first accounts can doubt the parents' concern for their children's lives, growth, and well-being. Yet had the first parents received different advice, they might have spent their time and talent helping their children understand their bodies and their situations, regardless of any ultimate decisions about surgical change.

As you are getting to know your new baby with an unusual appearance, separate your surprise, discomfort, and disappointment with her appearance from your fears for her future. At first your baby's face may seem so overwhelmingly different and distorted that you cannot imagine relating to her, and you may have trouble seeing those ways in which she looks like you, your partner, or other members of your biological families. Don't apologize for your initial negative response, because it can be a great joy to delight in the way your child looks. Not having that immediate gratification can pose a significant challenge for you as a parent. But remember that it is a different sadness and a different challenge from imagining that your child's life is ruined before it starts. Your child has other gifts to offer, and you can help her discover them.

Get to know your particular child. Look at her, touch her, get help learning her cues about what she wants. If her face has startling birthmarks, if her cleft lip is initially very distressing and interferes with your reading of her facial expressions, find all the other facets of her body, her movements, her sounds, her skin, her pleasure at being touched and held that feel ordinary and familiar and what you expected of your child.

Whatever your child's body looks like, however much it differs from the usual, your child has many features that are typical of other infants. As your child grows, there is every reason to expect that your child will be different in only some features. Do not let yourself, your doctors, your family, or anyone else insist that you focus on how your child differs from other children. That difference is only one facet of your child, and your time with her will help you discover all the ways that she is not different.

Next, remember that as uncommon as your child's impairment or disfigurement may be, other children and adults live with it, and other families are living with and loving their children whose bodies look like your child's unusual body. Along with Alice Dreger, I endorse having parents find others who have traveled your new road; they will tell you what no one else can about introducing your child to others and fending off curiosity, pity, or rudeness. While you are finding parents, get in contact with young people and adults who live with your child's atypical body, and hear their stories of strategies that work for them and ones that have failed them. Like others who have studied parents and children before you, they can tell you that time with your child is the best teacher and the best ally to forging empathy and mutual responsiveness.

Perhaps the most difficult work in parenting a child whose body is atypical and stigmatized comes in learning to recognize that the difference is simply a difference, not the flaw others perceive it to be. Throughout her chapter in this volume, Lisa Hedley wrestles with how she sees her daughter with achondroplasia. Is this a "flaw," as she sometimes describes it, or does LilyClaire look as she concludes, just the way someone who is a dwarf is supposed to look? Surgeons who insist on the need for appearance-normalizing surgery see this difference as bad, sad, dangerous for your child's acceptance and your child's future; you do not have to accept this characterization of your child's features. You don't have to love this difference, any more than you have to love every facet of your own physical self or the physical self of your partner. You may be correct in thinking that your child might have some unpleasantness and heartache because of how others respond to her, but you must be clear that the heartbreak stems from other people's cruelty, not from her flaw. Your child may not be statistically average, but she is morally equal to everyone else. As your child's first caretakers, you set a tone for your child and for the people who meet her in your company. Your son or daughter can learn from you to deserve to belong and to be included, and that sense of being worthy will help the boy or girl to become her or his own advocate.

Whether or not surgery can change your child's appearance, your child must have a self, a personality, a spirit, a curiosity, to bring to the world and to other people. As her parent, you begin to help her discover that self, and you can help her discover what she has to offer to others. You can teach her to reach out to other people, to let others know she wants to play with them, to be open and responsive to friendly overtures. As she grows older, you can show her that being liked by others does not require being exactly like others; it requires having a personality that offers something to others that they can enjoy. If people are stigmatized because they are seen as threats to group life, and feared to violate norms of reciprocity, one of the most important lessons you can teach your child is that she has things to offer others that they will enjoy and value. Children with typical bodies may have less difficulty in having pleasant interactions with other people, and they may have more opportunities for friendship, sociability, romance, and love. But they, too, must learn the same lesson: that after their face draws people to them, there must be a self that others will find a worthy friend and companion.

Perhaps a parent's deepest fear is that even if she loves her atypical child, no one else will see past that physical difference enough to know and love her. The father or mother may feel that a physical change will give the child opportunity for ordinary, static-free interaction that strengths of character can never achieve. Parents don't want to imagine a life of loneliness for their child, and they may understandably want less adversity for her even if they believe she has the psychological resources and fortitude to get through it.

Like Alice Dreger, Priscilla Alderson, and others, I am urging delay in changing a child's appearance until the child can voice her reactions to life with her body. I support collaborative decisions, whether they are for or against surgical alteration. I conclude by commenting on when and how that change may work well for parents and for the children who change their bodies to suit others' comfort.

Deciding Together about Surgery

Let us assume that the parents have been the good-enough parents everyone hopes children will have. They have loved their child and had fun with her. She knows that her face, or her genitals, or her body size differs from that of most other children and adults, and she appears to have incorporated this fact and gone about playing, bickering with her siblings, learning to share her toys, and learning to read. Margaret Little (1996) imagines a situation in which a small boy with atypical ears begs his parents for surgery, and they agree.

> Think of a young boy who has ears that stick straight out. Imagine further that he is one of the unfortunates who is teased mercilessly and constantly by his schoolmates and children of casual encounter. His parents have tried to comfort him and to offer him strategies for dealing with his tormentors, but to no avail. The taunting has begun to color his whole outlook on life: he becomes withdrawn, begins wetting the bed; his grades drop. His parents finally decide, with his enthusiastic support and relief, to request that a surgeon tuck his ears closer to his head. (164)

A *New York Times* story a year later makes clear that such hypothetical cases occur in real life: "'I was getting teased, called names like Dumbo and Big Ears,' said Scott, now 12, of Copiague, New York. 'I didn't feel that good about it. I wanted to look normal'" (Lambert 1997). And a heartwarming 1995 news story about surgery for a smile for 7-year-old Chelsey Thomas describes how the eleven-hour procedure would give her first chance at the pleasure of smiling (Associated Press 1995); a follow-up story (*Houston Chronicle* 1996) tells of the satisfaction she and her family have of seeing her smile as she blows out the candles on the cake at her eighth birthday. It is easy to understand how she and her family feel joy that she can now communicate pleasure, friendliness, and warmth in a spontaneous smile. Both children in these newspaper accounts are described as feeling relief and happiness with their changed appearance after the surgeries.

It appears that these two children were eager for the surgeries, and we can hope that the physical changes have continued to satisfy them and help them have the opportunity for easier social relationships than they experienced in their early lives. During our project deliberations, Emily Sullivan Sanford (this volume), a college student with achondroplasia, spoke about her decision to undergo the many surgeries and attendant hospitalizations and complications for lengthening her limbs and increasing her height by 11 inches. She recognized the reduced mobility that resulted from surgical complications, and she described herself as a "tall dwarf," fully aware that she will have the condition of achondroplasia forever.

If children report the kind of teasing, bullying, or unkindness that parents fear, and if they themselves start asking for help to deal with the responses coming their way, parents can raise the question with them of whether they would like to change their bodies as one strategy to deal with the problems they encounter. Parents and doctors need to make clear that surgery is not a cure-all; changing their bodies will minimize some differences from other people, but I have heard of no situation in which it would erase all of the stigmatized difference from others. Obviously, as Alderson (1993) points out, children should be told a good deal about what the procedures will be like, how many there will be, how well they will work, what the recovery will be like, and what they might look like after each procedure and after the contemplated surgical course is completed. They need to think about how much disruption to school, play, and ordinary life they want to undergo with the surgery, since most procedures are not one-time magical erasures of difference. If children perceive surgery as potentially helpful, they have a much greater chance of tolerating its complications, valuing what changes it brings, and making their peace with the fact that techniques are imperfect, change is not complete, and other people may still respond cruelly to remaining signs of difference.

If cleft lip surgery is typically effective in reducing the magnitude of visible difference, why do I say wait with it, as well as wait with more complex, less effective surgical correction? Imagine a 7-year-old boy or girl who is told about the possibility of such a surgery after months of teasing in school. Perhaps he will ask his mother: "If that's possible, why didn't you do it a long time ago?" The mother can say to her son, "I love you; we all love you in this family. We didn't need you to change in order for us to love you. We knew that if you wanted to change the way you looked, there would be time for you to make that decision. It is your body, not mine, that is getting changed if you do this surgery. You will have things done to you; I can help you think about what you want to do, and I can give you my advice and experience, but your body belongs to you. No one should touch it to hurt you, only to help you. If you want doctors to change your face, we can arrange that change, but it is your face and you have lived with it for these years. You get to decide whether you'll be happier if it is different from the way you have known it."

Many, perhaps most children, will opt for the surgery, but whether or not they change their faces, they will know that their parents didn't feel their bodies needed to be changed in order to live in the world. Children should get the chance to decide whether they think the treatment they are getting from others merits subjecting their bodies to invasive procedures. They will have a clear indication that parents, probably the most important people in their lives, do not need them to do this but will support them if they want to. They will have been accorded love and respect for their feelings and been assured that they are not alone in their lives, whichever way they decide.

Of course, in reality, parents and children are so intimately connected that children may choose what they think their parents want them to choose. In *Dwarfs: Not a Fairy Tale,* Emily Sullivan Sanford's mother wonders whether Emily underwent surgery because she, her mother, needed to have her accepted (Hedley 2001). Possibly neither Emily nor her mother will ever know for sure what mix of desire to please her parents, unhappiness with her situation, hope for an easier life, curiosity about what being taller would be like, or excitement about doing something controversial among people with achondroplasia all combined to influence her decision. But Emily perceives this surgery as something to which she committed herself, and she is thus able to live with all its results. If children hear from their parents and doctors that they are not what needs to change, that the world's response to them needs to change, they have a better chance at having a confident and competent self with which to make whatever decision they make about the battles they take on in their lives.

I close with the question I have been asked and have asked myself: What if surgical change were as simple and as effective as measles vaccine? Suppose a one-time surgery for a facial difference could entirely eliminate that difference, could give the child a face that no one would call atypical, disfigured? Suppose there were no other physical, cognitive, psychological impairments that went along with the facial disfigurement, and thus, once the surgery was done, there would be no impairment, no difference? The child would be normal. Would I counsel waiting in that case?

Just as there is nothing wrong with having a characteristic that is different from those most people have, there is nothing wrong with not having such a stigmatized feature. I don't see disability or difference as desirable in itself. If parents learned that a one-time, quick, safe procedure would change the child with the difference into the child they expected, I can certainly understand why they might say there was no reason to wait and every reason to bypass whatever emotional work is required to become the parent of a child with a startling difference.

Before they go ahead and change their child's body forever, they need to do much the same work Alice Dreger advises in her contribution to this book and that I have advised. They must ask themselves why they need their child to have a typical body.

They need to imagine what they will tell their child, or if they will tell their child that her body was surgically changed when she was an infant. Adoption practice has changed to include telling children that their social and psychological parents are not their birth parents. There is good reason to be cautious about what will happen to trust, openness, and mutuality in parent-child relationships if parents don't tell their child something that mattered to them about his early life (Bok 1989).

If they opt for surgery before their child can participate in making that decision, they should know, and should be ready to tell their child, that they were trying to protect their child against cruelty, prejudice, and discrimination. They may, as Margaret Little suggests, become complicitous with suspect norms by this decision, but they can minimize such complicity if they communicate to their child that avoiding bullying does not give her license to bully others for their differences. Teaching children integrity, concern for others, and respect for others ought to be at least as important as teaching children table manners and grammar. Whether or not there is surgery, much the same moral and psychological work needs to go on if parents are going to help children understand who they are and how they got to be the way they are. Early surgery, I am saying, carries its own risks and entails its own psychological work. It should not be perceived as an automatic response to a child's atypicality.

I am not convinced that any surgery undertaken by a parent for a child could ever be as simple, as psychologically uncomplicated as vaccinating a child against measles almost always turns out to be. If surgical change had no more psychological meaning than trying to learn how to be a good guest in a foreign country, I might be willing to say that parents could comfortably make that choice. But the change is contemplated because it has meaning to the professionals and the parents, and that meaning will eventually be communicated to the child. If parents decide their child's life will be better if surgery occurs during infancy, they must be ready to tell their child the story and to tell their child that they vaccinated her against smallpox, measles, and mistreatment. I can only hope that the child responds as well to the latter vaccination as most children respond to vaccines against disease. And I can only hope the vaccine will be as effective at preventing the mistreatment for which it was intended.

ACKNOWLEDGMENTS

In addition to all I learned from our project group deliberations, I owe special thanks to Alice Dreger and Erik Parens for generous encouragement and insights. Several members of a 2004 National Endowment for the Humanities (NEH) seminar gave up limited free time to let me present my ideas and get their wisdom. My student, Elana Katz, helped enormously through her research on a related project, and I also benefited greatly from discussing these ideas with Ann Eisenstein, Sara Mrsny, and Randi Stein. Last, the painstaking work of Lili Schwan-Rosenwald, Kyra Norsigian, and Saroj Fleming ensured the completion of this essay.

REFERENCES

Albrecht, G. L., and P. J. Devlieger. 1991. The disability paradox: High quality of life against all odds. *Social Science and Medicine* 48:977–88.

Alderson, P. 1993. *Children's Consent to Surgery.* Philadelphia: Open University Press.

American Academy of Pediatrics Committee on Bioethics. 1995. Informed consent, parental permission, and assent in pediatric practice. *Pediatrics* 95 (2):314–17.

Americans with Disabilities Act. 1990. Public Law No. 101 336, § 2.

Asch, A. 1998. Distracted by disability. *Cambridge Quarterly of Healthcare Ethics* 7(1):77–87.

Associated Press. 1995. Girl's surgery is performed for a smile, doctors hope. *New York Times,* December 16, section 1; page 8; column 1.

Basnett, I. 2001. Health care professionals and their attitudes toward decisions affecting disabled people. In *Handbook of Disability Studies,* edited by G. L. Albrecht, K. Seelman, and M. Bury, 450–67. Thousand Oaks, CA: Sage.

Bok, S. 1989. *Secrets: On the Ethics of Concealment and Revelation.* New York: Vintage.

Darling, R. B. 1979. *Families against Society: A Study of Reactions to Children with Birth Defects.* Beverly Hills, CA: Sage.

Davis, F. 1961. Deviance disavowal: The management of strained interaction by the visibly handicapped. *Social Problems* 9:120–32.

Davis, L. 1995. *Enforcing Normalcy: Disability, Deafness, and the Body.* New York: Verso.

Eagly, A. H., R. D. Ashmore, M. G. Makhijani, and L. C. Longo. 1991. What is beautiful is good, but . . . : A meta-analytic review of research on the physical attractiveness stereotype. *Psychological Bulletin* 110 (1):109–28.

Feingold, A. 1992. Good-looking people are not what we think. *Psychological Bulletin* 111:304–41.

Ferguson, P. 2001. Mapping the family: Disability studies and the exploration of parental response to disability. In *Handbook of Disability Studies,* edited by G. L. Albrecht, K. Seelman, and M. Bury, 373–95. Thousand Oaks, CA: Sage.

Frader, J., P. Alderson, A. Asch, C. Aspinall, D. Davis, A. Dreger, J. Edwards, E. K. Feder, A. Frank, L. A. Hedley, E. Kittay, J. Marsh, P. S. Miller, W. Mouradian, H. Nelson, and E. Parens. 2004. Health care professionals and intersex conditions. *Journal of Pediatric and Adolescent Medicine* 158 (5):426–28.

Francis, L., and A. Silvers, eds. 2000. *Americans with Disabilities: Exploring Implications of the Law for Individuals and Institutions.* New York: Routledge.

Frank, G. 1988. Beyond stigma: Visibility and self-empowerment of persons with congenital limb deficiencies. *Journal of Social Issues* 44 (1):95–118.

Frankel, C., and E. Juengst. 1991. Cosmetic surgery for a fatally ill infant. *Journal of Pediatric Ophthalmology and Strabismus* 28 (5): 250–54.

Gill, C. J. 2001. Divided understandings: The social experience of disability. In *Handbook of Disability Studies*, edited by G. L. Albrecht, K. Seelman, and M. Bury, 351–71. Thousand Oaks, CA: Sage.

Gliedman, J., and W. Roth. 1980. *The Unexpected Minority: Handicapped Children in America.* New York: Harcourt Brace Jovanovich.

Goffman, E. 1963. *Stigma: Notes on the Management of Spoiled Identity.* Englewood Cliffs, NJ: Prentice Hall.

Greenhouse, S. 2003. Lifetime affliction leads to a U.S. bias suit. *New York Times*, March 30.

Hahn, H. 1983. Paternalism and public policy. *Society* (March–April):36–46.

Harris, D. 1997. Types, causes and physical treatment of visible differences. In *Visibly Different: Coping with Disfigurement*, edited by R. Lansdown, N. Rumsey, E. Bradbury, T. Carr, and J. Partridge, 79–90. London: Oxford University Press.

Heatherton, T., R. E. Kleck, M. R. Hebl, and J. Hull, eds. 2000. *The Social Psychology of Stigma.* New York: Guilford.

Hebl, M. R., and R. E. Kleck. 2000. The social consequences of physical disability. In *The Social Psychology of Stigma*, edited by T. Heatherton, R. E. Kleck, M. R. Hebl, and J. Hull, 419–39. New York: Guilford.

Hedley, L. A. 2001. *Dwarfs: Not a Fairy Tale.* Home Box Office, a Division of Time Warner Entertainment Company.

Houston Chronicle News Services. 1996. Girl, 8, has birthday she can smile at. *Houston Chronicle*, June 30, section A; page 4.

Karen, R. 1994. *Becoming Attached: Unfolding the Mystery of the Infant-Mother Bond and Its Impact on Later Life.* New York: Warner.

Klein, S. D., and J. Kemp, eds. 2004. *Reflections from a Different Journey: What Adults with Disabilities Wish All Parents Knew.* New York: McGraw Hill.

Klein, S. D., and K. Schieve. 2001. *You Will Dream New Dreams: Inspiring Personal Stories by Parents of Children with Disabilities.* Kensington, OH: Kensington.

Lambert, B. 1997. Picture this: Big smiles after surgery. *New York Times*, October 18, section B; page 5; column 1.

Lefebvre, A., and I. Munro. 1986. Psychological adjustment of patients with craniofacial deformities before and after surgery. In *Physical Appearance, Stigma and Social Behavior: The Ontario Symposium (vol. 3)*, edited by C. P. Herman, M. P. Zanna, and E. T. Higgins, 53–62. Mahwah, NJ: Erlbaum.

Little, M. 1996. Cosmetic surgery, suspect norms, and the ethics of complicity. In *Enhancing Human Traits: Ethical and Social Implications*, edited by E. Parens, 162–76. Washington, DC: Georgetown University Press.

Lussier. A. 1980. The physical handicap and the body ego. *International Journal of Psycho-Analysis* 61:179–85.

National Organization on Disability. 1999. 1998 Harris Survey of Americans with Disabilities. www.nod.org.

Neuberg, S. L., D. M. Smith, and T. Asher. 2000. Why people stigmatize: Toward a biocultural framework. In *The Social Psychology of Stigma*, edited by T. Heatherton, R. E. Kleck, M. R. Hebl, and J. Hull, 31–61. New York: Guilford.

Note (no author). 1987. Facial discrimination: Extending handicap law to employment discrimination on the basis of physical appearance. *Harvard Law Review* 100:2035–45.

Ornstein, A., and P. Ornstein. 1984. Parenting as a function of the adult self: A psychoanalytic developmental perspective. In *Parental Influences: In Health and Disease,* edited by E. J. Anthony and G. Polluck, 183–232. Boston: Little, Brown.

Parens, E. 2005. Authenticity and ambivalence: Toward understanding the enhancement debate. *The Hastings Center Report* 35 (3):34–41.

Rogers-Salyer, M., A. Jensen, and R. Barden. 1987. Effects of facial deformities and physical attractiveness on mother-infant bonding. *Craniofacial Surgery First International Society of Cranio-Maxillo-Facial Surgery,* 481–85.

Rousso, H. 1984. Fostering healthy self-esteem. *Exceptional Parent* (December):9–14.

Ruddick, S. 1989. *Maternal Thinking: Toward a Politics of Peace.* Boston: Beacon.

Sandel, M. 2004. The case against perfection: What's wrong with designer children, bionic athletes, and genetic engineering? *Atlantic Monthly* 293 (3):50–60.

Schneider, J., and P. Conrad. 1980. In the closet with illness: Epilepsy, stigma potential and information control. *Social Problems* 28:31–33.

Scotch, R. K., and K. Schriner. 1997. Disability as human variation: Implications for policy. *Annals of the American Academy of Political and Social Science* 549:148–59.

Shakespeare, T., K. Gillespie-Sells, and D. Davies. 1996. *The Sexual Politics of Disability: Untold Desires.* New York: Cassell.

Shapiro, J. P. 1994. *No Pity: People with Disabilities Forging a New Civil Rights Movement.* New York: Three Rivers.

Stangor, C., and C. Crandall. 2000. Threat and the social construction of stigma. In *The Social Psychology of Stigma,* edited by T. Heatherton, R. E. Kleck, M. R. Hebl, and J. Hull, 62–87. New York: Guilford.

Stern, D. 2004. *First Relationship: Mother and Infant.* Cambridge, MA: Harvard University Press.

Stroman, D. W. 1982. *The Awakening Minorities: The Physically Handicapped.* Washington, DC: University Press of America.

Walters, E. 1997. Problems faced by children and families living with visible differences. In *Visibly Different: Coping with Disfigurement,* edited by R. Lansdown, N. Rumsey, E. Bradbury, T. Carr, and J. Partridge, 113–20. London: Oxford University Press.

Wasserman, D. 2000. Stigma without impairment: Demedicalizing disability discrimination. In *American with Disabilities: Exploring Implications of the Law for Individuals and Institutions,* edited by L. P. Francis and A. Silvers, 146–62. New York: Routledge.

Weiss, M. 1994. *Conditional Love: Parents' Attitudes toward Handicapped Children.* Westport, CT: Bergin and Garvey.

Wright, B. 1983. *Physical Disability: A Psycho-social Approach.* New York: Harper and Row.

CHAPTER SIXTEEN

What to Expect when You Have the Child You Weren't Expecting

Alice Domurat Dreger, Ph.D.

I feel that the most useful thing I can do in the context of this volume is to offer to parents a sort of guidebook to the experience of having a child with a noticeable anatomical difference in America today. I say a "guidebook" because, for many parents, having a child with an unusual anatomy is like suddenly finding yourself in a foreign country without knowing the language. And you realize pretty quickly that you're not an accidental tourist, you're an accidental permanent resident. Hallmark and Sprint and GE don't, in their misty commercials about newborn babies and mothers and fathers, suggest the possibility your kid might come out looking different from most kids. At most, intersex, achondroplasia, cleft lip, conjoined twinning, and the like are the silent ghosts that haunt pregnancies. When you get a prenatal sonogram, people don't ask, "Are you having a child with eleven toes, or intersex, or Down syndrome?" And though expectant parents seek sonograms because they fear something might be wrong, few if any are prepared when they find out something is. The fact is, even though this experience happens over and over, nobody gets you ready for it before it happens and people often act like it is a huge tragedy when it does happen. So you probably think you've got no training in this. Let me suggest otherwise, and try to make up for some of the gaps in training.

Before we get into the heart of the matter, though, I want to be clear I haven't personally experienced parenting a "different" child in any sustained way. I have only one child, a 3-year-old, and he has only occasionally looked wrong to other people, once for about a year when he was on the short side of the growth chart (a real social issue, I learned, for a boy), and once for a few days when an ugly rash covered his face, head, and neck. I *have* had a lot of conversations with parents who have had children with congenitally unusual traits, and a lot of conversations with adults who were born with unusual anatomical traits, and have received much feedback from them about what is helpful or useful or comforting for parents to know. So that is largely what I'm going on here. The medical specialists who treat intersex, cleft palate, achondroplasia, and other forms of socially challenging anatomies often function as if there is nothing to be learned by considering these conditions together. Each specialty tends to go off on its own and work on its little part of the pie. No doubt because they have good science training, medical specialists tend to be splitters, people who see each condition and even each case as fairly unique. But I'm a humanist (a historian by training), and from families coping with unusual anatomies, I've learned the value of lumping. So allow me to lump for a bit, to generalize about what you may experience, to generalize about what ideas you might want to consider.[1]

Now, American parents like you find themselves the subject of two daily dicta. The first is that you should do everything you can for your children—braces, tutors, antibiotic soap, organized soccer and baseball, cushy car seats with juice box holders in behemoth SUVs. The second is that even when (or especially when) the world rejects your children, you should accept them just as they are—nerdy, gay, dreamy, homely. Both of these dicta are understood as necessary manifestations of the mythical beast called Unconditional Love. If you really love your children *unconditionally,* you'll make whatever sacrifice you have to for them. If you really love your children *unconditionally,* you'll accept them fully, forgive them all their faults—nay, *love them for* all their faults.

As Lisa Hedley suggests in her contribution to this volume, this American ideology of parenthood makes it very hard to be a parent of a child born with an atypical anatomy, because there is an option presented to such parents that is not (yet) presented to most parents: the option of surgery to make the child look better. This option clearly speaks to the idea of doing everything you can for your child. But it also seems to negate the idea of accepting your child just as she is. After all, how are you supposed to pull off "I love you, now change"? It seems like opting for the surgery might be rejecting the child.

So when you choose surgery to change the way your child looks, are you rejecting him? A few adults whose parents chose appearance-normalizing surgeries for them do indeed feel that those surgeries meant their parents rejected some essential part of them.[2] This seems to be especially true where intersex is concerned, probably in large part because historically with intersex surgeries came a heavy veil of secrecy and shame.

But I think you'll find that most *surgeons* don't even consider this possibility, because they don't see these surgeries as rejections of your children. On the contrary, as heroic extensions of parents—as the pan-parents pediatric surgeons have become—surgeons see appearance-normalizing surgeries as they see all surgeries: as evidence of pure devotion to children. Surgeons understand the world can be cruel to people who look funny. Moreover, they believe it is not in their power to change society, and so they do what they can to help: they do surgery.

Most parents who choose normalizing surgeries for their children appear to reason the same way as surgeons (perhaps in part because surgeons do much of the on-the-fly counseling of these parents). If you choose an appearance-normalizing surgery for your child, chances are no other adult—at least no one in your inner circle—is going to suggest it means you are rejecting your child. Most people will see you as devoted, as being pragmatic and foregrounding the dictum of sacrifice to give the child the best life possible.

That's not to say you won't feel quietly conflicted about the surgery. These surgeries typically aren't done until the child is at least several months old, and some (especially follow-up surgeries) are often done when the child is several years old. As a consequence, by the time of the surgery—unless you're still grieving the loss of the normal child you expected to have, as some parents do for a long time (Ablon 1988)—you might find that you've come to see your child's anatomical difference as a fine, integral, even necessary part of her. Except for the fantasy time before your child came to you, when you imagined the standard-issue kid most parents imagine, you haven't known your child without this anomaly. It may not seem like an anomaly to you; it may seem normal to you and to the child, even if other people think of it as a deformity. So you may legitimately wonder if it makes sense to try to make that key characteristic go away. Joanne Green, who mothers three children born with clefts, talks about this conflicted feeling in her online essay, "The Reality of the Miracle: What to Expect from the First Surgery." She points out that "very few parents are initially thrilled with [cleft-lip] surgery. The baby will almost seem to be another baby. There will be a marked difference in the face. And it will take you a while to adjust to this new face. After all, you loved the old one!" (Green 1996).

Yet, alongside this voice of acceptance of the anomaly and doubt over appearance-normalizing surgery, your own experience and a lot of other people may tell you that the surgery has to be done, because it seems cruel to send a child into the world with a stigmatized body when something might be done about it. A lot of us can remember being teased or even tormented for having a florid pimple, very small or very large breasts, or a chubby physique. We can't imagine letting our own children go through such stigma if it seems preventable, even though most of us survived that teasing, even though some of those interactions may have shaped the stronger aspects of our personalities. Though we could, as adults, imagine putting ourselves through some degree of social challenge, we can't imagine having our children do that, so we may try to "save" them from it. (On this sort of reasoning, see Ellen Feder's chapter in this book.)

You may quite legitimately find yourself wondering: Why *do* people treat your child as if he is a shame just because he looks different? Why *do* strangers and familiars often treat you and your child with pity, even though you don't feel pitiful? Part of what's going on is that many people think children who look different are physically ill. Maybe your particular child is; maybe your child has a metabolic concern that diminishes or threatens her physical well-being. But even if your child has no underlying illness, some people may assume, because she looks different, that she is sick, and that therefore you and she mostly deserve pity. A lot of people don't know what to do when they encounter a sick or physically unusual child; our culture mythologizes childhood as being about health and innocence, so most people don't have a decent frame of reference for your child. As a result, you may spend a lot of your energy trying to explain the funny gray zone that you and your child inhabit—the zone of different-but-not-ill, or ill-but-essentially-well, or well-now-but-maybe-illness-coming-later. It's a zone most people can't tolerate very well, especially in children, especially as illness and anomalies become less and less visible in our culture.

You and your child may also be treated with shame because we live in a culture that categorizes people according to the way their bodies look. So we treat people who look old differently than people who look young. We treat people who appear to be women differently than people who appear to be men. When someone doesn't fit our categories neatly, we are often uncomfortable. That's in large part because identities are formed via relationships. I'm a mother because I have a child. I know I'm a woman because there are men and other women around me. If all people were white, or all were black, then there wouldn't be any racial identities. So when we meet someone whose gender seems to be uncertain, or someone who is of an ambiguous age, we find our own identities falling into some level of uncertainty. We're not sure how that relationship is supposed to go, the way we *are* sure when we know who we are and who the other person is.

So children who have socially challenging anatomical features necessarily cause other people around them to feel uncertain. Because of this, people often treat them the way they treat other people who have apparently violated a social norm: they treat them in such a way as to suggest they should be ashamed of themselves. They do this even though they don't mean to sometimes. You'll often find that once a stranger gets to know your child, the stranger will treat that child as she does other children; that's because she has gotten over the initial questions about identity and relationships. But, especially if you live in a suburban or urban area, there will be a lot of strangers, a lot of annoying shame attribution.

People may also treat you, the parent, as if you are shameful also because people tend to think that if a child has a congenital problem, it is the parents' fault. You must have done something wrong—especially if you are the mother. Unfortunately, this message is accidentally reiterated by health professionals who may want to know what happened during pregnancy, what your family history is. The message you may get is "we need to know what your problem is." You may find yourself getting pretty tired of explaining to yourself and others that this child isn't a tragedy; he isn't someone's fault. You end up sounding like you're Pollyanna-ish or self-deluded, even when you don't feel that way. And then you may end up running into people who want to pat your child on the head as if he were some sort of miracle totem; I wouldn't blame you if, like many parents I know, you find it especially annoying when people treat your child (and, by association, you) as a hero just for existing.

Chances are, unless you intentionally adopted a child with a birth anomaly, this isn't the identity you bargained for. For this reason, you may find yourself confused and disoriented, maybe even depressed or angry. It seems pretty unfair, because most parents don't have to go through this experience. Most get a window of many months or years before their children's identities start affecting them in ways that feel uncomfortable or shameful—most get to wait until their kid crashes the car or drops out of college or hooks up with the wrong kind of person. But you've gotten it right away, and you may feel strangely out of control.

For this reason, appearance-normalizing surgery may seem especially attractive. This kind of surgery seems to promise a return to the dream you had of parenting—of pride and certainty and uncomplicated love. If you're getting the message that this is all your fault, then surgery is going to seem even more like something you have to do, to prove you *are* a responsible, loving parent. You may feel like you have to publicly atone for your supposed sin, even if you know you didn't do anything wrong. And there are still more sources of pressure to choose surgery. There's that dictum I mentioned earlier, the one that says what it means to be a good parent is to do everything you can for your child. In America, that's understood largely in terms of acquisition—acquiring the best therapists and medicines for a child with ADD, acquiring braces for the child with crooked teeth, acquiring a good computer, acquiring dance and karate teachers. Because health care isn't understood as a basic right in this country, and because our medical system has been, at times, overly focused on profit for insurance companies, health care is seen as one more item of privilege to be acquired. So you may feel like, if you don't seek out the most intense medical interventions for your child, you'll be seen as poor or cheap. You may yourself believe (incorrectly) that the more health care interventions you and your child get, the better off you and your child will necessarily be.

You may also feel some pressure to do surgery because your health care providers talk about it a lot. Though they may talk about it just to make sure you know your options, the fact that they mention it a lot gives you the message they think it is an option you should be strongly considering. It's natural that you look to your medical providers to guide you. If they keep offering the surgery, you will probably get the sense that they think that is the way you should go. Surely, you may think, they wouldn't offer it if they thought your kid was okay without it; they don't offer all parents nose jobs for their children!

Finally, you may find surgery attractive because you think it will provide certainty when a lot of other things feel very uncertain. You may think it will make your child's identity certain—resolve the ambiguities built into her flesh—and by association make your child certain. In spite of the health care providers' citing you statistics about surgical risks, you may feel you owe it to your child to believe everything is going to be okay with this surgery. Focusing on the surgery may give you some definite way to think about the future, when everything else about the future feels so very unknown and indefinite.

So how are you supposed to decide about appearance-normalizing surgeries that are offered to you? First, wait. Wait until the initial shock of all this has worn off, until you can get to know this child—and yourself, as a parent—a little better. Wait until you are well enough to digest the flood of information coming your way. Wait until you get over any sensation of drowning, until you feel steady on your feet, steady enough to ask to talk to more people, including especially parents who have had this kind of experience (even if their child had a different anomaly) and adults who were born with this kind of body. Wait until you can start to sort out the real motivations for different treatment options, until you can get past the sensation that this is a medical emergency (because the kinds of conditions and surgeries we're talking about aren't). Wait until you can start realizing your strengths—your ability to love, to be uncertain together, to be your child's guardian—not just your points of weakness (Mouradian 2001). And if you find that you can't get to this point, then be as aggressive as you can in getting some help for yourself (Howe 1999). As they say before every commercial airplane flight, "Secure your own oxygen mask before assisting your child." One of the best things you can do for your child is to take care of yourself: lean on people to help you get the rest you need, find people who will take your ping-pong emotions seriously, be honest with yourself and others about how your life story has just changed without warning.

Then start to understand how what you're going through is in some ways like what most parents go through. You're just learning sooner than most that parenting isn't about certainty, it's about a faith in yourself and your child. Parents who have had a standard-issue child first often appear better able to handle a newborn child with an atypical trait because they realize the emotions they're feeling are actually something like what they went through before. They know that uncertainty comes with *all* parenting. They have faith in themselves that comes from experience. Forget Hallmark and Kodak; honest, experienced parents will tell you that nobody feels unconditional love for their kids all the time, nobody feels perpetually sure they can handle parenthood, nobody is prepared for how much your children change who you are. And know that almost every parent has moments of forbidden joy and pride about his children's oddities; it doesn't make you a bad person to find your child's difference kind of cool sometimes—it doesn't make you a freak to find this unusual experience as rewarding as it is trying.

That said, I hope you won't make your decisions concerning your child based mostly on what you need or what you want for yourself. Some people act as if the only axis along which parenting can run is the shame-pride axis; they find themselves spending most of their parenting energies trying to drag their child back to the pride end, whether that be through another surgery or another baseball trophy or admission to a prestigious school. They treat their children as mere enhancements to their own identities, even while they tell themselves they're doing it for their kids' sake. Though you are the chief guardian to your children, *you are not them*. They are entitled to their selves, I think, and it is not unreasonable that they would grow to see the right to decide what happens to their bodies as a major part of that entitlement.

You can—and I believe in many cases you should—wait until your child can participate in the decision about whether or not to use surgery to change the way she or he looks. If you decide to wait until your child can participate in the choice, it doesn't mean the surgeries will have to wait until the child is 18. The American Academy of Pediatrics (AAP) has endorsed the idea that even fairly young children can and should be allowed to be actively involved in decision making about their medical care. The AAP points out that encouraging children to do this helps them develop as moral decision makers (American Academy of Pediatrics 2001). It also signals to them that you, as a parent, trust them and value their feelings. It makes you a better parent.

As you go through the health care maze, chances are you (and then also your child) are going to become the expert on your child's condition. You may find that you know more than a lot of the professionals you consult—and there is no question you know a lot more about your particular child than they do. At the same time, sometimes you're going to see resistance on some professionals' part to your expertise. Sometimes you'll find the providers intentionally or unintentionally infantilizing you as they do your child, calling you "Mom" or "Dad"—funny how that makes you sound like a little kid in the medical setting!—as if you did not also have names and titles the way they know *they* do. Sometimes you'll want to fight their attitudes, but will be afraid to do so lest it come back to bite you or your child. Talking with other parents and nurses will often help here; they will be able to help you figure out how to navigate the maze, and will give you a chance to vent.

Working with mental health care providers—psychologists, psychiatrists, social workers—will also help. Relying on these folks doesn't make you a weakling or a nut or an inept parent, and it doesn't mean you don't love your child. I know you'll find added stigma by seeking mental health care, but you'll often find that some of these professionals can provide you with insights and resources you can't get anywhere else. I also know you'll probably find more funding (through insurance or elsewhere) available for surgeries and drugs than for mental health care. People in this country would be outraged if a child needed a surgeon and didn't have access to one, but they don't feel the same way about psychologists, psychiatrists, and social workers yet. Push anyway, and if you have it in you, push with other parents.

Keep in mind that your health care providers are not gods. They may seem that way sometimes, with all their knowledge and abilities, patience and kindness. The surgeons may seem especially heavenly or omnipotent. But be aware all your health care providers are dealing with their own identities in the same way you are, in their encounters with you and your children. When your surgeon says, "If this were my child, I'd do the surgery," he's not saying you should do the surgery. He's telling you about his own concerns about identity, about how he would parent this child, about his surgical mindset, and about his faith in his surgical technique. It doesn't mean you have to do it. Though a few (very few) medical professionals may want you to treat them like gods, none of them will do a better job for you and your child if you treat them that way. Treat them as humans, and understand they have limits just as you do—limits on their energy, their insight, their knowledge, their personal strengths.

Try hard to sort out what your child needs for medical reasons and what your child needs for social reasons, and then ask yourself if he really needs either. Try hard to find out what is known *statistically* (through peer-reviewed studies) about all the options, and take gaps in knowledge very, very seriously. Ask librarians at medical school libraries to help you find material and understand it. Be careful not to let one or two personal anecdotes completely color your decision making. (Stories will have a lot more power over you than statistics, but they shouldn't always.) Keep in mind, too, that all medical care comes with "side effects," many of which for you will show up front and center and not at all on the "side." This isn't just true for drugs and surgeries; it's also true for repeated clinic visits, which often give children the message that there is something wrong with them when there isn't, or the message that medicine is a major venue for daily life, which it doesn't have to be for everyone. Don't get into the habit of thinking the doctors will fix everything in your life. They won't, they can't, and they shouldn't.

Make sure you ask yourself and your surgeon, more than once: Given the risks, should you ever choose, on behalf of someone else (even your own child), a surgery offered purely for psychological and social reasons? Surgeons often tell me "you can't change society, so you have to change children's bodies," but clearly in many cases we *do* try to change society. We've tried to eliminate sexism that keeps girls down just because their bodies are different than boys, we've tried to eliminate racism that keeps some kids down just because their bodies are darker than others. So consider the possibility that, instead of changing your child's body, we should start expecting others to change their minds.

On that point, let me say this: I firmly believe we should all expect others to treat your children just as well as other children; your child should not be singled out for mockery, shame, dismissal, or pity because she looks different. *Your child's civil rights and status as a human being should not depend on the prevalence of her condition.* I think you, and I, and every person who considers himself a good person should maintain a very low tolerance for people behaving badly or excusing others' stupid behavior. But you have even more reason to do this: when you have a low tolerance for stupid behavior and excuses made for it, you not only evidence love for your children, you also show them the right way to be. My mother did this—she fiercely defended my younger brother, who is multiracial, when someone made a racist remark or assumption. And it gave us a clear message, not only that she (a white woman) thought Paul was fine, that she loved him intensely, but also that she believed people should indeed be judged by the content of their characters, not the color of their skin, and that good people stand up for this belief.

Does that mean if you choose an appearance-normalizing surgery for your child you're being "culturally complicit" (Little 1998)—supporting bad stereotypes about appearance? Maybe. The fact is, when you choose such a surgery, you're choosing it to align your child with a social norm that says appearance matters. Your intentions may be quite pure—truly in the best interest of the child—but the effect may be otherwise. If my parents had been able to choose a "whitening" for my brother, and had chosen to do that, though their intentions may have been good, they would have been ceding some power to racism. On the other hand, your declining surgery for your own child won't miraculously change society for the better, though it may be the case that people in your immediate environs develop better attitudes toward anatomical variation. In this sense, you and your child are in a hard position because—as my family was—your family is stuck on battle lines of politics and morality, and that's a hard place to try to live peacefully.

I don't think it unreasonable, regardless of your decision, for you to push people strong enough to do so to work to reduce the shame and pity attributed to people born with socially challenging traits. While there is a place for shame in the world—for example, I think it is appropriate to make someone feel shameful when she hurts another person unnecessarily—I don't think you or your child should be made to feel ashamed because he was born different. And I know a lot of your pain is going to come out of that wholly unnecessary shame attribution.

I also think it reasonable for you to find out as much as you can from people with firsthand knowledge about whether the trait with which your child has been born really is bad—whether it really needs "fixing." You may find, to your surprise, that people who have lived with it have chosen no interventions or minor interventions. Don't assume that just because *you* wouldn't want to live with that trait your child won't want to; it's no surprise that each of you would have a unique understanding of your bodies.

So you have to keep in mind the decision you make about your child will affect how she thinks, not only about herself, but about your relationship with her, and how she thinks about the meaning of appearance. As you think about who you want your child to become, think about whether you're modeling that outcome in your methods.

All of this leads to the question of what the goal of parenting is. And that's a hard question. I feel much more certain that I know what the goal of medicine is—to reduce suffering. But I don't think that the chief goal of parenting should be to reduce as much as possible the chances your child might suffer. When you take that as your goal, you make all sorts of presumptions about your child that you shouldn't, you waste resources (including your own energy) that might otherwise be better spent, you give your child a false sense of what it means to live as a human in this world.

I have to confess, I get this belief partly from the way my mother raised me. Though, as I noted above, my mother defended us against ignorant boors, she didn't think it was her job to do whatever she could to make sure her children would avoid social stigma and other forms of suffering. For instance, when I wanted a bra in seventh grade, to keep up with the other girls, my mother suggested I get back to her when I had something to hold up. When other parents were getting braces for their kids, my mother felt that, if my teeth worked to chew, it would be better to spend that money on my college education, her own financial security, or a worthy charity. Though I didn't necessarily appreciate my mother's decisions then, nowadays I think she was on to something.

And, I don't mean to sound unpatriotic, but I don't think it is a coincidence that my mother wasn't born and bred American. She didn't have the sense that the goal of parenting was to do all you can do for your children—or even that the goal was to love your children no matter what they do. She was one of those weird semi-feminist pious Roman Catholic European peasant-intellectual mothers. At the breakfast table she'd read Strunk and White's *Elements of Style* and Plato's *Republic* and Shakespeare's

Hamlet. While other parents in our Long Island suburban neighborhood seemed to spend a lot of their energy sheltering their children from "suffering"—getting them the latest fashions so they would be better accepted by their peers, or getting wandering eyes fixed so they wouldn't look weird, or hiding the looming mortality and seeping disability of grandparents—my mother's attitude was that children should be as clear as possible about as much of the world as possible, including about the portions of the world seeped in suffering. It wasn't that she thought we were inadequately grateful or that we should be wracked in guilt. (She never pulled the business of "Children in China would give anything to have what you have.") It was just that she saw strife and suffering as an inevitable part of life, just as she saw occasional peace and happiness as inevitable parts of life. When I would lament some decision of hers, declaring, "That isn't fair!" her response was inevitably, "Life isn't fair." She meant it as a simple description.

Her goal wasn't to make us suffer; that was always clear to me, even when I resented her decisions. Rather, it was just in her nature to be honest. In this sense, my mother was, and is, pretty much shameless. She didn't—or wouldn't, or couldn't—spend all of her time with us on the shame-pride axis. So she was shameless about the fact that we had to tube-feed and diaper-change my Parkinson's-ridden grandfather to keep him home with us, out of a nursing home. She also didn't see it as a point of pride—it just was the way it was. She was shameless about the fact that she had a multiracial, dark-skinned son in an otherwise white family and white neighborhood. But she also didn't think taking him in as her son made her a hero, a fountain of family pride. It was just the way it was. And this, from what I've seen, is a winning way to parent a child born with a socially challenging trait. (It is, in fact, a winning way to parent any child.) From what I've seen, this kind of approach—getting off the shame-pride axis and engaging with all of life together—allows both child and parent to spend much less of their energy apologizing for their existences, attempting to look like a hero, trying to hide what came . . . and much more of their energy being well together.

I came to understand my mother much better when I became a parent, but I also gained some insight into her even before that, from getting to know two undergraduate students, both of whom had facial anomalies. Because of my research and teaching on this subject, these two students separately came to me to tell me about their experiences, and later, when I was doing more of this work, they let me interview them. The difference of the first, Ruta Sharangpani, was that she was born with very little sight, noticeably cross-eyed, with one eye that shakes a lot. The difference of the second, whom I'll call Carole, was that she was born with a large hygroma (a cyst) on one side of her face. I use a pseudonym for Carole because she isn't "out" about her anomaly, though—like Ruta's—it is noticeable to anyone who sees her.

When Ruta was born, perhaps because Ruta's mother had had a close relative with the same anomaly as Ruta, or perhaps just because of her personality, Ruta's mother had a matter-of-fact, can-do attitude. According to Ruta, her mother made it clear she expected Ruta to do everything her sisters were also expected to do, except learn to drive. (Her blindness prevented this.) When I met Ruta's mother a few years ago, I could see this was true: Ruta's mother obviously expected Ruta, like her other daughters, to do well in the world, and saw no reason why Ruta's anomaly or disability should stand in the way of that. When Ruta was growing up, her parents helped her get access to technologies she needed to manage with very little sight, but they evinced no pity for her, no self-pity, and no shame about their daughter's anomaly. They also didn't think they should be considered heroes just for having Ruta. They didn't look to medicine to "fix" Ruta's issues; they didn't engage in what scholars call "medicalization" of their daughter's difference. Ruta is now in medical school, following in the footsteps of her oldest sister. She is a well-educated, confident, joyful person. She also has a strong disability rights-consciousness; that is, she has very little patience for people who try to limit others' rights because of their apparent anatomical impairments.

When Carole was born with a facial hygroma, a surgeon moved to take it off as soon as possible, not because it was causing any metabolic concerns but because it looked frightening. Unfortunately, that first surgery paralyzed part of Carole's face, inhibiting her ability to smile. The surgery also did not spell the end of the hygroma, which kept growing back. Carole's parents pursued surgery after surgery through Carole's childhood and adolescence, hoping she would eventually look normal. By the time I met Carole, the mother-daughter relationship in her case seemed to be weighted down by mutual guilt and frustration over Carole's situation, and Carole seemed to be still holding out some hope (though less than her mother) that another surgery would finally "fix" her face. In some ways, her identity seemed to be on hold, pending a surgical correction that will in all likelihood never happen—though Carole or her mother will always be able to find one more surgeon willing to give it a try. When last we met, Carole was fully qualified to be a teacher, but even in a state strapped for good teachers, she was only getting substitution work. Several people had tried to channel her into special education, figuring her own anomaly made that work appropriate to her, even though she had gotten high marks for her teaching in mainstream classrooms and wasn't interested or trained in special education. When last we spoke, about three years ago, unlike Ruta, Carole had little or no disability rights-consciousness, and seemed mostly confused by why she was having trouble getting a permanent job.

When I think about Ruta and Carole, both of whom grew up with ambitious parents in upper-middle-class Michigan suburbia with stigmatizing facial anomalies, I can't help but feel the differences in their lives stem from the way their parents understood their anomalies. I don't say this to blame the mother in Carole's case, as too often happens. But what I do notice is what a big difference parental attitudes—particularly maternal attitudes—have made for these two women. I find myself wishing that the medical profession could figure out a way to help more parents achieve the mentality of Ruta's mother—a mentality that refuses to fantasize that medicine can fix everything, a mentality that says pride in or shame about our children should not stem from our feelings about their anatomies, a mentality that acknowledges the uncertainty of all parenting. Instead, very often the medical profession, in its desire to help, fosters the mentality of Carole's mother—the mentality that hopes medicine will reconstruct for us children of whom we can finally feel unequivocal love and acceptance.

This is why the intersex advocacy group I have worked with as a volunteer—the Intersex Society of North America (www.isna.org)—has the mission that it does: building a world free of shame, secrecy, and unwanted genital surgeries for people born with atypical reproductive anatomies. The order of those concerns is not random; it is clear from everything I've read by people born with unusual anatomical traits, and by their parents—as well as innumerable conversations I've had—that in families dealing with socially challenging anatomical traits, *shame is the biggest problem,* with secrecy a close second. That is why I believe that the most important thing you are going to have to do as a parent is to reject, reduce, and sometimes absolutely fight the shame attributed to you and your child, including that attributed by some well-meaning health care providers, grandparents, and strangers.[3] The only way to do this is to know that you and your child have nothing to be ashamed of. Once you reach that point—and chances are you'll reach that point and then have to go back to it again and again—you can clear the decks of the ship that is your family. You will still have great uncertainty in your life. Children, even when they're grown, are all about uncertainty. But you will have become certain of one thing: your child is not a tragedy, and neither are you.

NOTES

1. Some of the themes in this article are more fully developed in Dreger (2004).

2. Max Beck, who was born with atypical genitalia and whose parents elected for a corrective genital surgery, recalls realizing "What I knew myself to be was too horrible; I wasn't a viable fetus." See Preves (2003, 74–75). Deborah Kent, who is blind, writes about how the fear of blindness among her family sometimes feels like rejection of her: "I will always believe that blindness is a neutral trait, neither to be prized nor shunned. Very few people, including those

dearest to me, share that conviction. My husband, my parents, and so many others who are central to my life cannot fully relinquish their negative assumptions. I feel that I have failed when I run into jarring reminders that I have not changed their perspective. In those crushing moments I fear that I am not truly accepted after all." Kent (2000, 62).

3. For a perfect example of a health team attributing shame while trying to help, see www.cleft.org, which claims on its homepage that "Any child with a correctable facial deformity which goes uncorrected—for any reason—is always and forever a tragedy, for if it is not then life itself has become one."

REFERENCES

Ablon, J. 1988. *Living with Difference: Families with Dwarf Children*. New York: Praeger.

American Academy of Pediatrics Policy Statement. 2001. Informed consent, parental permission, and assent in pediatric practice (RE9510). *Pediatrics* 95:314–17. (www.cirp.org/library/ethics/AAP/).

Dreger, A. C. 2004. *One of Us: Conjoined Twins and the Future of Normal*. Cambridge, MA: Harvard University Press.

Green, J. 1996. *The Reality of the Miracle: What to Expect from the First Surgery*, available at www.widesmiles.org. (www.widesmiles.org/cleftlinks/WS-162.html).

Howe, E. G. 1999. Intersexuality: What should careproviders do now? In *Intersex in the Age of Ethics*, edited by A. D. Dreger, 221–23. Hagerstown, MD: University Publishing Group.

Kent, D. 2000. Somewhere a mockingbird. In *Prenatal Testing and Disability Rights*, edited by E. Parens and A. Asch, 57–63. Washington, DC: Georgetown University Press.

Little, M. O. 1998. Cosmetic surgery, suspect norms, and the ethics of complicity. In *Enhancing Human Traits*, edited by E. Parens, 162–76. Washington, DC.: Georgetown University Press.

Mouradian, W. E. 2001. Deficits versus strengths: Ethics and implications for clinical practice and research. *Cleft Palate Craniofacial Journal* 28 (May): 255–59. See www.isna.org.

Preves, S. E. 2003. *Intersex and Identity: The Contested Self*. New Brunswick, NJ: Rutgers University Press.

Page numbers in *italics* refer to illustrations.

Ablon, Joan, 218

abnormal, definition of, 96

acceptance. *See* love and acceptance

accepting love, 242

accommodations to others' preferences, 227–28

achondroplasia: disclosure of, 40; experience as mother of child with, 43–48; experience as person affected with, 30–32; impact of, 30. *See also* limb-lengthening procedure

acquisition and parenting, 257

adolescence: anatomical difference and, 17–19; androgen insensitivity syndrome and, 5; appearance concerns in, 146; medical examinations during, 7–8; parent-child-surgeon triangle in, 137; YQOL-R collaborative study and, 149–50

agency of children, 167. *See also* assent for surgery from child; involvement of child in decisions about surgery

AIS (androgen insensitivity syndrome), 3–4, 207n. 8

Alderson, Priscilla: on children's awareness, 34, 136; on decision making, 213, 229, 246; on disclosure, 247

Alsop, Peter, "It's Only a Wee Wee", 202–3

ambiguous voices, 167–68

ambivalence: about surgery, 255; of appearance concerns, 229–31; dealing with, 100–101; of parents, 25–26, 43–47; in relationship between what is normal and what is desired, 92–93; resolving, 101–5

American Academy of Pediatrics (AAP): on ambiguous genitalia, 206; "Informed Consent, Parental Permission, and Assent in Pediatric Practice," xxiii–xxiv, 213, 214, 259

Americans with Disabilities Act, 219, 233

androgen insensitivity syndrome (AIS), 3–4, 207n. 8

anomaly: definition of, 96; normalizing, 100–101; simple compared to questionable variations, 96–97; social intolerance of, 97; stigma attached to, 99; visible compared to invisible, 92

anxiety and disability, 234

appearance concerns: age of awareness of, 14; ambiguous genitalia and, 199–200; ambivalence of, 228, 229–31; cultural norms and, 231–37, 261–62; psychological outcome and, 146

Asch, Adrienne, xxix, 220

Aspinall, Cassandra, 220

assent for surgery from child, 120–21, 213

attachment, 148

authenticity, 181

Bacon, Francis, 184–85

Beauchamp, T., 172

Beck, Max, 265n. 2

Bellah, Robert, *Habits of the Heart,* 85–86

bell curve, 94, *95,* 123

Benhabib, Seyla, 171

Bestand, 52–54, 57, 58, 63

best interests of child, determining, 217

Better than Well (Elliott), 180–81

Biddle, Jeff, 183

bioethics: consumer-protection, 69, 70, 82, 84; role of, 78; Socratic, 69–70, 82–85, 165 birth of disabled child: discovery of disability and, 217–19; feeling of crisis after, 22, 23; grief after, 43, 218; shock and, 23, 61. *See also* expectant parents, experience as

body: as *Bestand*, 57, 58; fixing, 68; integrity of, 241; pleasing others and, 230–31; as project, 71–72; willingness to reshape to conform to demands of field, 75–76. *See also* appearance concerns

body modification, traditional, 72, 75

body projects, choice of, 78

Borgmann, Albert, 181

Bourdieu, Pierre: field and, 75–76; *habitus* and, 99–100, 190, 191–92, 205

Canguilhem, George, *The Normal and the Pathological*, 94, 96, 98

capital, 75–76

caring for self, 68–69

Changing Faces (charitable group), 150

Chase, Cheryl, xvi

childcare, practice of, 176–78

children, definition of, 157

Children with Special Health Care Needs (U.S. Department of Health and Human Services), 127

choice: coercion and, 195–96; framework of, 78. *See also* decision making

cleft lip and palate, 117, 120, 126–27, 247. *See also* craniofacial deformity; craniofacial surgery

Clinical Standards Advisory Group (CSAG) study, 143–44

clitoral recession, 208n. 9

clitorectomy, 206, 207–8n. 9

clitoromegaly, 189

coercion in decision making, 27, 195–96. *See also* pressure

Colombia, 216–17

common sense, 55, 191–92, 204

community, 105

competence, 158, 161–62

conformity in 1950s, 91

congenital adrenal hyperplasia, 207n. 5

consumer-protection bioethics, 69, 70, 82, 84

consumption ethic, 180–81

context of surgery, 70–72

control, presumption of, 186–87

cosmetic operation, 120

Cox, Lynne, 95–96

craniofacial deformity: approaches to, 263–65; practical interventions for, 150; terminology of, 114

craniofacial surgery: developing evidence base for, 143–45; longitudinal study of, 147–48; moral justification for, 80–82; primary cleft lip, xxix, 20; psychological outcomes and, 145–47; quality of life and, 132–33; rating evidence and, 142–43; tension between goals in, 113–14; variables to address in outcome studies, 145; YQOL-R collaborative studies and, 149–50

crisis: feeling of when bearing child with anatomical difference, 22, 23; meeting with surgeon and, 126

Davis, Kathy, 87n. 4

Davis, Lennard, 94, 106–7, 237

decision making: by affected person, 20–21, 27–28, 123–24; for child, 27, 135–36; delay of, 30; dialogue and, 82–85; on end to surgery, 80–81; framework of choice and, 78; Heideggerian point and, 61–62; holding open, 84, 258–59; interdisciplinary team care and, 127–28, 138; legal standard for, 212–13; limb-lengthening procedure and, 33–35, 37–38, 77; more just, benign, and efficacious ways for, 170–72; perspective of affected adult and, 219–21; research on, 159–63; responsibility for, 168–70; as shared, 20–21; surgical, 117–21, 127–28. *See also* informed consent; involvement of child in decisions about surgery

deformity, difference compared to, 122–23. *See also* craniofacial deformity

Delgado, Richard, 179

desire for normal/normality, 105–8

developing evidence base in craniofacial care, 143–45

devices, transformation of things into, 181–82

dialogue: on appearance-altering surgery, 235–36; significance of, 82–85; with surgeon, 118–19

difference: affirming, 220–21; appreciating and destigmatizing, 228–29; crisis, and bearing child with, 22, 23; deformity compared to, 122–23; eliminating compared to accepting, 18–19; flaw compared to, 245; injustice and, 236–37; intolerance of, 99; normalizing, 203–4; physical illness and, 256; sexual, 191, 204–5

Difference in the Family, A (Featherstone), 104

disability: anxiety and, 234; moral model of, 95; parental discovery of, 217–19

disability rights, 78

disclosure of medical condition: achondroplasia and, 40; to child, 31, 247, 248–49; to friends, 10; informed consent and, 163–65

discrimination, 233–35

discussions of health care, including child in, 26

distress and research, 161

diversity affirmation, 113, 116–17

domination, parents as agents of, 197–98, 200–201

Dreger, Alice, xvi, 219–20, 243, 244, 246

Durkheim, Emile, 70

dwarf, 31

Dwarfs: Not a Fairy Tale (documentary, Hedley), 41, 248

Edwards, James, 163, 166, 167

ELL (extended limb-lengthening). *See* limb-lengthening procedure

Elliott, Carl, xiv, 84, 180–81

emotional counseling: for child, 5, 199; for parent, 4, 11, 260

emotional growth, fostering of, 177

end to surgery, deciding on, 80–81

enframing (*Gestell*), 54–55

Enhancing Human Traits project, xiv

erasure, techniques of, 55–57

ethical considerations: bioethics, role of, 78; consent and competence, 158; consumer-protection bioethics, 69, 82, 84; first-order, 59–60; Heidegger and, 58; limb-lengthening procedure and, 34; philosophy, technology, and, 59–66; Socratic bioethics, 69–70, 82–85, 165

Eurocleft study, 143, 144

evidence and master narratives, 180

expectant parents, experience as, 22–23, 253. *See also* birth of disabled child

explanation of self, 47–48

facts, as realities to be faced, 65

Faden, R., 172

family and *habitus*, 102–3

fear, and temptation to fix, 61–62, 218, 244, 245–46

Featherstone, H., *A Difference in the Family*, 104

Feder, Ellen, 99–100

feeding problems, 126–27

feet, surgery on, 72–76

"Female Genital Mutilation," 208–9n. 17

feminism, 19

field, 75–76

first-order ethical disputes, 59–60

Foucault, Michel, 83

Frader, Joel, xxvii

Francis, L. P., 95

Frank, Arthur, 163, 167–68, 185

Frank, Gelya, 239

functional objection: to intersex surgery, 79; to technoluxe, 74

gender issues, 196–97

genitalia, atypical: American Academy of Pediatrics on, 206; appearance concerns and, 199–200; studies related to, 189–90. *See also* intersex surgery

Gestell, 54–55

goal of parenting, 262–65

gods: health care providers as, 260; humans as becoming, 64–65

Goffman, Erving, 87n. 6, 87n. 8, 234

"Good Country People" (O'Connor), 91, 106

good enough parenting, 238

good life, understanding of: appearance and, 228, 229–37; medicine, using in pursuit of, 84–85; Scientific Fix master narrative and, 187–88; Socratic bioethics and, 69; Ugly Outcast master narrative and, 182–83. *See also* quality of life

grace, 187

Green, Joanne, 255

grief, after birth of disabled child, 43, 218

Habits of the Heart (Bellah et al.), 85–86

habitus, 99–100, 102–3, 191–92, 205

Hahn, H., 234

Hamermesh, Daniel, 183

Hastings Center Surgically Shaping Children project, The, concerns of, xiv–xv; experience of, 68; hard lesson of, 83–84; recommendation of, xxix; strands of inquiry of, xv; surgeon role in, 113; surgery chosen for, xiii–xiv

health, definition of, 141

health care: as acquisition, 257; including child in discussions of, 26

Hedley, LilyClaire, 43–48, 163, 188

Hedley, Lisa: *Dwarfs: Not a Fairy Tale* (documentary), 41, 248; on "flaw," 245; involvement of child in decision making and, 218–19; on limb-lengthening surgery, 98; on parenthood, 254; questioning and repositioning of, 83; Scientific Fix master narrative and, 187–88

Hegi, Ursula, *Stones in the River*, 95, 108

Heidegger, Martin: on Being of things, 52–53; on *Bestand*, 52–54, 57; ethics and, 58; on *Gestell*, 54–55; on order and ordering, 61; on *Seinsvergessenheit*, 59; on techniques of erasure, 55–57; on technology, 52, 73

herd instinct, 100, 107

historicizing ourselves, 62

homosexuality, 97

hormone replacement therapy, 4, 5–6

how to live, conceptions of, 178–79

humanism: of Heidegger, 58; medicine in cause of democratic, 76

humiliation: craniofacial surgery and, 81; foot surgery and, 73, 75, 82–83; suffering and, 58

hypospadias, 208n. 16

ideal: normal compared to, 94–95, 106–7; normalization and, 123

idealized child, dealing with loss of, 43, 218

identification, failure of, 199–201, 205

identity: achondroplasia and, 29, 32, 211–12; appearance and, 19–20; desire for recognition and acceptance of, 103; explanation of self and, 47–48; limb-lengthening procedure and, 33–35, 40–42; raising child and, 25–26, 43, 46; shared starting place and, 18

"If we *can* do it, eventually we *will* do it" refrain, 62–63

incorporating perspective of affected adults into decision making, 219–21

individualism, 107–8

infantilizing of young people, 162–63

informed consent: American Academy of Pediatrics policy statement on, xxiii–xxiv, 213, 214, 259; disclosure and, 163–65; doctrine of, 213–14; intersex surgery and, 80, 205; for non-life-threatening conditions, 214–17; research on, 159–63; risks, uncertainty, and, 135; voluntariness and, 172. *See also* decision making

initial consultation with surgeon, 116–17

injustice and difference, 236–37

instrumental rationality, 181–82

integrity, 186–87

intellectual growth, fostering of, 177

interdisciplinary team care, 126–28, 138

internalization of norms, 103–4

intersex, definition of, 207n. 7

Intersex Society of North America (ISNA), xvi, 79, 238, 265

intersex surgery: anger of adults who have undergone, 204; benefactor of, 204–6; in Colombia, 216–17; imperative of normality and, 190–92; limitations of, xxviii; Mary's story, 198–201; moral justifications for, 78–80; parents and, 192–93; Ruby's story, 193–98; Sarah's story, 201–4

intimacy, family, 170

involvement of child in decisions about surgery: achondroplasia and, 30; age and, 136; assent and, 120–21, 213; benefits of, 219; craniofacial, 123; delay and, 228–29; example of, 27–28; guidance for, 246–49; health care jargon and, 38; information sharing and, 163–65; intersex, 123–24; levels of, 165–68; respect and, 170–72; responsibility and, 168–70; working group and, xxix

isolation of parents, 193, 218

"It's Only a Wee Wee" (Alsop), 202–3

judgment of value, normal as, 94–100

Kant, I., 163

Kent, Deborah, 265–66n. 2

Kessler, Suzanne, 189–90, 206, 208n. 11

Kramer, Peter, xiv, 73

Kuklin, Susan, *Thinking Big*, 31, 42

La Leche League, 208n. 12

legal witness, child as, 161

leukemia, 129

Levine, Suzanne, 73, 76

life, as project, 71–72

limb-lengthening procedure: advantages of, 39–42; decision making and, 33–35; description of, 46; experience with, 29, 35–39; language of moral justification for, 76–78; seduction of, 45–46

Lindemann, Hilde, 163, 228, 232. *See also* Nelson, Hilde

Listening to Prozac (Kramer), 73

Little, Margaret, 235–36, 246, 249

Little People of America, 77, 220

liver transplant, 129–30

Locke, 163

longevity, 98

love and acceptance: achondroplasia and, 30–31, 33, 34, 41; demonstrating, 243–46; desire for normality and, 104–8; experiences with family and, 13–14, 15; lies and, 11; in parent-child relationship, 16–17, 237–43. *See also* unconditional love

lucidity, 186

Lussier, A., 239

Mandela, Nelson, 86–87n. 1

markings on body, traditional, 72, 75

Marsh, Jeffrey, 80

master narratives: description of, 179–80, 187; Scientific Fix, 184–88; Self-Absorbed Consumer, 180–82; Ugly Outcast, 182–84, 187–88; "vulnerable child," 163; Women's Place in Society, 183–84

Maternal Thinking (Ruddick), 176, 243

May, William, 242

medical condition: difference in perspective between persons with same, 41–42; severity of, and need to trust, 128–29; support from others with same, 8–10, 32; as tragedy, 11–12. *See also* disclosure of medical condition; secrecy about medical condition

medical management of cases, 7–8

medical product lines, 74

medical uncertainty, 133–35, 258

membership: body markings and, 72, 75; in minority, 40, 41–42

memory, communities of, 85–86

mental health care providers, 260

micropenis, 189

midget, 31

minority, membership in, 40, 41–42

models of care, 126–30

modernity, 78

momentum and decision to end surgery, 81

Money, John, 193, 206–7n. 3

moral justifications for surgery: craniofacial, 80–82; intersex, 78–80; limb-lengthening, 76–78

moral model of disability, 95

Mouradian, Wendy, xiv, 164

Mueller, Gillian, 33, 77

Nelson, Hilde, 59. *See also* Lindemann, Hilde

neoliberalism, 82

neoliberal medicine, 70–71, 73, 76

Nietzche, F., 56, 84, 100–101, 107

Nisbett, Richard, 179

Noel, Madame, 87n. 4

norm. *See* statistical norm

norma, 94

normal, definition of, 93–96

Normal and the Pathological, The (Canguilhem), 94, 96, 98

"normal childhood," legal conceptions of, 214–15

normalcy/normality: ambiguity and, 93; avoiding tyranny of, 101–5; desire for, 43, 90–93, 104–5; imperative of, 190–92; as judgment of value, 96–100; love, and desire for, 104–8; stranger's gaze and, 104; as tyrant, 108; as undesirable, 101

normalization: of difference, 203–4; ideal and, 123; limb-lengthening surgery as form of, 77–78; parental decision-making related to, 217–19

normalizing anomalous, 100–101

normalizing surgery: desire of parents for, 13–16; moral worry about, 182; risk-benefit analysis of, 221

normal life, 90–91

normative framework, "thick," 177–78

O'Connor, Flannery, "Good Country People," 91, 106

ogive curve, 94, 95

O'Keeffe, Georgia, 30

One of Us: Conjoined Twins and the Future of Normal (Dreger), xxviii

ordering of things, and technology, 53, 54–55, 56, 61–66

Orlan, 71

Ornstein, A., 237, 238

Ornstein, P., 237, 238

outcome assessment in craniofacial care: developing evidence base and, 143–45; longitudinal study, 147–48; overview of, 141; psychological and psychosocial, 145–47, 148, 150–51; quality of life measures, 148; rating evidence, 142–43; variables to address, 145; YQOL-R and, 149–50

outcomes and appearance, 231–37

pain: alleviation of, and medical profession, 118; experience of, 36–38; psychological, dealing with, 35–36. *See also* suffering

parens patriae, 215

parental empathy, 237–38

parent education, 240

parents: acquisition and, 257; ambivalence of, 25–26, 43–47; authority of, 161, 212–13; desire for normalizing surgery and, 13–16; difference in perspective between child and, 26–28; discovery of disability by, 217–19; efforts to protect child by, 16–17, 255; emotional counseling for, 4, 11, 260; experience of, 92, 102–3; as experts on child's condition, 259–60; failure of identification and, 199–201, 205; fundamental obligations of, xiv; goal of, 262–65; good enough, 238; intersex surgery and, 192–201; isolation of, 192, 218; relationship with, and child's sense of self, 16–17, 237–43; responsibility of, 29, 48; shame-pride axis of, 259, 263; support for, 11, 196–97, 244; surgeon, child, and, 136–38; surgery decision and, 23–24, 120–21, 213, 214, 259; vulnerability of, 126, 136–38, 190, 195–96. *See also* expectant parents, experience as; permission for surgery from parents; power relationship between parents and children

Partridge, James, 150

Pellegrino, E. D., 131

permission for surgery from parents, xxiii–xxiv, 120–21, 213, 214, 259

perspective: of affected adults, incorporating into decision making, 219–21; difference between child's and parent's, 26–28; difference between persons with same medical condition, 41–42; religious, 63–64

philosophy and ethical quandaries, 59–66

Piaget, J., 136, 159

post–World War II period, 91

power relationship between parents and children: as asymmetrical, 176; conceptions of how to live and, 178–79; domination and, 197–98, 200–201; master narratives and, 180, 185

prenatal testing and disability rights project, xiii

prescriptive, master narratives as, 179–80

pressure: to choose surgery, 257–58; to conform, 25. *See also* coercion in decision making

primary care model, 126

primary cleft lip surgery, xxix, 20

property rights over children, 164, 179

protectionist bioethics, 69, 70, 82, 84

psychological outcomes, 145–47

psychological pain, dealing with, 35–36

psychosocial function, 115, 123, 124

psychosocial outcomes, 145–46, 148, 150–51

psychosocial support, 127, 169

quality of life: craniofacial outcome and, 132–33; definition of, 118, 132, 148; Durkheim on, 70; measures of, 148–50. *See also* good life, understanding of

questionable variations, 96–97

rape, medical examination compared to, 7–8, 194–95

reality, medicine and, 81

recommendation for surgery, implications of, 237

reconstructive operation, 120

rejection: by others, concerns about, 15, 183; surgery and, 254–55

religious perspective, 63–64

research methods with children, 159–61

resource allocation objection to technoluxe, 74–75

respect for views of children, 170–72

responsibility for surgical decision, 127–28

restaurant script, 179

restitution narrative, 185

risk, developmental model for, 147–48

risk-benefit analysis for surgery, 119, 142–43, 221

Ross, Lee, 179

Rousso, Harilyn, xxvii, 239

Ruddick, Sara, *Maternal Thinking*, 176, 243

rush to surgery, 23–24

salience, indicators of, 60–61

Sandal, Michael, 242

Sanford, Emily Sullivan, 85–86, 219, 247, 248

scars, 85–86

science: medicine and, 133; technology and, 51

Scientific Fix, master narrative of, 184–87. *See also* surgical fix, seduction of

Scott, E., 136

secrecy about medical condition: in families, 4–5, 265; by hospital staff, 202; intersex surgery and, 6–7, 79, 197

seeing, as perspectival, 56, 65–66

Seinsvergessenheit, 59

Self-Absorbed Consumer, master narrative of, 180–82

self-confidence, postsurgical, 235

self-esteem: psychological well-being and, 233; reinforcing, as moral justification for surgery, 79; surgery and, 240

self-expression, 181

self-fulfillment, 181

self-image, secrecy about medical condition and, 7

self-regard and norms, 105

self-respect, 184, 186

sense of self and parent-child relationship, 16–17, 237–43

sexual relationships, 10–11

shame: difference and, 256–57; in families, 265; intersex surgery and, 79; motivation behind surgery and, 15–16

shame-pride axis of parenting, 259, 263

Sharangpani, Ruta, 263–65

Shklar, Judith, 58

shock: dealing with when seeing child, 23; temptation to fix and, 61

side effects of medical care, 260

Silvers, A., 95

"sketches of landscapes," 66

socialization, 177–78, 200, 240–41. *See also* master narratives

social skills training program, 150

social stigma, 98

socioemotional tasks, 147–48

Socrates, 83

Socratic bioethics, 69–70, 82–85, 165

sonograms, 253

Speltz, M. L., 147–48

standing-reserve, 73. See also *Bestand*

state interest in child rearing, 212–13, 214, 215–16

statistical norm, 94, 95, 96, 98, 123

Stern, D., 238

stigma: definition of, 87n. 8; protecting child from, 255; as source of exclusion and danger, 98, 99; sources of, 234–36

Stones in the River (Hegi), 95, 108

suburban housing, rationale behind, 181

success of surgery, 79

suffering: alleviation of, and medical profession, 118; human, and evil, 58; medical intervention and, 85; parenting and, 262–63; scars and, 85–86. *See also* pain

support: from others with same medical conditions, 8–10, 32; for parents, 11, 196–97, 244; psychosocial, 127, 169

surgeon: decision making of, 117–21; detachment and, 131–32; disclosure of uncertainty and, 134–35; initial consultation with, 116–17; paternalistic role of, 121, 124; personality of, 121–22; questioning, 261; relationship between parent, patient, and, 136–38; relationship between patient and, 125; trust and, 130

surgery: comparing, 114–15; conflating concerns about, xxviii–xxix; context of, 70–72; elective nature of, 212; on feet, 72–76; limitations of, xxviii, 185, 241, 242; moral justifications for, 76–82; normalizing, 13–16, 182, 221; pressure to choose, 257–58; reconstructive versus cosmetic, 119–20; risk-benefit formula and, 119, 142–43, 221; success of, 79; technology and, 57–60; vulnerability and inequality in setting of, 130–32. *See also* craniofacial surgery; intersex surgery; involvement of child in decisions about surgery; surgeon

surgical fix, seduction of, 43–48, 68–69, 236–37, 260

survey research about children, 159

Taylor, Charles, 71–72, 85, 181

teasing, 16

technology: concepts of, 51–57; corrective surgery on children and, 57–60; ethical quandaries and, 60–66; Heidegger on, 73; science and, 51

technoluxe: definition of, 74; dialogue and, 82–83; moral justifications for surgery and, 76–82; objections to, 74–75

terminology, 114–15, 122–24

testicular feminization syndrome, 6

Thinking Big (Kuklin), 31, 42

Thoreau, H. D., 65

"to fix" verb, 116–17

tool, explicit attention to, 56–57

tragedy, medical condition as, 11–12

transforming love, 242

trust: of infants, 240; between physician, patient, and family, 125; severity of medical condition and, 128–29; vulnerability and, 130–32, 197–98

truth: Heidegger on, 52; philosophy and, 60–61

trying to hold her/his own, 76

twins, conjoined, 219–20

"twisted ovaries" lie, 4–5, 7

Ugly Outcast, master narrative of, 182–84, 187–88
uncertainty, medical, 133–35, 258
unconditional love, 254, 259

value, normal as judgment of, 94–100
values, advertising and, 180–81
variables to address in outcome studies, 145
victim complex, 37
vital functions, 115
vocabularies, 55
Vogue (magazine) story on "flawless foot," 72–74
voluntariness in consent, 172
vulnerability: of parents, 126, 136–38, 190, 195–96;
    trust and, 128–32, 197–98
"vulnerable child" master narrative, 163

Walker, Margaret Urban, 186–87
ways of revealing things, 56
Weiss, Meira, 238
Winkler, Mary, 171
Wittgenstein, L., *Philosophical Investigations*, 66
Wolfe, Alan, 84
Women's Place in Society, master narrative of,
    183–84

young people, infantilizing of, 162–63
Youth Quality of Life Instrument Research tool
    (YQOL-R), 149–50